# 501 HUMAN
# DISEASES

# 501 HUMAN DISEASES

## David F. Mullins, PhD

Vice President for Institutional Research,
Advancement, Technology, and Accreditation

East Mississippi Community College

**THOMSON**

**DELMAR LEARNING**    Australia   Canada   Mexico   Singapore   Spain   United Kingdom   United States

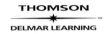

**THOMSON**

**DELMAR LEARNING**

### 501 Human Diseases
by David F. Mullins, PhD.

**Vice President, Health Care Business Unit:**
William Brottmiller

**Editorial Director:**
Cathy L. Esperti

**Acquisitions Editor:**
Marah Bellegarde

**Editorial Assistant:**
Jadin Babin-Kavanaugh

**Developmental Editor:**
Deb Flis

**Marketing Director:**
Jennifer McAvey

**Health Care Channel Manager— Education:**
Tamara Caruso

**Marketing Coordinator:**
Chris Manion

**Production Manager:**
Barbara A. Bullock

**Art and Design Specialist:**
Alexandros Vasilakos

**Production Coordinator:**
Jessica McNavich

**Project Editor:**
Ruth Fisher

**Library of Congress Cataloging-in-Publication Data**

Mullins, David F.
  501 human diseases / David F. Mullins.
    p. ; cm.
  Includes index.
  ISBN 1-4018-2521-4
  1.  Diseases—Dictionaries.
  [DNLM: 1.  Internal Medicine—Handbooks. 2.  Signs and Symptoms—Handbooks.  WB 39 M9596f 2006]  I. Title: Five hundred one human diseases. II. Title.
  RC41.M85 2006
  616'.003—dc22
                              2005011618

### NOTICE TO THE READER

Publisher does not warrant or guarantee any of the products described herein or perform any independent analysis in connection with any of the product information contained herein. Publisher does not assume, and expressly disclaims, any obligation to obtain and include information other than that provided to it by the manufacturer.

The reader is expressly warned to consider and adopt all safety precautions that might be indicated by the activities described herein and to avoid all potential hazards. By following the instructions contained herein, the reader willingly assumes all risks in connection with such instructions.

The publisher makes no representations or warranties of any kind, including but not limited to, the warranties of fitness for particular purpose or merchantability, nor are any such representations implied with respect to the material set forth herein, and the publisher takes no responsibility with respect to such material. The publisher shall not be liable for any special, consequential, or exemplary damages resulting, in whole or part, from the reader's use of, or reliance upon, this material.

*This book is dedicated to the hope that most people read it for interest's sake alone. For those who suffer from disease, my thoughts have been on you as I wrote each paragraph. Here is wishing you a speedy recovery.*

# Contents

# xii Contents

# Preface

There has been an explosion in the number and need for health care professionals in the United States and around the world. Advances in modern transportation make it possible for people to be halfway around the world in only hours, and every traveler carries microorganisms along for the ride. The increasing number of multidrug-resistant diseases, the risk of bioterrorism, and the high rate of immunosuppressing diseases worldwide give rise to a number of diseases in the United States that were, heretofore, so rare as to be relatively obscure. *501 Human Diseases* addresses the need for a cursory knowledge of human diseases, including those that have global significance but perhaps occur less often in the United States.

## DEVELOPMENT OF THE BOOK

*501 Human Diseases* developed from a need for brief explanations of diseases. Over the past few years, an ever-increasing number of diseases have influenced the world and caused great speculation concerning their effects on the public. These events have made a rudimentary understanding of many diseases a must for health care professionals as well as for the general public. Advances in medicine, ranging from cloning, to stem cell research, to the Human Genome Project, have brought disease and its treatment and diagnosis to the forefront of the world's attention.

*501 Human Diseases* is designed as a reference guide to diseases and their causes. This book should be used as a reference for understanding the influence of specific diseases, their treatment, and their diagnosis. *501 Human Diseases* can also be used to identify common disease characteristics of specific diseases, including signs, symptoms, and likely outcomes of the disease.

This book was developed with the health care professional and the general public in mind. *501 Human Diseases* is medically accurate, but use of medical jargon is limited and explained, while still maintaining scientific integrity. *501 Human Diseases* is designed to be a companion reference guide for learners in health care professions, health care practitioners, and the general public. This book is intended to provide only the most basic information concerning diseases so that learners, practitioners, and the public can quickly find accurate and timely information concerning diseases, their signs and symptoms, their treatments, and tests used in their diagnosis. *501 Human Diseases* is intended to be a springboard rather than a destination.

## ABOUT THE AUTHOR

David F. Mullins began his undergraduate education at Purdue University and received his BS from the Cincinnati College of Mortuary Science. He also holds both an MS in Higher Education Administration and a PhD in Sociology from Mississippi State University. Dr. Mullins began his career as a firefighter and emergency medical technician in aircraft crash rescue, and he has also trained in hazardous materials management and mass fatality response. In addition, he is a licensed funeral director and embalmer and an instructor of mortuary science. Currently, he is Vice President for Institutional Research, Advancement, Technology, and Accreditation at East Mississippi Community College, where he also authored *Microbiology and Pathology for Mortuary Science* and *The Illustrated Guide to Anatomy and Physiology: An Introductory Text for the Study of Embalming and Disease.*

## ACKNOWLEDGMENTS

The author and Thomson Delmar Learning would like to acknowledge the following individuals for their review of the manuscript and their helpful suggestions.

Carole Berube, MA, MSN, BSN, RN
    Professor Emerita in Nursing
    Instructor in Health Sciences
    Bristol Community College
    Fall River, Massachusetts

Susan S. Erue, RN, BSN, MSEd, PhD in progress
    Assistant Professor
    Iowa Wesleyan College
    Division of Health and Natural Sciences
    Mount Pleasant, Iowa

Marsha Hemby
    Department Chair, Medical Assisting
    Pitt Community College
    Greenville, North Carolina

Linda Scarborough, RN, CMA, CPC, BSM
Healthcare Management Technology Program Manager
Lanier Technical College
Oakwood, Georgia

Pamela K. Terry, PhD, CHES, CADP
Associate Professor
Community Health and Health Services Management
Western Illinois University
Macomb, Illinois

# How to Use 501 Human Diseases

During my early EMT training, I remember an instructor who chastised me for asking a question about how to treat a patient suffering a heart attack. She quickly corrected me by saying that patients do not have "heart attacks." She insisted that I use terms like myocardial infarction, arrhythmia, tachycardia, brachiacardia, atrial fibrillation, ventricular fibrillation, coronary artery occlusion, and the like, to precisely describe the specific disorders affecting the diseased heart. My response then, and my response now, is that 99 percent of the people just need to know they are having a heart attack. That is what they tell their family, that is what they tell their friends, and that is what they tell themselves.

## MEDICAL TERMINOLOGY AND COMMUNICATION

Health care practitioners need two sets of vocabulary, in my opinion. The most important set of vocabulary is the medical terminology used to diagnose and treat the patient's illness. This is the vocabulary set essential to effectively communicate with other health care professionals.

The second vocabulary set is the straight-talk express. This is the vocabulary set necessary for effective communication, which requires that a message first be encoded by the sender and then decoded by the recipient. If the recipient cannot decode the message, the message was not communicated. Understanding the intended message is the key to communication.

For example, a physician might tell another physician that a patient exhibits dysphagia, pleural effusion, and dyspnea due to mesothelioma. The same physician needs to be able to tell the patient that lung cancer is making it hard to swallow and breathe. The cancer is also producing fluid in the chest that makes it even harder to swallow and breathe.

This book was written from years of experiencing the mystification of allied-health students and the general public by medical jargon. The fact is, as I perceive it, that medicine is mostly about common sense and vocabulary. Although medical terminology is necessarily specific, it need not marginalize those who have the most to gain from its thorough understanding. How can patients participate in their own care if they do not understand their illness?

*501 Human Diseases* is written for learners, practitioners, and the general public. Learners absolutely need to master the vocabulary presented in their textbooks, but they also need to understand what that vocabulary means. Given the urgent need for more health care professionals due to the aging population, medicine must become more accessible to learners. Practitioners rarely can afford patients the time necessary for a thorough explanation of their condition in easily understood terms. This book can help practitioners by providing patients with plain and easy-to-read information that can encourage patients to understand their illness and actively participate in their own care. The key, in my opinion, to relieving anxiety is knowing what to expect. This book provides that information.

## DISEASES AND CONTENT

The diseases in this book were selected from the Centers for Disease Control and Prevention (CDC) Web sites. Some of these diseases do not presently occur in the United States, but may occur in the future due to bioterrorism, increased travel, and importation of foreign goods. Other diseases are extremely rare in the United States and are not covered in many medical texts, which is why they are included here. Still others are genetic diseases that may soon be eradicated due to advances brought about through cloning, stem cell research, and the Human Genome Project.

This book is designed to be a springboard to further information. I am not a physician, and this book is not designed for diagnosis. Nor is it a traditional reference text that provides specific information about a particular disease. Bother *Taber's* and *Mosely's* medical encyclopedias are excellent resources for that type of information. In contrast, *501 Human Diseases* is a general guide to diseases, which is why the diseases are listed alphabetically. Each presentation includes a brief description of the disease, the signs and symptoms of the disease, potential treatment options, and some of the tests that might be completed as part of the diagnosis and treatment of the disease. I present the information in this way because it answers the questions I have received through the years in the order in which most people usually ask them.

With the speed at which medicine is advancing, it is not possible to list every possible drug and every possible test that might be prescribed or conducted. The descriptions of the diseases and their signs and symptoms will not change, but treatment and diagnosis are changing rapidly. With access to the Internet, it is my belief that readers of this book will find better information concerning treatment and testing from reliable Web sites. Such information will be the most current and hopefully the most accurate. This book is a springboard to that information. In addition, it provides a thumbnail sketch of numerous diseases. Its true value lies in its ability to point the reader in the direction of a fuller understanding of the technical materials written for highly educated practitioners in other sources.

Personally, because I am allergic to aspirin and have a low tolerance for many drugs, I use the Internet to find the latest information before I take new medication. I want to know possible side effects and how the medication works in my body. I also want to know what interactions the drug may have with other medications I may be taking. The Internet offers descriptions of procedures, graphics, and access to others who have taken the medication or had the same test. Often, Web sites will provide insights into how to better tolerate the medicine or make the test more comfortable.

## RELIABLE INTERNET WEB SITES

Unfortunately, many Web sites are not reputable. Using the Internet does not guarantee accuracy. When searching for information, look for government Web sites (which end in .gov), organizations (which end in .org), and educational institutions (which usually end in .edu). The list of Web sites included in the appendix of this book is a good place to start.

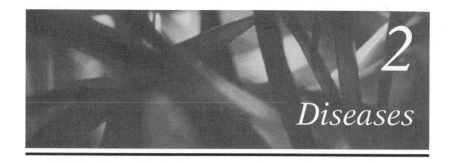

*2*

*Diseases*

## AARSKOG SYNDROME

### Description

Aarskog syndrome is an extremely rare X-linked, recessive genetic disorder. Although females may exhibit Aarskog syndrome, the disease is most severe in males. Aarskog syndrome is caused by mutations in a gene called *FGDY1* found on the short arm of the X chromosome (Xp11.22) (MCA/MR, 1999; NORD, 2005).

### Signs and Symptoms

Aarskog syndrome is characterized by a rounded face, a widow's-peak hairline, wide-set eyes, drooping eyelids, a small nose with nostrils tipped forward, underdeveloped midportion of the face, delayed eruption of teeth, and a mildly sunken chest. Children also exhibit a short stature, delayed puberty, inguinal hernias, and protruding navels (belly buttons). Persons with Aarskog syndrome have short, webbed fingers and toes, a simian crease in the palm, and an incurving fifth finger. They also have a wide groove above their upper lip, a crease below their lower lip, and moderate mental deficiency. The top portion of their ear is folded over slightly.

### Treatment

There is no specific treatment for Aarskog syndrome. Orthodontic treatment is used to treat some facial abnormalities. The effect of growth hormones in the treatment of Aarskog Syndrome is still being studied in trials (Stewart, 2004a).

### Testing

X-rays and genetic testing are used to diagnose Aarskog syndrome.

## AASE SYNDROME

### Description

Aase syndrome is a rare, idiopathic (cause is obscure or unknown), inherited disorder that may be detected in early infancy. The primary characteristic is anemia, which is caused by underdevelopment of the bone marrow. Bone marrow produces red blood cells, which are illustrated in

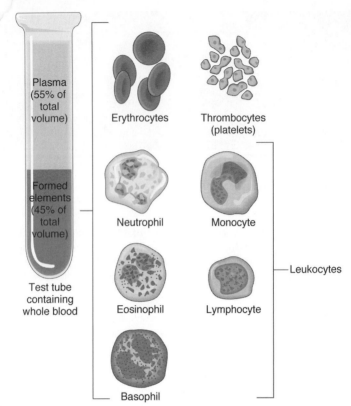

**Figure 2-1** Components of blood

Figure 2-1. Aase syndrome may also be known as anemia triphalangeal thumbs, or it may be called Aase-Smith syndrome (Albuisson, 2003).

## Signs and Symptoms

Aase syndrome is characterized by anemia, heart defects, slowed growth, skin pallor, delayed closure of the fontanelles, narrow shoulders, cleft palate, deformed ears, and droppy eyelids. Persons with Aase syndrome are unable to extend their joints. They also have triple jointed thumbs, absent or small knuckles, and decreased skin creases at the finger joints (Stewart, 2003a).

## Treatment

There is no specific treatment for Aase syndrome. Treatments may include bone marrow transplants, blood transfusions, and the use of corticosteroids (NORD—Aase, 2003).

## Testing

Tests used in the diagnosis of Aase syndrome include Complete Blood Count (CBC), echocardiogram, X-rays, and bone marrow biopsies.

## ABRUPTIO PLACENTAE

### Description
Abruptio placentae, which is also known as ablatio placentae, is the sudden, premature detachment of the placenta from a normal uterine site of implantation. It occurs in approximately 1 out of 120 births, and the risk of occurrence increases in future pregnancies. Abruptio placentae occurs when bleeding and a hematoma form in part of the uterus that forms the placenta. The hematoma can compress the vessels supporting fetal blood supply. If the muscular wall of the uterus ruptures, abruptio placentae can be fatal to the fetus and the mother.

### Signs and Symptoms
Abruptio placentae is characterized by vaginal bleeding, abdomoninal or back pain, and uterine tenderness. Other symptoms may include abnormal uterine contractions and premature labor. Fetal distress is common, and the fetal death rate is about 15 percent (Gaufberg, 2004).

### Treatment
Treatment consists of monitoring both the mother and the fetus. If either becomes unstable, immediate cesarean delivery may be necessary. In less severe cases, amniotic fluids and pooled blood may be removed through needle aspiration to reduce pressure.

### Testing
Abruptio placentae is observable via ultrasound.

## ABSCESS

### Description
An abscess is a localized collection of pus that is walled off by a membrane that results from invasion of a pus-causing microorganism. Skin abscesses are often caused by *Staphylococcus aureus* bacteria in skin wounds, and abscesses are more prevalent after impaling or penetrating injuries that drive infectious microorganisms into deep tissues. Figure 2-2 illustrates a variety of skin lesions that can develop into abscesses.

### Signs and Symptoms
Abscesses can disrupt the surrounding tissues' ability to function due to the resulting inflammation. If the microorganisms in the abscess spread, a fatal infection can develop.

### Treatment
Abscesses are treated with antibiotics. Severe abscesses may need to be drained.

### Testing
There is no specific test for abscesses, but cultures of lesions and pus may be used to identify the cause of the infection.

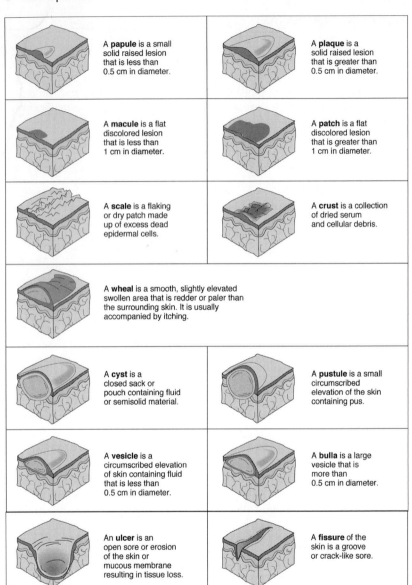

**Figure 2-2** Skin lesions

## *ACANTHAMOEBA* INFECTION

### Description

*Acanthamoeba* are amoebas, and many can infect humans (e.g., *A. culbertsoni,*
*A. polyphaga, A. castellanii, A. healyi, A. hatchetti, A. rhysodes*). *Acanthamoeba*
are found in soil, freshwater, seawater, hot tubs, HVAC units, dialysis units,

and contact lens paraphernalia. *Acanthamoeba* enter the skin through a wound, the nose, or the eyes (DPD, 2004).

## Signs and Symptoms
Amoebas travel throughout the body, especially the lungs and central nervous system. Through improper storage, handling, and disinfection of contact lenses, *Acanthamoeba* can enter the eye. *Acanthamoeba* cause a serious, often deadly, infection called granulomatous amebic encephalitis (GAE). Symptoms include headaches, stiff neck, nausea and vomiting, tiredness, confusion, loss of balance, seizures, and hallucinations.

## Treatment
Eye and skin infections are treated with propamidine isethionate and neomycin-polymyxin B-gramicidin. Keratoplasty—a type of eye surgery—is necessary in severe infections. Although most cases of brain infection with *Acanthamoeba* have been fatal, recovery has occurred with amphotericin B treatment.

## Testing
In central nervous system infection with *Acanthamoeba*, diagnosis is made by microscopic examination of cerebrospinal fluid, stained smears of biopsy specimens (e.g., brain tissue, skin, cornea), or corneal scrapings. Cultivation of the causal organism, and its identification by direct immunofluorescent antibody, may be used in diagnosis.

## ACANTHOSIS NIGRICANS

### Description
Acanthosis nigricans results in velvety, light-brown or black markings on the neck, under the arms, or in the groin (Levine, 2002). Acanthosis nigricans is associated with obesity and high levels of insulin production. Acanthosis nigricans is most prevalent in people with darker skin pigmentation, and persons with ovarian cysts.

### Signs and Symptoms
Eating starches and sugars raises insulin levels, which causes acanthosis nigricans by activating insulin receptors in the skin that excite the epidermis to grow abnormally. Acanthosis nigricans may become malignant.

### Treatment
There is no specific treatment for acanthosis nigricans. Treatment includes Retin-A, 20 percent urea, alpha hydroxy acids, and salicylic acid prescriptions. The prognosis for patients with malignant acanthosis nigricans is poor.

### Testing
Diagnosis of acanthosis nigricans is based on physical exam, but a skin biopsy may be needed. If no clear cause of acanthosis nigricans is obvious,

it may be necessary to search for one with blood tests, endoscopy, or X-rays to identify underlying causes.

## ACHALASIA

### Description

Achalasia is an idiopathic disorder of the sphincter at the inferior end of the esophagus (Sawyer, 2003). In cases of achalasia, there is low pressure in the esophageal sphincter, due to a neuromuscular dysfunction. Achalasia is characterized by a failure of the smooth muscles of the esophagus to coordinate with the lower esophageal sphincter. People with achalasia are more prone to cancers of the esophagus.

### Signs and Symptoms

The sphincter remains closed when the esophagus attempts to pass food into the stomach. This lack of coordination between the muscles of the esophagus and the sphincter muscles is accompanied by weak or absent peristalsis, which is the circular and longitudinal contraction of muscles that moves the food through the esophagus into the stomach. The lack of movement of swallowed food particles results in increased secretions from the upper esophagus that can be aspirated into the airway.

### Treatment

The four main classes of drugs used in the treatment of achalasia include calcium channel blockers, anticholinergic agents, nitrates, and opioids. Achalasia may also be treated with a balloon to dilate the esophagus and disrupt the muscle fibers of the lower esophageal sphincter. Botulinum toxin (Botox) can be used to relax the muscles of the esophagus.

### Testing

Achalasia is diagnosed with a barium swallow performed under fluoroscopic guidance. Endoscopy, supplemented by biopsy, excludes other diseases. A barium swallow (aka: upper GI) is a series of X-rays used to examine the upper digestive tract. The organs do not appear on X-rays, but barium does appear, showing the outline of the organs.

## ACHONDROPLASIA

### Description

Achondroplasia is a genetic disorder of bone growth caused either by inheritance or genetic mutation and resulting in a condition known as dwarfism. Achondroplasia is accompanied by deformed joints and poor muscle tone, which can result in sudden death—often during sleep. Deaths result from compression of the upper end of the spinal cord, which interferes with breathing. The compression is caused by abnormalities in the size and structure in the foramen magnum of the skull, which is the hole through which the spinal cord passes, and the vertebrae in the neck.

## Signs and Symptoms

The average overall height of an adult with achondroplasia is about four feet tall. Persons with achondroplasia have shortened arms and legs, but their torso is nearly normal size. Their upper arms and thighs are more shortened than their forearms and lower legs. They also may have a large head with a prominent forehead. Their nose usually has a flat bridge. The hands of achondroplasia patients are short with stubby fingers and a separation between the third and fourth fingers resulting in a trident hand.

## Treatment

There is no specific treatment for achondroplasia. Deformities may be treated surgically.

## ACNE

## Description

Acne is the term for blackheads, whiteheads, and pimples on the skin. Acne can cause serious and permanent scarring.

## Signs and Symptoms

Acne starts between the ages of 10 and 13 and usually lasts 5 to 10 years. Men are more likely than women to have severe, long-lasting forms of acne. Women are more likely to have acne caused by cosmetics and hormonal changes associated with menstruation. Acne lesions are common on the face, but also occur on the neck, chest, back, shoulders, scalp, and extremities.

## Treatment

Due to the commercialization of acne treatment, many treatments are not medically sound and are not proven effective. Medically approved treatments for severe acne include corticosteroids, isotretinoin, antibiotics, oral contraceptives, and topical retinoids.

## Testing

Acne is diagnosed based on physical exam. No tests are required.

## ACRODERMATITIS

## Description

Acrodermatitis is an idiopathic skin condition in children associated with viral infections. In Italian children, acrodermatitis is seen in conjunction with hepatitis B, but this is rare in the United States. Acrodermatitis is also associated with Epstein-Barr virus infections, cytomegalovirus, coxsackieviruses, parainfluenza virus, respiratory syncytial virus, and some live virus vaccines.

## Signs and Symptoms

The lesions of acrodermatitis are small, coppery-red, flat-topped, firm bumps that appear in crops or long lines. The lesions appear symetrically on the body. The rash does not itch, and it appears on the face, arms, legs, and buttocks. This is one of the few rashes that appears on the palms and soles. Generalized enlargement of the lymph nodes and liver may be present.

## Treatment
Acrodermatitis is self-limiting and is, therefore, not treated.

## Testing
Tests used in the diagnosis of acrodermatitis include skin biopsy, liver function tests, hepatitis virus serology, hepatitis B surface antigen test, screening for EBV antibodies, and bilirubin level tests (Drayer, 2003a).

## ACROMEGALY

### Description
Acromegaly appears slowly over time and is caused by overproduction of human growth hormone within the anterior portion of the pituitary gland. In most cases of acromegaly in adults, the overproduction of growth hormone is caused by a benign tumor of the pituitary gland known as an adenoma.

### Signs and Symptoms
Acromegaly is a chronic disease characterized by elongation and enlargement of bones of the extremities and certain head bones, especially the forehead and the jaws (see Color Plate 1). Other symptoms include abnormal growth of the hands and feet, enlargement of the nose and lips, thickening of the face, protrusion of the brow and lower jaw, increased space between the teeth, and high blood pressure. In addition, acromegaly may cause deepening of the voice due to enlarged sinuses and vocal cords, sleepiness, moodiness, and snoring due to upper airway obstruction. Persons with acromegaly often have impaired vision in combination with diabetes mellitus. Changes to the skin may include thickening of the skin, excessive sweating, and skin odor. In women, acromegaly can cause a discharge from the breasts and abnormalities of the menstrual cycle; men may become impotent.

### Treatment
Treatments for pituitary adenoma related to acromegaly include surgery, drug therapy, and radiation therapy. The drugs used inhibit the production of human growth hormone.

### Testing
In cases of acromegaly, human growth hormone levels are tested. The level of insulin growth factor 1 is elevated. Radiological tests are used to identify pituitary tumors.

## ACTINOMYCOSIS

### Description
Actinomycosis is a chronic infection of the face and neck due to the presence of bacteria in the nose and throat. Actinomycosis produces abscesses

and open draining sinuses that discharge sulfur granules. Actinomycosis is caused by *Actinomyces israelii,* which are bacteria in the nose and throat. Actinomycosis is not contagious, but it can develop into meningitis if not treated (Wener, 2004a).

## Signs and Symptoms

*Actinomyces* is an opportunistic pathogen that produces disease when it is introduced into the facial tissues by trauma, surgery, or infection. It is a cause of dental abscesses after tooth extraction, and the infection may progress to the underlying bones where it can cause osteomyelitis. *Actinomyces* forms an abscess, producing a hard, reddish-purple lump. The abscess ruptures, producing a draining sinus tract. Actinomycosis may also occur in the chest, abdomen, or other areas of the body (Johnson, 2003; Mahon & Manuselis, 2000).

## Treatment

Antibiotics are effective in the treatment of actinomycosis. Penicillin is the preferred treatment. Surgical drainage of the lesion may be required, but full recovery is expected with treatment.

## Testing

Microscopic inspection of drained fluid indicates the presence of sulfur granules and *Actinomyces.* A tissue or fluid culture also indicates the presence of *Actinomyces.*

# ADDISON'S DISEASE

## Description

Addison's disease is a rare hormone disorder, occurring when the adrenal glands fail to produce enough cortisol and aldosterone. Addison's disease is also known as chronic adrenal insufficiency or hypocortisolism. About 70 percent of reported cases of Addison's disease are autoimmune disorders of the adrenal cortex. Tuberculosis accounts for about 20 percent of cases of primary adrenal insufficiency in developed countries. Other causes of adrenal insufficiency include chronic fungal infections, metastasis of cancer cells to the adrenal glands, and amyloidosis.

## Signs and Symptoms

Addison's disease is characterized by weight loss, muscle weakness, nausea, vomiting, and diarrhea. Low blood pressure may result in dizziness and fainting, and persons with Addison's disease may also experience sudden, penetrating pain in the back, abdomen, and legs. Persons with a light complexion may develop a bronze darkening of the skin; persons with a dark complexion may develop milky-white patches on the skin.

## Treatment

Replacement therapy with corticosteroids will control the symptoms of Addison's disease. A combination of glucocorticoids and mineralocorticoids are given. With adequate replacement therapy, most people with Addison's disease are able to lead normal lives.

## Testing

The diagnosis of Addison's disease includes tests for low cortisol levels, low serum sodium levels, increased potassium levels, and radiological examination of the abdomen.

## ADENOCARCINOMAS

### Description

The World Health Organization defines adenocarcinoma as a malignant epithelial tumor with tubular, acinar, or papillary growth patterns, and mucus production by the tumor cells. Basically, this definition implies that adenocarcinomas look like the tissues of a gland, and they can produce fluids. Adenocarcinoma is the most common type of lung cancer, especially among women and nonsmokers. It is among a family of cancers known as non–small-cell carcinomas. Adenocarcinomas are most likely to occur in the lungs, esophagus, colon, or salivary glands. Adenocarcinomas may result from scars caused by previous diseases and trauma to the lungs. Color Plate 2 is a photograph of an ulcerated adenocarcinoma of the colon.

### Signs and Symptoms

The majority of adenocarcinomas occur at the periphery of the lung and often cause no symptoms until they are advanced. Patients, therefore, may have no idea that they have cancer, until it has spread throughout their body and is beyond treatment. Adenocarcinomas frequently lie just below the pleural membranes that surround the lungs. The pleural surface is puckered over the tumor. The combination of the black pigmentation and the mucus secreted by the tumor gives it a glistening, pale gray color.

### Treatment

Adenocarcinomas are treated with chemotherapy, radiation therapy, and surgery.

### Testing

Testing for adenocarcinoma includes tissue biopsy and radiological exams of the chest.

## ADENOVIRUS INFECTIONS

### Description

Adenoviruses cause respiratory illness, but they may cause gastroenteritis, conjunctivitis, cystitis, and rash illness as well. Under conditions of crowding and stress, adenovirus infection can cause a disorder known as acute respiratory disease (ARD).

### Signs and Symptoms

Adenovirus infection is characterized by symptoms similar to those of the common cold, pneumonia, and bronchitis. Adenovirus can be transmitted by direct contact, fecal-oral transmission, and occasionally waterborne transmission.

## Treatment
Most adenovirus infections are mild and require only symptomatic treatment.

## Testing
Testing for adenovirus infection includes cultures and tests for the presence of antibodies in the blood.

## ADRENAL CRISIS

### Description
Acute adrenal crisis is a medical emergency caused by a lack of cortisol. The adrenal glands produce three types of hormones, all of which are called corticosteroids. Cortisol is a glucocorticoid, which is a corticosteroid that maintains glucose regulation, suppresses the immune response, and is released as part of the body's response to stress. Adrenal crisis occurs if the adrenal gland is deteriorating, if there is pituitary gland injury, or adrenal insufficiency is not adequately treated. Risk factors for adrenal crisis include infection, trauma, surgery, adrenal gland or pituitary gland injury, and premature termination of treatment with steroids such as prednisone or hydrocortisone.

### Signs and Symptoms
Patients may experience dizziness, weakness, sweating, abdominal pain, nausea, vomiting, headache, low blood pressure, dehydration, fever, chills, darkening of the skin, and rapid heart rate. Other symptoms include joint pain, weight loss, loss of appetite, skin rash, and confusion. Excessive sweating on the face and palms, as well as confusion or coma, may also occur.

### Treatment
In adrenal crisis, hydrocortisone must be given immediately. If infection is the cause of the crisis, antibiotic therapy may be needed. If not treated early, adrenal crisis is fatal.

### Testing
Tests used in the diagnosis of adrenal crisis include an adrenocorticotrophic hormone (ACTH) or Cortrosyn stimulation test for cortisol, tests of fasting blood sugar levels, serum potassium levels, and tests of serum sodium levels.

## AFRICAN SLEEPING SICKNESS

### Description
In the United States, 21 cases of East African trypanosomiasis have been reported since 1967 in travelers to Africa. There are approximately 20,000 cases of both East and West African sleeping disease reported each year worldwide. The disease is spread by the tsetse fly, which is a bloodsucking

fly found only in Africa. A bite by the tsetse fly is often painful and can develop into a red sore.

## Signs and Symptoms

East African trypanosomiasis is caused by the protozoa *Trypanosoma brucei rhodesiense* (Figure 2-3). Fever, severe headaches, irritability, fatigue, swollen lymph nodes, and aching muscles and joints are symptoms of East African sleeping sickness. A skin rash may also be present. Progressive confusion, personality changes, slurred speech, and seizures occur when the infection invades the central nervous system. If left untreated, death occurs within several weeks or months.

West African trypanosomiasis, also called Gambian sleeping sickness, is caused by the protozoa *Trypanosoma brucei gambiense*. Symptoms include fever, rash, swelling around the eyes and hands, severe headaches, extreme fatigue, and aching muscles and joints. Swelling of the lymph nodes on the back of the neck results in Winterbottom's sign. Once the central nervous system becomes involved, personality changes, irritability, loss of concentration, progressive confusion, slurred speech, and seizures occur. Sleeping for long periods of the day and having insomnia at night is a common symptom of West African sleeping disease. If left untreated, death occurs within several months to years.

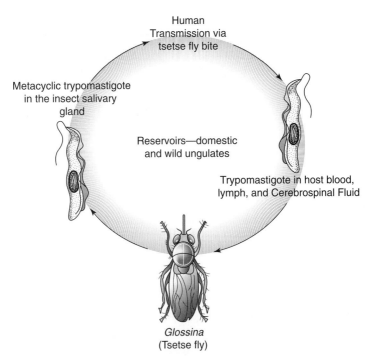

**Figure 2-3** Life cycle of *Trypanosoma brucei gambiense* and *Trypanosoma brucei rhodesiense*

## Treatment

Anthelmintic drugs used in the treatment of trypanosomiasis include suramin, melarsoprol, eflornithine, and pentamidine isethionate.

## Testing

Tests for trypanosomiasis include blood smears, blood composition, and examination of aspirates from affected lymph nodes or lesions.

## AICARDI SYNDROME

### Description

Aicardi syndrome is a rare genetic disorder that is believed to be inherited on the X chromosome, although it may also occur randomly through sporadic mutation. It is characterized by spasms in infants and mental retardation. The brain does not have a completely developed corpus callosum, which in healthy persons connects the left and right hemispheres of the brain. This defect results in seizures. The brain may also be undersized. The ventricles, which produce and circulate the brain in cerebrospinal fluid, may be enlarged. There may also be cysts in the brain that cause gaps in the brain tissue. Worldwide, there are less than 500 cases of Aicardi syndrome (Aicardi Syndrome Foundation, 2004; Goldenring, 2004a; NINDS Aicardi, 2005).

### Signs and Symptoms

Children are diagnosed with Aicardi syndrome between the ages of three months and five months. Diagnosis is based on female sex (or XXY genotype male), lesions of the retina or optic nerve, infantile seizures, and absence of the corpus callosum.

### Treatment

There is no specific treatment of Aicardi syndrome, except to treat symptoms.

### Testing

Tests for Aicardi syndrome include eye exams, Computer Tomography (CT) scan of the head, Magnetic Resonance Imaging (MRI) scan of the head, Electroencephalogram (EEG), and genetic testing.

## AIDS

### Description

Acquired Immune Deficiency Syndrome (AIDS) is a contagious disease that compromises the immune system. AIDS is caused by the human immunodeficiency virus (HIV). HIV is capable of becoming multidrug-resistant. It is estimated that in 2000, 10 percent of newly HIV-infected persons throughout Europe were infected with drug-resistant strains of the virus (McNeil, 2003).

According to the National Center for HIV, STDs, and TB Prevention (1998), in 1984, three years after the first reports of AIDS, researchers discovered the human immunodeficiency virus type 1 (HIV-1). In 1986, a second type of HIV, called HIV-2, was isolated from AIDS patients in West Africa. In persons infected with HIV-2, immunodeficiency develops more slowly and is milder.

HIV is a retrovirus that affects T cells within the immune system. It attacks the RNA of the T cell, causing the T cell to alter its DNA structure to that of HIV. The result is that when infected T cells replicate, the T cell creates more HIV. AIDS is the final stage of HIV infection. The average incubation period for AIDS development is 10 years from the point of initial infection.

## Signs and Symptoms

AIDS is characterized by diseases called opportunistic infections, which are caused by microbes that do not cause illness in healthy people. Figure 2-4 identifies some of the diseases common to AIDS. *Pneumocystis carinii* is a fungus that causes pneumonia in AIDS patients but is rarely

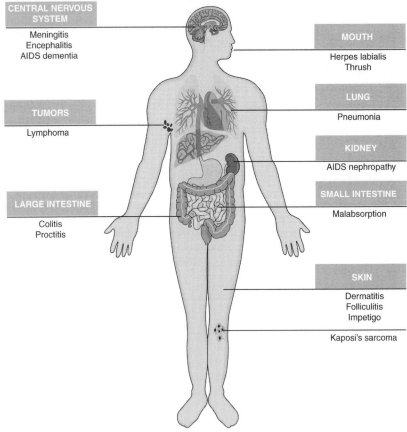

**Figure 2-4** Diseases associated with AIDS

symptomatic in healthy individuals. *Toxoplasma gondii* is a protozoon that infects AIDS patients causing encephalitis. *Cytomegalovirus* causes fever, encephalitis, and blindness. Herpes simplex viruses and the varicella-zoster virus, which causes chicken pox and shingles, can be fatal as well. *Mycobacterium tuberculosis* can cause severe cases of tuberculosis. Kaposi's sarcoma is a common skin and blood vessel cancer found in cases of HIV infection. Fungi such as *Histoplasma capsulatum,* which cause pulmonary infections, *Cryptococcus neoformans,* which cause meningitis, and *Candida albicans,* which cause overgrowths in the esophagus and respiratory tract, can all be fatal.

### Treatment

There is no cure for AIDS. However, a variety of chemotherapeutic agents are lengthening the lives of HIV-infected individuals.

### Testing

Blood tests used to diagnose HIV infection measure levels of antibodies and include the Enzyme Immunoassay (EIA), the Enzyme-Linked Immunosorbent Assay (ELISA), and the Western blot test.

## ALBINISM

### Description

Albinism is a failure to produce melanin pigment due to genetic defects. In Type 1 albinism, a genetic defect in tyrosinase, which is the enzyme responsible for breaking down tyrosine, leads to failure in converting amino acid to melanin. Type 2 albinism, which allows a slight pigmentation at birth, is due to a defect in the P gene.

### Signs and Symptoms

Albinism is characterized by absence of pigment from the hair, skin, or iris of the eyes. Patients exhibit patchy absences of skin color and patches of light-colored hair. The patient's eyes may not track properly, and they may exhibit sensitivity to light and poor vision (Hart, 2004a; NOAH, 2002).

### Treatment

There is no treatment for albinism. The skin and eyes must be protected from the sun.

### Testing

Genetic testing is used to diagnose albinism. An electroretinogram test, to determine brain waves produced by light shined in the eye, can reveal dysfunction of the visual system in ocular forms of albinism.

## ALKAPTONURIA

### Description

Alkaptonuria is a rare disease in which the body does not have enough of an enzyme called homogentisic acid oxidase (HGAO). Because normal amounts of the HGAO enzyme are missing, homogentisic acid (HGA) is not used and builds up in the body. Some is eliminated in the urine, and the rest is deposited in body tissues, where it is toxic. The result is ochronosis, a blue-black discoloration of connective tissue including bone, cartilage, and skin caused by deposits of ochre-colored pigment (Roth, 2003).

### Signs and Symptoms

Patients with alkaptonuria are usually not aware of the disease until about age 40. The earliest sign of the disorder is the tendency for diapers to stain black. Upon contact with the air, urine will turn black. There may be a slate-blue or gray discoloration in the whites of the eyes or in the ear cartilage. Calcifications may be palpable in these areas, particularly in the cartilage of the ear. Arthritis and heart disorders are also common.

### Treatment

No medications are known to be useful in treating alkaptonuria. Vitamin C is recommended for older children and adults because it is an antioxidant that helps retard the formation of deposits in the cartilage.

### Testing

For infants, young children, and asymptomatic young adults, evaluation by simple urine testing can be done. Homogentisic acid can be identified in urine using gas chromatography-mass spectroscopy.

## ALPORT SYNDROME

### Description

Alport syndrome is an inherited disorder involving kidney damage, bloody urine, hearing loss, and eye defects (Devarajan, 2004). The disease involves the basement membrane of the kidney, the cochlea of the inner ear, and the eyes. These disorders are due to a mutation in type IV collagen genes. Alport syndrome is rare, and the genetic defect is typically found on the X chromosome.

### Signs and Symptoms

In women, the disorder is usually mild, with minimal or no symptoms. Women, even if they have no symptoms, can transmit the gene for the disorder to their children. In men, the symptoms are more severe and progress faster. Alport syndrome causes chronic glomerulonephritis, which is an inflammation of the kidneys, although initially there are no symptoms. End-stage renal disease is present by the age of 40. Alport syndrome is characterized by abnormal urine color, bloody urine, hearing loss, loss of vision, cough, swollen legs, and swelling around the eyes.

### Treatment

There is no treatment to prevent the progression of Alport syndrome. High blood pressure must be controlled. Eventually treatment is necessary for chronic renal failure and end-stage renal disease, requiring dialysis and renal transplant.

## Testing

There are no specific physical characteristics of Alport syndrome during a normal physical, except for the presence of bloody urine. Urinalysis may indicate blood, protein, and other abnormalities. Blood urea nitrogen (BUN) and creatinine are elevated. There may be a decrease in the red blood cell count in the hematocrit. Audiometry may show nerve deafness. A renal biopsy will indicate chronic glomerulonephritis.

## ALSTRÖM SYNDROME

### Description

Alström syndrome is an inherited disease. Although intelligence is not affected, patients may be both deaf and blind. They may also be obese and have diabetes mellitus (Newmark, 2003a). Alström syndrome is rare, and it is more common in Holland and Sweden than in the United States. The mutated gene is *ALMS1*, but how this gene causes Alström syndrome is unkown.

### Signs and Symptoms

Alström syndrome is characterized by sensitivity to light, nobbling eye movements, congestive heart failure, blindness, hearing loss, diabetes, liver failure, fibrous lesions in the lungs, and renal dysfunction leading to failure (Alström Syndrome International, 2005).

### Treatment

There is no specific treatment for Alström syndrome, except to treat the symptoms.

### Testing

Tests used in the diagnosis of Alström syndrome include eye exams, blood tests (e.g., chem-20, serum triglycerides, hyperglycemia), tests of thyroid function, hearing tests, and echocardiogram.

## ALVEOLAR HYDATID DISEASE

### Description

Alveolar hydatid disease is caused by *Echinococcus multilocularis*, which is a tapeworm found in foxes, coyotes, dogs, and cats. Although human cases are rare, infection in humans causes tumors to form in the liver, lungs, brain, and other organs (see Color Plate 3). If left untreated, alveolar hydatid disease can be fatal. Alveolar hydatid disease is found worldwide, but in North America, *E. multilocularis* is found primarily from eastern Montana to central Ohio, as well as in Alaska and Canada. Animals become infected when they eat rodents carrying *E. multilocularis*. The tapeworm matures in the intestine of the infected animal and lays eggs there; then the infected animal passes the eggs in its feces. The animals are not harmed by the tapeworm, nor do they have symptoms of alveolar hydatid disease.

## Signs and Symptoms

Alveolar hydatid disease is caused by tumorlike tapeworm larvae growing in the body. Because the larvae are slow-growing, infection with alveolar hydatid disease may not produce any symptoms for many years. Pain or discomfort in the upper abdominal region, weakness, and weight loss may occur. Symptoms are similar to those of liver cancer and cirrhosis of the liver.

## Treatment

Surgery is the most common form of treatment for alveolar hydatid disease, although removal of the parasite mass is not a cure. After surgery, medication is needed to keep the cyst from growing back.

## Testing

Blood tests indicate the presence of the parasite in cases of alveolar hydatid disease.

## ALZHEIMER'S DISEASE

## Description

Alzheimer's is an idiopathic disorder for which there is currently no cure. Alzheimer's usually begins after age 60, although it is possible for younger people to develop this disease. The disease is named after Dr. Alois Alzheimer, a German doctor who, in 1906, noticed changes in the brain tissue of a woman who died of an unusual mental illness. He found clumps of starchlike material, known as amyloid plaques, and tangled bundles of fibers, known as neurofibrillary tangles, in her brain. Patients also exhibit a reduction in the amount of necessary chemicals, referred to as neurotransmitters, in the brain that allow communication between cells.

## Signs and Symptoms

Alzheimer's disease involves parts of the brain that control thought, memory, and language. At first, the only characteristic of Alzheimer's disease may be mild forgetfulness. As the disease progresses, individuals may forget how to do simple tasks like brushing their teeth or combing their hair, and they may begin to have problems speaking, understanding, reading, or writing. In latter stages of Alzheimer's disease, people become anxious or aggressive and may wander away from home. Patients experience sundowning and become more demanding, restless, upset, suspicious, or disoriented, and they may hallucinate at night. Sundowning results from a lack of light, which fails to stimulate certain areas of the brain, exacerbating the manifestations of dementia.

## Treatment

Although there is no cure for Alzheimer's disease, some medicines (i.e., Aricept) may help control behavioral symptoms such as sleeplessness, agitation, wandering, anxiety, and depression.

## Testing

There is no test to diagnose Alzheimer's disease while a person is living.

# AMEBIC DYSENTERY

## Description
Amebic dysentery, which is also known as amebiasis, is caused by the protozoon *Entamoeba histolytica*. The cyst form of *E. histolytica* is found in food and water, and they are spread through the fecal-oral route to humans. Stomach acid destroys the vegetative cells but does not affect the cysts they form. The cysts enter the intestine, where the cyst's wall is digested and the vegetative form is released. The cells multiply in the epithelial cells of the colon. The typical mucous and bloody bowel movements indicate the protozoa's ability to feed on red blood cells and tissues of the gastrointestinal tract. *Entamoeba histolytica* may also infect tissues outside the digestive tract. Color Plate 4 is a photograph of the right flank of the torso of a person with an *E. histolytica* infection. Amebiasis occurs in the United States primarily among male homosexuals who have many sexual partners, and among poor migrant workers. Worldwide there are approximately 30,000 deaths annually resulting from amebiasis.

## Signs and Symptoms
The symptoms of amebiasis are mild, but they may include chronic diarrhea. In cases of ulcerative colitis, peritonitis may also occur. Amebiasis can be fatal.

## Treatment
Oral antiparasitic medications are used to treat amebiasis and are determined by the severity of infection.

## Testing
Tests for amebiasis include stool cultures, serology, and sigmoidoscopy.

# AMYOTROPHIC LATERAL SCLEROSIS

## Description
Amyotrophic lateral sclerosis (ALS) is a progressive, fatal, neurological disease that belongs to a class of disorders known as motor neuron diseases. Although ALS was first reported in a woman in 1869, it received the name Lou Gehrig's disease for a baseball player who died from it in 1941.

## Signs and Symptoms
ALS is the result of the degeneration of specific nerve cells in the central nervous system that control voluntary movement. The degeneration of these motor neuron cells results in the weakening and eventual atrophy of the muscles they control. The deterioration of the muscles leads to paralysis. The signs and symptoms of ALS, which depend on the affected muscles, include tripping and falling, loss of motor control in the hands and arms, speech impairment, difficulty swallowing, breathing impairment, fatigue, and sever muscle twitching and cramping.

## Treatment
There is no cure for amyotrophic lateral sclerosis. ALS is usually fatal within five years. Riluzole may prolong life, but it is not a cure.

## Testing

Neuromuscular examination reveals weakness beginning in one limb or in a proximal group (shoulders or hips). Muscle tremors, spasms, twitching, or atrophy may also be present. Atrophy and twitching of the tongue are also common. Some patients have difficulty controlling laughing or crying, and their gag reflex is abnormal. An electromyogram (EMG) indicates nonfunctional motor nerves; yet sensory nerves function normally.

## ANALGESIC NEPHROPATHY

### Description

Analgesic nephropathy involves damage to the kidneys caused by overexposure to medications, especially over-the-counter medications containing phenacetin, acetaminophen, aspirin, or ibuprofen. Analgesic nephropathy can occur by taking the equivalent of three pills per day for six years. This frequently occurs as a result of self-medication, often for chronic pain. Analgesic nephropathy occurs in about 4 out of 100,000 people, mostly women over 30 years of age. The incidence has decreased significantly since phenacetin is no longer widely available in over-the-counter preparations.

### Signs and Symptoms

Although there may be no symptoms, analgesic nephropathy is characterized by fatigue, abdominal and back pain, changes in urine output, blood in the urine, confusion, bleeding disorders, digestive upset, and swelling.

### Treatment

Analgesic nephropathy is treated by the severity of kidney failure. This may include dietary changes, fluid restriction, dialysis, or kidney transplant. The damage to the kidney may be temporary or chronic (Agha, 2003a).

### Testing

Tests used in the diagnosis of analgesic nephropathy include blood toxicology screen for salicylate (e.g., aspirin), a urinalysis, CBC, examination of material passed in the urine, and an Intravenous Pyelogram (IVP) (Franklin, 1984).

## ANAPHYLAXIS

### Description

Anaphylaxis is a sudden, severe, and whole-body allergic reaction. Histamine and other substances are released causing constriction of the airways, resulting in difficulty breathing and abdominal pain, cramps, vomiting, and diarrhea. Histamine also dilates the blood vessels causing low blood pressure, and histamine causes fluid to leak from the bloodstream into the tissues causing lowered blood volume. The combination of low blood pressure and low blood volume results in shock. Pulmonary swelling and hives can interfere with breathing. Prolonged anaphylaxis can cause heart arrhythmias. Common causes of anaphylaxis include insect bites, horse serum used in some vaccines, food allergies, and drug allergies (e.g., polymyxin, morphine, X-ray dye). Pollens and other inhaled allergens rarely cause anaphylaxis.

## Signs and Symptoms

Anaphylaxis is characterized by sudden difficulty breathing, confusion, slurred speech, rapid and weak pulse, and cyanosis. Other symptoms may include hives, generalized itching, nausea, vomiting, diarrhea, abdominal pain, skin redness, and cough. Reactions may begin with a tingling sensation or metallic taste in the mouth. A drop in blood pressure may cause fainting. Symptoms begin within minutes and last not more than an hour (Sampson et al., 1992).

## Treatment

Anaphylaxis is an emergency condition that may require cardiopulmonary resuscitation (CPR). People with known severe allergic reactions may carry an Epi-Pen or other allergy kit, and should be assisted if necessary. Emergency interventions may include endotracheal intubation, which is placing a tube through the mouth into the airway, or emergency tracheostomy or cricothyrotomy, which are surgeries to place a tube directly into the trachea through the neck (Figure 2-5). Epinephrine should be given by injection without delay. Antihistamines (e.g., diphenhydramine) and corticosteroids (e.g., prednisone) are used to reduce symptoms.

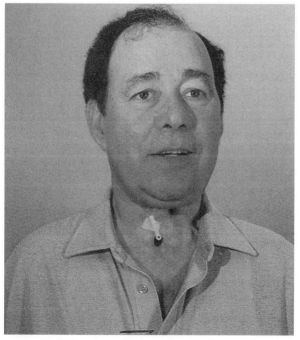

**Figure 2-5** Laryngeal stoma

Anaphylaxis can result in death, but usually responds well to immediate treatment (Accetta, 2004).

## Testing

Testing for the specific allergen that caused anaphylaxis is postponed until after treatment.

## ANEMIA

### Description

Anemia is not a disease, it is a symptom of other diseases. Anemia is a blood disorder in which the capacity of the blood to transport oxygen is decreased, usually because the total number of red blood cells is diminished. The two broad categories of anemia are primary anemia and secondary anemia. Primary anemia includes those types of anemia in which there is a decrease in the production of red blood cells; secondary anemia includes those anemias in which there is an increased loss or destruction of red blood cells. Generally speaking, anemia results from bleeding or from decreased levels of red blood cells, due to either their increased destruction or decreased production in the body. Anemia results from internal bleeding, vitamin deficiencies, decreases in red blood cell production, or increases in red blood cell destruction by the spleen.

### Signs and Symptoms

Possible symptoms of anemia include fatigue, chest pain, skin pallor, increased heart rate, and difficulty breathing.

### Treatment

There are a wide variety of types of anemia, and each is treated by its cause. In some cases, blood transfusions and erythropoietin will correct anemia.

### Testing

Red blood cell counts and hemoglobin level tests are used to diagnose anemia. Other tests are specific to the type of anemia suspected.

## ANENCEPHALY

### Description

Anencephaly is a birth defect in which the brain is grossly malformed (Best, 2002). The cause of anencephaly is not known. It has been linked to maternal diabetes and hyperthermia in early development.

### Signs and Symptoms

The top portion of the brain (i.e., cerebellum and cerebrum) is missing or greatly reduced, but the lower portion is present. Anencephaly is apparent at birth due to the absence of the cranial vault and portions of the cerebrum and cerebellum. Facial structures are generally present and appear relatively normal. The skull occasionally is covered by skin, but usually it is not. Babies are frequently stillborn, and spontaneous abortion during pregnancy is common.

### Treatment

Anencephaly is always fatal, and there is no treatment or cure available.

### Testing

There is no test for diagnosing anencephaly although imaging may be performed to determine the extent of the defect.

## ANEURYSM

### Description

An aneurysm is the abnormal enlargement or bulging of an artery caused by damage to or weakness in the blood vessel wall. Although aneurysms can occur in any blood vessels, they almost always form in an artery. There are several areas in which aneurysms are more common in the body than others. Although most fatal aneurysms occur in the abdominal aorta or in cerebral arteries of the brain, aneurysms may occur in the thoracic aorta of the chest or in the large arteries of the lower extremities. They are known as peripheral aneurysms when they occur in the extremities. The rupture of an aneurysm can cause bleeding and may lead to sudden death. Figure 2-6 is a photograph of a ruptured aortic aneurysm.

### Signs and Symptoms

Most people are unaware that they have an aneurysm. Symptoms of an aortic aneurysm may include pain in the back, abdomen, or groin. Most aortic aneurysms are detected during a physical exam for other health reasons.

The symptoms of a cerebral aneurysm differ from the symptoms of an aortic aneurysm. Common characteristics of cerebral aneurysms include headaches, drowsiness, neck stiffness, nausea, vomiting, mental confusion, and dizziness.

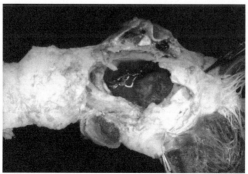

**Figure 2-6** A ruptured aortic aneurysm.
(Courtesy of the CDC, Susan Lindsley)

## Treatment

Small aneurysms rarely rupture and can be treated by medications like beta-blockers that lower blood pressure. Large aneurysms, however, may require surgical removal. During surgery, the damaged portion of the artery is replaced with a flexible tube called a graft.

## Testing

Aneurysms can be detected by imaging tests and angiograms. An angiogram is an X-ray used to produce images of the inside of blood vessels.

## ANGIOMAS

### Description

An angioma is a benign tumor that consists of vessels. These tumors can be located anywhere on the body (see Color Plate 5).

### Signs and Symptoms

Some of the different types of angiomas include spider angiomas, cherry angiomas, and senile angiomas. Benign tumors of blood vessels are known as hemangiomas; benign tumors of lymph vessels are known as lymphangiomas. Port-wine stains, or birthmarks, are hemangiomas of the capillaries.

### Treatment

Angiomas may be removed by spraying liquid nitrogen on the skin, which freezes the tissue. Although infrequent, angiomas may recur after removal. Angiomas are mainly treated for cosmetic reasons.

## ANGIOSARCOMAS

### Description

Angiosarcomas are uncommon cancers that grow rapidly, arising from cells derived from vessels. Angiosarcomas are aggressive, spreading throughout lymph nodes and the rest of the body. Angiosarcomas are more frequent in skin and soft tissue but may occur in any region of the body, including the liver, breast, spleen, bone, or heart.

### Signs and Symptoms

Angiosarcomas have a high mortality rate owing to their biological properties. Often, the cancer is advanced by the time signs and symptoms appear. Malignant tumors of blood vessels are known as hemangiosarcomas, and malignant tumors of lymph vessels are known as lymphangiosarcomas.

### Treatment

Treatment for angiosarcomas can include chemotherapy, radiation therapy, and surgery.

## Testing

As with most soft tissue tumors, angiosarcomas are diagnosed through radiological examinations. Additional tests may include biopsy and needle aspiration.

## ANGIOSTRONGYLIASIS

### Description

Angiostrongyliasis is caused by *Angiostrongylus cantonensis,* which is a worm that infects rats. Humans can become infected with *A. cantonensis* by eating raw or undercooked snails, slugs, freshwater prawns, frogs, or crabs. Infection is more prevelant in cultures in which eating snails is more common. Although most cases of *A. cantonensis* infection occur in Southeast Asia, the Pacific Islands, and the Caribbean, a few cases have occurred in the United States in Hawaii and Louisiana. *Angiostrongylus cantonensis* is not spread from contact with infected persons, nor is it spread through contact with contaminated cat feces. The infection is typically self-resolving without medical treatment (Ohio State University, 1996).

### Signs and Symptoms

Symptoms of *A. cantonensis* infection are typically mild and last about two weeks, but a rare type of meningitis known as eosinophilic meningitis may develop. Symptoms include headache, stiff neck, tingling or painful feelings in the skin, low-grade fever, nausea, and vomiting (*Angiostrongylus cantonensis infection,* 2004).

### Treatment

Antibiotic treatment for angiostrongyliasis is rare because the parasite dies over time without treatment. No drug has proven to be effective for the treatment of *A. cantonensis* or *A. costaricensis* infections. Relief of symptoms for *A. cantonensis* infections can be achieved by the use of analgesics, corticosteroids, and careful removal of the cerebral spinal fluid at frequent intervals.

### Testing

In eosinophilic meningitis the cerebrospinal fluid is abnormal (e.g, elevated pressure, proteins, and leukocytes). In abdominal angiostrongyliasis, eggs and larvae can be identified in tissue biopsies.

## ANISAKIASIS

### Description

Anisakiasis is a parasitic infection caused by ingestion of *Anisakis simplex* or *Pseudoterranova decipiens.* The adults stages of these roundworms reside in clusters within the mucosal layer of the stomach of marine mammals. The occurrence of anisakiasis is most common in areas of the world with high rates of eating raw fish or squid like Japan, the Pacific Coast of South America, and the Netherlands (*Anisakiasis,* 2004).

## Signs and Symptoms

The symptoms of anisakiasis begin within hours after ingestion of the parasite, and include violent abdominal pain, nausea, and vomiting. The larvae may be coughed up as well. If the larvae infect the intestines, the victim can experience an eosinophilic granulomatous response that mimicks the symptoms of Crohn's disease.

## Treatment

The treatment for anisakiasis is surgical or endoscopic removal of the parasite.

## Testing

Testing for anisakiasis includes gastroscopic examination during which the larvae are visualized and removed. Examination of biopsied tissue may also be conducted.

## ANKYLOSING SPONDYLITIS

### Description

Ankylosing spondylitis is an idiopathic, chronic inflammatory condition affecting axial joints including the spine and sacroiliac joints. It causes eventual fusion of the spine, and peripheral joints may become involved (Schaffert, 2003).

### Signs and Symptoms

The signs of ankylosing spondylitis normally appear in a person's late teens or 20s. The large joints of the lower extremities are more commonly involved in the juvenile form of ankylosing spondylitis. The disease is marked by a gradual onset of low back pain that worsens in the morning and abates during the day. The pain is lessened with activity and worsens during periods of rest, which helps distinguish ankylosing spondylitis from mechanical low back pain. In about a quarter of the cases, proximal joints are involved in the disease; small joints are rarely involved. Pain and stiffness of the rib cage and chest pain may also occur.

### Treatment

The goal of treatment is to control pain and decrease inflammation, primarily through nonsteroidal anti-inflammatory drugs. Sulfasalazine, steroids, and immunosuppressive agents also are used. No particular drug is superior for treating ankylosing spondylitis.

### Testing

Testing indicates low-grade anemia associated with chronic diseae. Antinuclear antibody (ANA) and rheumatoid factor (RF) are within reference ranges. Although not always present, HLA-B27 antigen is positive most of the time. X-ray of the pelvis shows sacroiliitis or fusion of sacroiliac joints.

## ANTHRAX

### Description

Anthrax is a disease common in livestock around the world. Animals become infected by spores found on plants they eat (Figure 2-7). The three forms of human anthrax include cutaneous, inhalation, and gastrointestinal anthrax. Each of these forms of anthrax results from wound contamination or the inhalation or the ingestion of spores. In the United States, there are typically less than five anthrax cases per year. Worldwide, however, several thousand cases are reported annually. Anthrax is of recent interest as a biological weapon (Anthrax, 2003 and 2002).

To become infected with any form of anthrax, the individual must be exposed to the spores of *Bacillus anthracis*. The bacterium is a gram-positive rod found singly or in chains; however, its gram staining changes with age or nutritional stress. It is an aerobic and facultative bacterium that forms spores aerobically. It is nonmotile, unlike other species of the genus *Bacillus*. The unique capsule on *B. anthracis* protects it from the body's phagocytic cells. In other words, *B. anthracis* changes are based on environmental conditions. It requires oxygen, but it can adapt to the available level of oxygen in the environment. It can also become dormant until good environmental nutrition becomes available.

### Signs and Symptoms

Cutaneous anthrax lesions usually remain localized, but they may spread to the lymph glands. If a septic infection occurs, its symptoms are fever, malaise, and headache, although in normal cases of cutaneous anthrax septic infection does not develop. Inhalation anthrax has similar symptoms lasting about three days before a sudden phase of respiratory

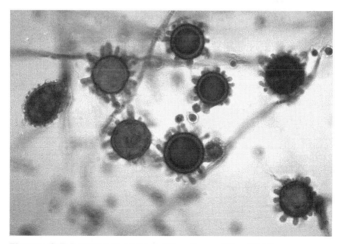

**Figure 2-7** Bacterial spores (Courtesy of the CDC)

distress occurs. The severe phase of inhalation anthrax may take only 24 hours before death occurs.

## Treatment
Anthrax is typically treated with a broad array of antibiotics. Anthrax is not a contagious disease.

## Testing
Anthrax is diagnosed by isolating *B. anthracis* from blood, skin lesions, or respiratory secretions.

## AORTIC COARCTATION

### Description
Coarctation of the aorta is a narrowing of the aorta most commonly found near the left subclavian artery, which is in the left shoulder (Shah, 2002). Aortic coarctation usually occurs when the middle layer of the arterial wall folds around the aorta. The aorta may be deformed along its length, it may be in segments, or it may be twisted. The deformed aorta has layers consisting of thickened ridges that protrude into the inside of the aorta (i.e., the aortic lumen). Aortic coarctation disrupts the flow of blood, is assocated with aneurysms, and causes the death of the neighboring blood vessels.

### Characteristics
Infants may experience congestive heart failure, severe acidosis, or poor circulation in the lower body. Most adults have no symptoms, although they may experience hypertension, headache, nosebleed, leg cramps, muscle weakness, cold feet, or neurological changes. The left arm may be smaller than normal.

### Treatment
Coarctation is treated with surgery to correct the deformed aorta.

### Testing
Testing for coarctation may include normal X-rays, barium esophagram, echocardiogram, MRI, cardiac catheterization, and electrocardiogram.

## APERT SYNDROME

### Description
Apert syndrome is a genetic disease that is also known as acrocephalosyndactyly. Apert syndrome can be inherited and is characterized by premature closure of the seams between the skull bones, resulting in a triangular shape to the head. Apert syndrome is caused by mutations in the fibroblast growth factor receptor 2 gene. The face is distinctive. There may be webbing between the fingers and toes. The bones in the hands and feet eventually fuse.

## Signs and Symptoms

Apert syndrome is characterized by limb deformities, early closure of fontanelles resulting in ridges along the suture lines, underdevelopment of the midface, bulging eyes, delayed soft spot closure, short stature, hearing loss, mental retardation, and ear infections. Fusion or severe webbing of adjacent fingers and toes occurs, resulting in what is referred to as mitten hands (Kaplan, 1991; Stewart, 2003b).

## Treatment

Treatment consists of surgery to correct the skull, midface, and palate.

## Testing

Apert syndrome is diagnsoed with imaging tests, and a genetic test for mutations in the fibroblast growth factor receptor 2 gene can confirm the diagnosis.

## APLASTIC ANEMIA

## Description

Aplastic anemia is not a single disease, but a group of closely related disorders characterized by the failure of the bone marrow to produce all three types of blood cells: red blood cells, white blood cells, and platelets. Chemicals such as benzene and arsenic may cause destruction of bone marrow. X-rays and ionizing radiation may damage the bone marrow as well. Aplastic anemia may be inherited or can result from a viral infection.

## Signs and Symptoms

Underproduction of white blood cells causes unexplained infections. Underproduction of platelets causes excessive bleeding. And fatigue results from an underproduction of red blood cells.

## Treatment

Severe cases of aplastic anemia require immediate treatment to stabilize the disease until a stem cell transplant can be performed. Patients with mild or moderate symptoms often receive blood transfusions, platelet transfusions, and drug therapy.

## Testing

Diagnosis of aplastic anemia is based on a CBC. Aplastic anemia is strongly suspected when two or three of the cell counts are extremely low. A definitive diagnosis is made if a marrow biopsy shows a great reduction in the number of cells in the marrow itself.

## APPENDICITIS

## Description

Appendicitis is inflammation of the appendix, which is a small, wormlike structure attached to the cecum on the lower right side of the abdomen. If untreated, an inflamed appendix can burst, causing a potentially fatal infection of the abdomen known as peritonitis. Appendicitis may occur after a viral infection or when the opening connecting the large intestine and appendix becomes blocked. Appendicitis is considered an emergency, due to the risk of rupture.

## Signs and Symptoms
The characteristics of appendicitis include pain in the lower-right side of the abdomen, nausea, vomiting, constipation, diarrhea, low-grade fever, abdominal swelling, and loss of appetite.

## Treatment
Appendicitis is treated by an appendectomy, which is surgery to remove the appendix.

## Testing
A physical exam to determine location and response to pain (e.g., McBurney's sign, rebound tenderness, guarding, psoas sign, Rovsing's sign) and an abdominal CT scan with rectal contrast are used to diagnose appendicitis.

## ARTERIOSCLEROSIS

### Description
Arteriosclerosis is a disease of the arterial vessels marked by thickening, hardening, and loss of elasticity in the arterial walls. There are three forms of arteriosclerosis: atherosclerosis; sclerosis of arterioles; and calcification of the medial layer of the arteries, which is a rare disorder known as Mönckeberger's calcification. Arteriosclerosis is found in the large and medium-sized arteries in the body, which include the aorta, carotid arteries, iliac arteries, coronary arteries, and the femoral arteries. The presence of a large quantity of plaque causes the artery to be hard, inelastic, and brittle.

### Signs and Symptoms
Symptoms include leg pain, especially in the calves and feet; numbness or pain in the foot or toes when at rest; and ulcers or gangrene on the foot or toes. The problem is common in diabetics.

### Treatment
Arteriosclerosis is treated with exercise, medications, and—rarely—surgery.

### Testing
Testing for the presence of arteriosclerosis may include checking for an abnormal whooshing sound called a bruit. Testing also includes EKG, chest X-ray, ultrasound, CT scan, angiograms, and an exercise stress test. An ankle/brachial index may also be conducted to compare blood pressure in the ankle with that of the arm.

## ARTERITIS

### Description

Arteritis is an idiopathic, inflammatory disease that affects the arteries. The arterial system is illustrated in Figure 2-8. The most common causes are infections. For example, arteritis may accompany infectious respiratory diseases like aspergillosis, pneumonia, and tuberculosis. Lesions may appear in the inflamed arteries of the respiratory system. Arteritis may accompany autoimmune diseases like systemic lupus erythematosus, rheumatoid arthritis, and inflammatory bowel disease. Two diseases characterized by arteritis include Takayasu's arteritis and temporal arteritis.

### Signs and Symptoms

Typically, temporal arteritis afflicts the large arteries in the head, resulting in a severe headache that develops suddenly at the temples or back of the head. The blood vessels in the temple may feel swollen and bumpy to the touch, and the scalp may feel painful when the hair is brushed. Double vision, blurred vision, large blind spots, or blindness may develop. The jaw, chewing muscles, and tongue may hurt when eating or speaking.

### Treatment

Corticosteroids such as prednisone are prescribed to reduce inflammation. Medications that suppress the immune system, such as cyclophosphamide or methotrexate, are occasionally prescribed to minimize the dose of steroids needed.

### Testing

Biopsy of the artery is the most likely confirmation of specific forms of arteritis.

## ARTHRITIS

### Description

Arthritis is inflammation of the joints. There are many forms of arthritis, which all have different causes ranging from infections to excessive use of a particular joint. For some people, arthritic pain lasts only a few months and goes away without causing any noticeable damage. Others have moderate forms marked by periods of symptom flare-up and periods of remission. Still others have a severe form of the disease that is active most of the time, lasts for many years or a lifetime, and leads to serious joint damage and disability.

### Signs and Symptoms

There are numerous forms of arthritis, but they are all characterized by redness, swelling of the joints, lack of flexibility of the joints, hardening and stiffening of the joints, loss of function, and disfigurement of the joints.

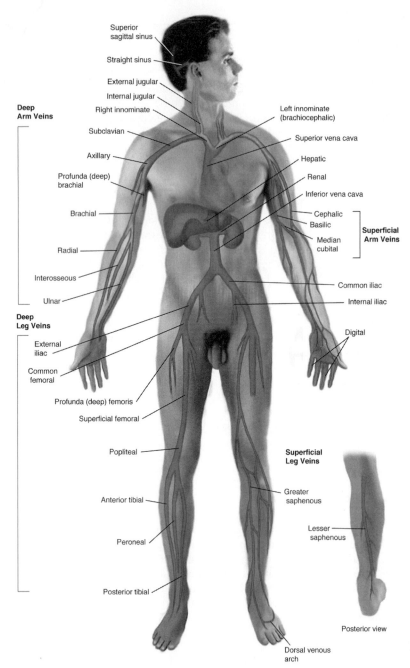

Superior sagittal sinus

Straight sinus

External jugular

Internal jugular

**Deep Arm Veins**

Right innominate

Subclavian

Axillary

Profunda (deep) brachial

Brachial

Radial

Interosseous

Ulnar

**Deep Leg Veins**

External iliac

Common femoral

Profunda (deep) femoris

Superficial femoral

Popliteal

Anterior tibial

Peroneal

Posterior tibial

Left innominate (brachiocephalic)

Superior vena cava

Hepatic

Renal

Inferior vena cava

Cephalic

Basilic

Median cubital

**Superficial Arm Veins**

Common iliac

Internal iliac

Digital

**Superficial Leg Veins**

Greater saphenous

Lesser saphenous

Posterior view

Dorsal venous arch

**Figure 2-8** Arterial system

## Treatment

There is no cure for arthritis. Disease-modifying antirheumatic drugs are used to slow the course of disease. Biologic response modifiers are new drugs that block the action of inflammation, triggering cellular proteins (i.e., cytokines) that trigger inflammation. Three of these drugs—etanercept (Enbrel), infliximab (Remicade), and adalimumab (Humira)—reduce inflammation by blocking the reaction of TNF-$\alpha$ molecules. Anakinra (Kineret) blocks a protein called interleukin 1 (IL-1) that is seen in excess in patients with arthritis. Surgical procedures include joint replacement, tendon reconstruction, and synovectomy.

## Testing

Arthritis can be difficult to diagnose in its early stages for several reasons. There is no single test for the disease, and symptoms differ greatly. Tests include rheumatoid factor, CBC, Erythrocyte sedimentation rate (ESR), C-reactive protein, and X-rays to determine the degree of joint destruction.

## ASBESTOSIS

### Description

Asbestosis is a pneumoconiosis resulting from the inhalation of asbestos, which is a crystalline form of silica that has a fibrous structure. The extremely fine strands of asbestos are capable of reaching far down the respiratory tract, where they interact with the immune system (i.e., macrophages) to cause fibrous lesions, which may develop into cancer. Asbestos was once used in flame-retardant materials, insulation, roofing shingles, floor tiles, siding, and joint compounds. Asbestos must be inhaled to cause asbestosis.

### Signs and Symptoms

Asbestosis is characterized by difficulty breathing, cough, tightness in the chest, and chest pain. Other possible symptoms include nail abnormalities and clubbing of the fingers.

### Treatment

There is no cure for asbestosis, but asbestos must be avoided. Treatments of symptoms include respiratory treatments to remove secretions from the lungs, and medications to thin secretions. Oxygen may also be needed.

### Testing

Diagnosis is based on imaging tests of the chest and lung function tests.

## ASCARIASIS

### Description

Ascariasis is a disease caused by infection with the ascarid worm, which can grow to over 12 inches in length and lives in the small intestine. Ascariasis occurs in impoverished regions of the world exhibiting substandard sanitation and hygiene. Infection also occurs in rural areas of the southeastern United States. The most likely source of ascarid egg ingestion is from infected pig manure. Humans may ingest contaminated pig manure if it is used as fertilizer in gardens. Infected humans can also pass ascarid eggs in their feces, so contact with contaminated human feces may also lead to infection (*Ascaris infection*, 2004).

## Signs and Symptoms

Ascariasis is typically asymptomatic, although abdominal pain may occur in cases of advanced infection. As the immature worms migrate through the lungs, coughing and labored breathing may occur. The intestines may become blocked with worms. The overriding sign of disease, if present, is malnutrition.

## Treatment

Treatment includes medications that kill intestinal parasitic worms (e.g., albendazole or mebendazole).

## Testing

Testing includes examination of feces for parasites and ova, abdominal X-rays, and a CBC.

## ASHERMAN'S SYNDROME

### Description

Asherman's syndrome is the presence of adhesions as a result of scar formation after uterine surgery. Typically, it occurs after repetitive dilatation and curettage (D & C) procedures are performed. Asherman's syndrome is more likely in the presence of an infection in the uterus during the D & C. Adhesions can also form in the uterus after infection with tuberculosis or schistosomiasis. These infections are rare in the United States, and Asherman's syndrome is even less common. The lesions associated with Asherman's syndrome do not usually contain blood vessels, which aids in their treatment (P. Chen, 2004a).

### Signs and Symptoms

Asherman's syndrome is characterized by lack of menstruation, infertility, and recurrent miscarriages. These symptoms are more likely to indicate Asherman's syndrome, as opposed to other conditions, if they occur suddenly after a D & C or other uterine surgery.

### Treatment

Surgical treatment includes removing adhesions or scar tissue from the uterus. This procedure, known as hysteroscopy, can usually be performed with small instruments and a camera through the cervix. After scar tissue is removed, the uterine cavity must be kept open to prevent recurrence of the adhesions. This is done by placing a small balloon inside the uterus for several days. Estrogen replacement therapy may also be used while the uterus heals. Antibiotic treatment may be needed as well. Some surgeons avoid the use of energy-generating instruments like lasers to remove adhesions from the uterus; they use scissors instead.

## Testing

Asherman's syndrome is diagnosed by a pelvic exam. Transvaginal ultrasounds and hysteroscopy may reveal scar tissue in the uterus. Lab tests for tuberculosis or schistosomiasis may be necessary. Other imaging tests used in the diagnosis of Asherman's syndrome include sonohysterography and hysterosalpingograms (Klein & Garcia, 1973).

## ASIATIC CHOLERA

### Description

Asiatic cholera, also known as epidemic cholera, is caused by *Vibrio cholerae*, which is a bacterium found in contaminated seafood, usually from the Gulf coast of the United States. Cholera is more common in Asia and is endemic in India. When untreated, cholera has a 50 percent mortality rate in comparison to treated cases, where the mortality is near 1 percent.

### Signs and Symptoms

*V. cholerae* grows in the small intestine producing a poison that results in the secretion of chlorides, bicarbonates, and water. These high levels of electrolytes and water cause rice-water stool (see Color Plate 6). The loss of between three and five gallons of fluid and electrolytes from the intestines each day causes fatal shock. The blood becomes extremely viscous due to the loss of fluids, causing failure of the organs. Fever is not a typical symptom of cholera.

### Treatment

Treatment replaces fluid and electrolytes lost through diarrhea. Pharmaceutical treatment may include tetracycline and other antibiotics.

### Testing

Gram stain, stool culture, and blood culture are positive for *V. cholerae*.

## ASPERGER SYNDROME

### Description

Asperger syndrome, which was labeled autistic psychopathy in 1944 by Hans Asperger, is an idiopathic disorder related to autism. Asperger syndrome may be a mild form of autism. Although Asperger syndrome may be genetic, some theories suggest a prenatal infection. Although people with Asperger syndrome exhibit marked deficiencies in social skills, many have above-average intelligence. Generally, there is no language development delay; however, patients often are unable to properly use language socially. They lack an understanding of the rhythmic and intonational aspects of language (Blackman, 2004a).

## Signs and Symptoms

Children with Asperger syndrome fail to use body language, fail to develop peer relationships, are unable to share in other people's happiness, and lack social and emotional reciprocity. There is no delay in cognitive development, in the development of age-appropriate self-help skills, or in curiosity about the environment. Asperger patients are often inflexible about specific nonfunctional routines or rituals, and they may exhibit persistent preoccupation with parts of objects. There is often an unusually intense preoccupation with narrow areas of interest, such as obsession with train schedules, phone books, or collections of objects. Asperger syndrome may also include repetitive self-injurious behavior. Patients may also exhibit extremely rich vocabularies although they fail to comprehend language pragmatics (OASIS, 2005).

## Treatment

There is no cure or specific treatment for Asperger syndrome.

## Testing

There is no specific test for Asperger syndrome.

## ASPERGILLOSIS

### Description

Aspergillosis is a disease found among gardeners and farmers. It is caused by a fungus present in decaying vegetation and manure. *Aspergillus fumigatus* spores spread through ingestion or inhalation (Figure 2-9). Other forms of aspergillosis can be caused by *A. flavus*, which is a mold found on corn, peanuts, and grains; *A. glaucus*, which is a bluish mold found on dried fruit; and *A. niger*, which forms black spores in the ear canal. The immunocompromised are most at risk for contracting aspergillosis (*Aspergillosis*, 2002).

### Signs and Symptoms

Aspergillosis is an infection of the mucous membranes resulting in lesions in the bronchi, lungs, ear canal, skin, eyes, nose, or urethra. Nodules may form in the kidney, lungs, or liver. Aspergillosis is accompanied by fever, cough, and chest pain. The fungi may then disseminate to other organs, including the skin, bones, and brain, where the disease may cause fatal brain lesions.

### Treatment

Depending on the severity of disease and the degree of involvement of the lung tissue, surgical excision of tissues infected with fungus may be necessary. Severe aspergillosis is treated with intravenous amphotericin B, itraconazole, or other antifungal medications.

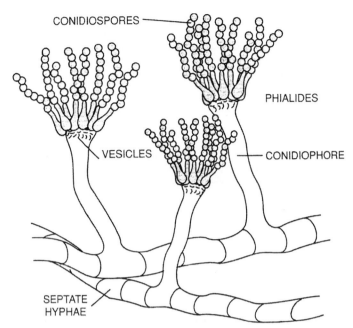

CONIDIOSPORES

PHIALIDES

VESICLES

CONIDIOPHORE

SEPTATE
HYPHAE

**Figure 2-9** *Aspergillus fumigatus*

## Testing

Aspergillosis is diagnosed through chest X-rays, CT scan, sputum stain and culture, biopsy, aspergillus antigen skin test, and aspergillosis antibody tests.

## ASPIRATION PNEUMONIA

### Description

Aspiration pneumonia is an inflammation of the lungs and bronchial tubes caused by inhaling food, liquids, or secretions, from the mouth into the lungs. A lung abscess may result from aspiration pneumonia. Persons with an altered mental status, altered level of consciousness, or abnormal swallowing reflexes are at the highest risk. Aspiration of vomit can produce acute respiratory distress. Aspiration pneumonia may be caused by drug or alcohol ingestions, including drugs for general anesthesia, brain traumas, meningitis, and diseases of the throat.

### Signs and Symptoms

Aspiration pneumonia is characterized by the sudden onset of coughing and difficulty breathing associated with eating, drinking, or vomiting. It may also include altered mental status, cyanosis, expectoration (discharge from throat or lungs) of putrid materials, fever, chest pain, abdominal pain, loss of appetite, and weight loss. Aspiration pneumonia may also cause alterations in heartbeat, crackles and bronchial rales primarily in the right lung, and decreased breath sounds. A condition known as egophony, in which the patient's voice is modified as to resemble the bleating of a goat, may be heard when applying the ear to the patient's chest. When the patient says "e," it is heard as an "a" through a stethoscope placed on the chest.

## Treatment
Aspiration pneumonia is treated with antibiotics, and acute respiratory distress may be fatal.

## Testing
Tests for aspiration pneumonia may include bronchoscopy, thoracentesis, chest X-rays, and CBC. Bronchial samples may be needed for antibiotic therapy but are not always necessary.

## ASTHMA

### Description
Asthma is a condition in which the bronchi are hypersensitive to stimuli. Not unlike an allergic reaction, the mucous lining of the bronchi become irritated, and the bronchi proceed to swell shut, causing a reduction in airflow. Attacks often cause the individual to hunch forward in an attempt to inhale. Asthma attacks may be caused by allergens such as pollen, dust, mold spores, or animal dander. Respiratory tract infections may also cause asthma attacks. Certain foods such as eggs, shellfish, and chocolate may bring about an asthma attack. Increased fatigue adds to the likelihood of an attack.

### Signs and Symptoms
Individuals with asthma have a characteristic wheezing sound accompanied by shortness of breath. It usually begins suddenly, resolves spontaneously, is periodic, worsens at night or early morning, and is aggravated by exposure to cold air, exercise, or heartburn. The wheezing is normally relieved by bronchodilators. Other symptoms include a nonproductive cough and intercostal retractions, which occur when the muscles between the ribs attempt to expand the rib cage to force more air into the lungs. More severe disease characterisitics include severe anxiety, rapid pulse, cyanosis, sweating, decreased consciousness, nasal flaring, chest pain, and coughing up blood. It may also take twice as long to exhale as to inhale.

### Treatment
Treatment includes controlling exposure to potential allergens. Long-term control medications include inhaled steroids (e.g., Azmacort, Vanccril, AeroBid, Flovent), leukotriene inhibitors (e.g., Singulair, Accolate), long-acting bronchodilators (e.g., famoterol, Serevent), cromolyn sodium (Intal) or nedocromil sodium, and combinations of anti-inflammatories and bronchodilators, using either separate inhalers or a single inhaler

(Advair Diskus). Medications to control attacks may include short-acting bronchodilators (e.g., Proventil, Ventolin, Xopenex) and corticosteroids (e.g., prednisone, methylprednisolone).

### Testing
Tests for asthma include pulmonary function tests, peak flow measurements, chest X-rays, allergy tests, arterial blood gas, and eosinophil counts.

## ATELECTASIS

### Description
Atelectasis is commonly referred to as a collapsed lung. Atelectasis is the loss of lung volume due to inadequate expansion of air spaces, which results in inadequate oxygen and carbon dioxide exchange within the lungs. The result is that blood is not able to eliminate carbon dioxide and refresh itself with the oxygen it needs. There are two categories of collapsed lung: obstructed and nonobstructed (described next).

### Signs and Symptoms
Obstructive atelectasis is the most common type of collapsed lung, and it results when the trachea or bronchi become blocked. Causes of obstructive atelectasis include choking on a foreign body, tumors in the airway, fungal respiratory infections, or the presence of excessive amounts of mucus that plug the airway. Examples of diseases associated with mucous blockage include bronchial asthma, chronic bronchitis, cystic fibrosis, paralysis, and amyotrophic lateral sclerosis. Depending on the level of obstruction, the entire lung, a single lobe, or a segment of the lung may collapse.

Nonobstructive atelectasis can be caused by loss of contact between the parietal and visceral pleurae, compression, loss of surfactant, and replacement of lung tissue by scarring. Congestive heart failure can cause the accumulation of fluids resulting in nonobstructive lung collapse, or it may be caused by blood or air within the pleural cavity. Penetrating trauma, such as gunshot wounds or stab wounds, may allow air to leak from inside the lung into the pleural space. The trapped air between the outside and inside of the lung prevents the lung from fully expanding and causes it to collapse. This condition is referred to as a pneumothorax. If blood becomes trapped in the same space, the condition is referred to hemothorax.

### Treatment
The goal of treatment is to re-expand the lung and remove secretions. This may be accomplished by positioning the patient on the unaffected side to allow re-expansion of the lung, removal of any obstruction by bronchoscopy, encouragement of deep breathing for incentive spirometry, percussion of the chest, and positioning the patient for postural drainage. The collapsed lung usually reinflates gradually once the obstruction has been removed, although residual scarring or damage can occur.

### Testing
Tests for atelactasis include chest X-rays and bronchoscopy.

## ATHEROSCLEROSIS

### Description
Atherosclerosis is a process in which deposits of fatty substances—cholesterol, cellular waste, calcium, and other substances—build up in the inner lining of an artery, forming plaque (see Color Plate 7). It usually affects large and medium-sized arteries and is common among the elderly. Although plaque can become large enough to block arteries, it is most dangerous when its integrity is challenged allowing the possibility of fragmentation. If fragile plaque ruptures, the pieces of plaque each become a floating embolus that can cause blood clots. If the embolism blocks an artery that supplies blood to the heart, the resulting acute cardiac failure can lead to sudden death. If the artery leads to the brain, a stroke may occur that may also lead to sudden death. Obstruction of the arteries of either the upper or lower extremities can lead to gangrene (Atherosclerosis, n/d).

### Signs and Symptoms
Atherosclerosis is a slow, complex disease that typically starts in childhood and progresses with age. Potential causes of damage to the arterial walls are believed to include elevated levels of cholesterol and triglyceride in the blood, high blood pressure, smoking tobacco, and diabetes. Hypertension, obesity, family history of cardiovascular diseases, and physical inactivity all predispose individuals to atherosclerosis. Symptoms are based on the affected artery, but may include chest pain, periods of inability to function, strokes, fainting, pain, and numbness or tingling.

### Treatment
Treatment of atherosclerosis often includes medications and diet to reduce fats and cholesterol levels. Exercise and weight loss are also recommended. Medications include cholestyramine, colestipol, nicotinic acid, gemfibrozil, probucol, atorvastatin, and lovastatin. Aspirin, ticlopidine, clopidogrel, or anticoagulants may be used to reduce the risk of clot formation. Balloon angioplasty and stenting may be used to open occluded arteries. Endarterectomy or a bypass graft may be required in severe cases.

### Testing
Atherosclerosis may not be diagnosed until symptoms develop. Atherosclerosis may be noted by a reduced or absent pulse in the affected artery and by the presence of a bruit, which is a whooshing or blowing sound heard over the affected artery with a stethoscope. Other common tests include ankle/brachial indices, Doppler study, ultrasonic duplex scanning, CT scans, magnetic resonance arteriography, arteriography, intravascular ultrasound, and cardiac stress testing.

## ATRIAL MYXOMA

### Description
Atrial myxomas are the most common primary benign heart tumors. Unlike atrial myxoma, most tumors of the heart are due to secondary

metastasis, which means they have spread from another site. Atrial myxomas occur in the heart wall and on the cardiac septum. Atrial myxomas are more common in women, and most occur in the left side of the heart (Sharma, 2004a).

## Signs and Symptoms
People who have atrial myxomas experience breathing difficulties that worsen with activity, while lying flat, and during sleep. Other signs and symptoms include dizziness, fainting, heart palpitations, chest pain, cough, fever, weight loss, joint pain, Raynaud's phenomenon, swelling, and clubbing of the fingers.

## Treatment
Most atrial myxomas are benign and can be removed by surgical resection.

## Testing
Two-dimensional echocardiography is used to diagnose myxomas.

## AUTISM

### Description
Autism is a physical condition linked to abnormal biology and neurochemistry in the brain. Autism is idiopathic, but genetic factors seem to be important. For example, identical twins are more likely than fraternal twins or siblings to both have autism. Autism may also be linked to abnormalities along the digestive tract, indicating that diet may be a cause. Proteins in foods like wheat and milk may cause leakiness in the gut that introduces substances into the brain. Several major studies have found no connection between the mumps measles rubella (MMR) vaccine and autism.

### Signs and Symptoms
Most autistic children are diagnosed between 18 months and two years of age. They have difficulties in verbal and nonverbal communication, social interactions, and pretend play. In some, aggression toward others or themselves may be present. Some children with autism appear normal before age two and then suddenly regress and lose language or social skills. Autistic persons may perform repeated body movements, show unusual attachments to objects, or have unusual distress when routines are changed. Individuals may also experience sensitivities in the senses of sight, hearing, touch, smell, or taste (Autism Society of America, 2005; Hart, 2004b).

### Treatment
There is no cure for autism. A variety of effective therapies are available, including applied behavior analysis, medications, music therapy, occupational therapy, physical therapy, sensory integration, speech therapy, and vision therapy. In addition, there have been case reports of children with autism seeing improvement in behavior by following a gluten-free or a casein-free diet. Not all experts agree that dietary changes will make a difference, and not all reports studying this method have shown positive results.

## Testing

There is no biological test for autism, so diagnosis is based on specific criteria in the *Diagnostic and Statistical Manual IV*. The diagnostic evaluation of autism includes a complete physical and neurologic examination, as well as the use of a specific diagnostic instrument such as the Gilliam Autism Rating Scale, the Pervasive Developmental Disorders Screening Test—Stage 3, the Childhood Autism Rating Scale, or the Autism Diagnostic Observation Schedule—Generic. Children with known or suspected autism will often have genetic testing and metabolic testing.

## B VIRUS ENCEPHALOMYELITIS

### Description

B virus encephalomyelitis is a fatal disease of the brain and meninges surrounding the brain caused by B virus, which is also known as cercopithecine herpesvirus 1 (CDC, 2002). B virus is commonly found among macaque monkeys. Infected monkeys exhibit no signs of disease. B virus encephalomyelitis is rare in humans, but is estimated to be fatal in 80 percent of untreated patients. Similar to hepatitis B virus in humans, monkey B virus is transmitted through contact with monkey secretions.

### Signs and Symptoms

Initial signs of infection include skin lesions, itching, pain, or numbness near the exposure site (e.g., bite or scratch).

### Treatment

The most critical period for the prevention of B virus infection is during the first few minutes after exposure. Immediately wash the skin. Three orally administered drugs—acyclovir, valacyclovir, and famciclovir—are currently available for treatment of B virus infection.

### Testing

B virus is classified as a Biosafety Level 4 biologic agent, which also includes the Ebola virus and Marburg viruses. Cultures must be sent to a facility that has expertise with B virus.

## BABESIOSIS

### Description

Although it is a common nonhuman animal infection, babesiosis can also be a rare but fatal human disease transmitted by infected ticks. In the United States, babesiosis occurs mainly in northeastern coastal areas, especially in New York and Massachussetts, although cases have been reported in California, Georgia, Missouri, Washington, and Wisconsin. Babesiosis is caused by the *Babesia* parasite, which is a protozoan that can infect deer ticks, which also spread Lyme disease. Concurrent infections of babesiosis and Lyme disease may occur. Babesiosis has also been known to occur as a result of transfusion of contaminated blood (*Babesiosis*, 2004).

## Signs and Symptoms

*Babesia* is a parasite that attacks the red blood cells. The symptoms of babesiosis, if present, may include fatigue, loss of appetite, fever, drenching sweats, muscle pain, and headache. Symptoms may last for several months, and they may appear up to 12 months after tick-bite exposure. Severe complications of babesiosis include dangerously low blood pressure, liver disorder, hemolytic anemia, and kidney failure.

## Treatment

Although it may be fatal, most cases of babesiosis are asymptomatic and resolve without medical treatment.

## Testing

Babesiosis is diagnosed through testing for the presence of *Babesia* in the red blood cells.

## BACILLARY ANGIOMATOSIS

### Description

Bacillary angiomatosis is caused by infection with *Rochalimaea* bacteria, and it is one disease used by the CDC to define the presence of AIDS in HIV-positive patients. If a person has HIV and a low T-cell count (specifically CD4+ T-lymphocytes), and the person has bacillary angiomatosis, the person is considered by the CDC to have AIDS. Bacillary angiomatosis can be spread through contact with cats (Schwartz, 2004).

### Signs and Symptoms

Bacillary angiomatosis is characterized by the presence of a rash that is similar in appearance to Kaposi's sarcoma, a type of cancer found in AIDS patients. The rash is present both externally and internally. The rash is purple to bright red, and it does not turn white when pressed lightly with the finger. As the number of lesions increases, other symptoms such as fever, weight loss, vomiting, sweats, chills, and loss of appetite develop.

### Treatment

Bacillary angiomatosis is treated with antibiotics, but if left untreated, it can be fatal.

### Testing

Diagnosis of bacillary angiomatosis is based on physical examination and blood culture.

## BACILLARY DYSENTERY

### Description

Bacillary dysentery, which is also known as shigellosis, is caused by a group of anaerobic, gram-negative rods known as *Shigella* species. The *Shigella* bacteria are found only in the intestinal tracts of humans, apes, and monkeys. The disease is spread via the fecal-oral route by flies, fingers, and contaminated food or water. Young children in day care centers; the impoverished who live in overcrowded, inadequate housing; and, people who participate in anal-oral sex are at a higher risk of contracting shigellosis. There are approximately 20,000 to 25,000 cases of dysentery reported in the United States each year. If untreated, the mortality rate of dysentery can be as high as 20 percent (*Shigellosis*, 2003).

### Signs and Symptoms
Shigellosis is noted by the presence of acute abdominal pain or cramping, watery diarrhea, vomiting, nausea, acute fever, and the presence of blood, mucus, or pus in the diarrhea. The blood and mucus result from damage to the colon by the *Shigella* toxin, although the bacteria remain in the small intestine. Symptoms and signs appear approximately 24 to 48 hours after ingestion of the microorganism. Patients may have up to 20 bowel movements per day.

### Treatment
Bacillary dysentery usually lasts two to three days. Treatment is designed to counter the effects of dehydration. Antidiarrheal medications are contraindicated because they may prolong the course of the disease. Antibiotics may be indicated for patients who are severely symptomatic. Sulfamethoxazole-trimethoprim (Bactrim), ampicillin, ciprofloxacin (Cipro), or chloramphenicol (Chloromycetin) are frequently used.

### Testing
Tests for bacillary dysentery include stool cultures, CBC, and tests for the presence of white blood cells in stool.

## BACTERIAL VAGINOSIS

### Description
Bacterial vaginosis is a vaginal infection in which the normal balance of *Lactobacillus* bacteria in the vagina is altered by the presence of anaerobic bacteria (e.g., *Prevotella, Mobiluncus, G. vaginalis, Mycoplama hominis*). The cause of this bacterial alteration is not fully understood; however, it has been related to having multiple sex partners, douching, and using an interuterine device (IUD) for contraception (*Bacterial vaginosis*, 2004 and 2002).

### Signs and Symptoms
Bacterial vaginosis is the most common vaginal infection in women of childbearing age. As many as half of the women with bacterial vaginosis may not report symptoms, which include pain; itching; burning; and a grayish-white, thin, malodorous vaginal discharge, especially after intercourse. Although bacterial vaginosis rarely causes complications, it has serious risks, including increased susceptibility to sexually transmitted diseases, development of pelvic inflammatory disease, and complications of pregnancy.

**Treatment**

Antibiotics used to treat bacterial vaginosis include metronidazole and clindamycin.

**Testing**

Testing of vaginal discharge may be conducted through wet mount, Whiff test, measurement of vaginal pH, Gram staining, oligonucleotide probes, cultures, and pap testing.

## BALANITIS

**Description**

Balanitis is an inflammation of the foreskin and head of the penis, usually caused by poor hygiene in uncircumcised men. Balanitis may be caused by an infection. Sometimes it is caused by inflammation due to soap. Reiter's syndrome and other diseases can cause balanitis (Gilbert, 2003a).

**Signs and Symptoms**

Balanitis is characterized by redness of the foreskin or penis, rashes on the head of the penis, foul-smelling discharge, and painful penis and foreskin.

**Treatment**

Treatment depends on the cause of the balanitis. Infectious balanitis is treated with antibiotics, steroids, and, in severe cases, circumcision.

**Testing**

Balanitis can be diagnosed by examination alone, but additional tests such as skin culture for infectious microorganisms are often needed. Occasionally, a skin biopsy is required.

## BALANTIDIASIS

**Description**

Balantidiasis is a parasitic infection caused by *Balantidium coli*, which is a large, ciliated protozoon (Chijide, 2002). *B. coli* is the largest human protozoan parasite, and it releases hyaluronidase, which aids it in its ability to colonize the mucosa of the large intestine. *Balantidium coli* is often present in pigs, rodents, and nonhuman primates, which shed the infective cysts in their feces. Humans become infected through ingestion of these cysts.

**Signs and Symptoms**

Balantidiasis is characterized by persistent diarrhea, dysentery, abdominal pain, and weight loss. These symptoms may be severely debilitating.

**Treatment**

Balantidiasis is treated with antibiotics like tetracycline, iodoquinol, and metronidazole. The worldwide distribution of *B. coli* is approximately

1 percent, but epidemics have occurred in psychiatric hospitals in the United States.

## Testing

Diagnosis of balantidiasis is based on detection of trophozoites in stool specimens or in tissue biopsies collected during endoscopy.

## BARRETT'S ESOPHAGUS

### Description

Barrett's esophagus is a disorder in which incorrect tissue (i.e., columnar epithelium) replaces the healthy lining of the esophagus (i.e., squamous epithelium). Barrett's esophagus is the most common cause of esophageal cancer. The rate of esophageal cancer is increasing in the Western world, and it has a poor prognosis, mainly because individuals present with late-stage disease. Barrett's esophagus is an acquired condition, secondary to the leaking of stomach acid into the esophagus (i.e., chronic gastroe-sophageal reflux damage) (Srinivas, 2004).

### Signs and Symptoms

Barrett's esophagus is characterized by heartburn, excessive salivation associated with acid exposure, difficulty swallowing, and a sensation of a lump in the throat. Heartburn and acid regurgitation often occur after eating, especially after large meals.

### Treatment

Although cancer can develop in patients with short-segment Barrett esophagus, the rate of occurrence is not known. Until the risk of cancer is specifically defined, endoscopic surveillance is not recommended in those with short-segment Barrett's esophagus. After esophagectomy, balloon dilatation may be performed with fluoroscopic guidance, if the esophagus becomes narrowed.

### Testing

Barrett's esophagus is diagnosed with a double-contrast esophagography. Other imaging tests include nuclear medicine technetium-pertechnetate scanning, endoluminal ultrasonography, and CT scanning.

## BARTTER'S SYNDROME

### Description

Bartter's syndrome is thought to be caused by a defect in the kidney's ability to reabsorb potassium, which results in an excess of potassium in the body. The exact cause of Bartter's syndrome is not known. In some cases it may be genetic, and the condition is congenital.

### Signs and Symptoms

This disease usually occurs in childhood. Symptoms include muscle cramping and weakness, constipation, increased frequency of urination, and growth failure. Other symptoms include enlarged cells in the kidney, alkalosis related to reduced potassium, and increased production of the hormone aldosterone. Although increased blood pressure is a sign of kidney disease, blood pressure is not elevated in cases of Bartter's syndrome.

## Treatment

Bartter's syndrome is treated by keeping the blood potassium level above 3.5 mEq/L. This is achieved through a diet rich in potassium, salt, and magnesium supplements. The long term prognosis for patients with Bartter's syndrome is not certain. Infants who experience severe growth failure typically grow normally with treatment, but kidney failure is possible (Graham, 2002).

## Testing

The diagnosis of Bartter's syndrome is made by finding low levels of potassium in the blood. Other tests include measures of blood chloride, blood pH, and levels of the hormones renin and aldosterone. Tests also indicate high levels of potassium and chloride in the urine. These same signs and symptoms can also occur in people who have taken excessive amounts of diuretics or laxatives. Urine tests can be done to exclude these causes. In Bartter's syndrome, a biopsy of the kidney may show overgrowth of cells in the kidney's juxtaglomerular apparatus, but this is not found in all patients, especially in young children (Frassetto, 2004).

## BASSEN-KORNZWEIG SYNDROME

### Description

Bassen-Kornzweig syndrome is an inherited disorder that affects both sexes, but predominantly males. It is due to mutations in one of two genes: apolipoprotein B (APOB) or microsomal triglyceride transfer protein (MTP). Bassen-Kornzweig syndrome causes the body not to make lipoproteins, resulting in an inability to properly digest fat, underdeveloped nerves, poor muscle coordination, and other nerve disorders.

### Signs and Symptoms

Bassen-Kornzweig syndrome is characterized by a failure to grow in infancy, fatty stools, frothy stools, foul-smelling stools, protruding abdomen, poor muscle coordination, slurred speech, curvature of the spine, and progressive vision loss.

### Treatment

There is no cure for Bassen-Kornzweig syndrome. It is treated with large doses of vitamin supplements containing the fat-soluble vitamins (vitamin A, vitamin D, vitamin E, vitamin K) and medium chain triglycerides. Severe forms of the disease lead to irreversible neurologic disease before age 30.

### Testing

Tests used in the diagnosis of Bassen-Kornzweig syndrome include CBC, cholesterol studies, fecal examination, eye exams, tests for apolipoprotein B in the blood, genetic testing for mutations in the APOB or MTP genes, and nerve conduction velocity testing.

## *BAYLISASCARIS* INFECTION

### Description
*Baylisascaris* is an intestinal roundworm that can infect a variety of animals—including raccoons, dogs, and humans—which pass the eggs in their feces. The eggs are resistant to most environmental conditions and, with adequate moisture, can survive for years. Humans become infected when they ingest infective eggs in soil, water, or on objects that have been contaminated with animal feces. Once in the body, the eggs hatch into larvae, which travel through the muscles and organs. Fewer than 25 cases were diagnosed in the United States in 2003, and they were found in Oregon, California, Minnesota, Illinois, Michigan, New York, and Pennsylvania. *Baylisascaris* infection was fatal in 5 of those cases (*Baylisascaris infection,* 2004).

### Signs and Symptoms
Symptoms of *Baylisascaris* infection include nausea, fatigue, liver enlargement, loss of coordination, loss of muscle control, coma, and blindness.

### Treatment
There is no curative treatment for *Baylisascaris* infection at this time. Prevention of *Baylisascaris* infection includes avoiding direct contact with raccoons, their feces, and avoiding or disinfecting surfaces contaminated by raccoon feces.

### Testing
Diagnosis of *Baylisascaris* infection is made by ruling out other infections.

## BEDSORES

### Description
Bedsores are preventable pressure sores that are technically known as decubitus ulcers. With proper care, bedsores should not occur. Bedsores occur when a person's weight compresses tissue between the bed or wheelchair and a superficial bone. The compressed tissue receives inadequate blood flow, and it becomes necrotic and infected.

### Signs and Symptoms
Bedsores are classified by stage of development as described in Table 2-1. Bedsores do not skip stages. A stage 3 or stage 4 bedsore began as a stage 1 wound but was not diagnosed or treated.

### Treatment
Bedsores need to be treated immediately. Begin by relieving the pressure through the use of mechanical devices such as pillows, special foam cushions, and sheepskin. Improve nutrition and other underlying problems

**Table 2-1** Stages and Treatment of Bedsores

| Stage | Description | Treatment |
| --- | --- | --- |
| Stage 1 | This is the initial stage, in which the skin is unbroken, red, and superficial. | Improved nutrition, including the prevention of dehydration, is the first step toward prevention of bedsores. The cause of the pressure should also be removed. Padding is also available to help cushion the area and reduce pressure. |
| Stage 2 | A partial layer of the skin is injured, and a blister is probably present. | The wound is cleaned and covered to prevent infection. |
| Stage 3 | The bedsore extends through all layers of the skin and is at a high risk of infection. | A bedsore at this stage requires medical treatment, which includes antibiotics and pharmaceuticals that aid in the healing process. |
| Stage 4 | The bedsore has reached the underlying muscle and bone. The bedsore is necrotic and infected. | The surgical removal of the necrotic tissue is likely, and aggressive treatment of the infection is required to keep it from becoming a fatal blood poisoning. Amputation of the affected area may be necessary. |
| Stage 5 | This is an older classification, in which the wound is extremely deep, possibly involving organs. | The treatment is the same as stage 4 bedsores. |

that may affect the healing process. If the pressure ulcer is at stage 2 or worse, clean and care for open ulcers to prevent infection. Keep the area clean and free of dead tissue. A common treatment is to rinse the affected area with salt water to remove necrotic tissue. The sore should be covered with special gauze dressing made for pressure ulcers. Do NOT massage the area of the ulcer, as it may damage deeper tissue. Donut-shaped or ring-shaped cushions are also NOT recommended because they interfere with blood flow. Monitor the ulcer for signs of infection, which include a foul odor and inflammation of the ulcer.

## BEJEL

### Description
Bejel, which is also known as endemic syphilis, is a bacterial infection caused by *Treponema* bacteria, which also cause sexually transmitted syphilis. Bejel, which is caused by *T. pallidum endemicum*, is typically spread among children, most commonly in the Middle East and the southern Sahara desert

regions. In Europe, cases have been diagnosed in children who have moved from endemic areas. In one study, 12 percent of children younger than five years old in Niger had been infected. High rates of infection are also observed in Mali, Burkina Faso, and Senegal (Fine, 2002).

## Signs and Symptoms

Primary lesions are painless, white ulcers in the mouth. The secondary stage begins while the primary lesion is still present or after a latent period. Secondary lesions may be in the mouth or be present in a variety of rashes. If untreated, bejel may cause disfiguring skin lesions as well as deformities of the bone and cartilage. A condition known as gangosa may occur late in the disease because the nasopharyngeal cartilage is destroyed. The eyes may also be affected.

## Treatment

If left untreated, bejel may cause significant disfigurement, pain, and disability. With penicillin therapy, cure rates of 95 to 97 percent are possible.

## Testing

Treponemes cannot be easily and readily cultured. The current tests for bejel are direct microscopic identification when lesions are present, nontreponemal tests used for screening, and treponemal tests used for confirmation. Confirmation of diagnosis depends on dark-field examination and serologic testing.

## BELL'S PALSY

### Description

Bell's palsy involves damage to the facial cranial nerve, which controls movement of the muscles of the face (Campellone, 2004a). Statistics indicate that the disorder affects approximately 2 in 10,000 people. The cause is often not clear, although herpes infections, sarcoidosis, diabetes, and Lyme disease may be involved. Bell's palsy may also be due to inflammation of the facial nerve where it travels through the bones of the skull. Other causes, such as head injury and tumor, need to be excluded.

### Signs and Symptoms

Bell's palsy is characterized by pain around the ear that may precede weakness of facial muscles by one or two days. Other symptoms may include loss of taste, sensitivity to sound on the affected side, headache, facial stiffness, a feeling of the face being pulled to one side, facial droop, difficulty grimacing, facial paralysis on the affected side, and drooling. Dry eye also may occur due to inability to close the eye on the affected side.

### Treatment

There is no specific treatment for Bell's palsy, and often no treatment is necessary. Corticosteroids or antiviral medications may reduce swelling and relieve pressure on the facial nerve. These drugs must be given early, preferably within 24 hours of the onset of paralysis. Surgical procedures to decompress the facial nerve have not been shown to routinely benefit people with Bell's palsy. Approximately 60 to 80 percent of cases resolve completely within a few months, but Bell's palsy may be permanent (Lambert, 2005).

## Testing

If there are no other abnormalities upon phyiscal examination, no imaging studies are usually done. Blood tests for sarcoidosis or Lyme disease may be considered under some circumstances. If there is no improvement in the facial paralysis after several weeks, an MRI is done to rule out other causes of the dysfunction. An EMG and nerve conduction studies may also be done to determine the severity of nerve damage.

## BENIGN PROSTATIC HYPERPLASIA

### Description

Benign prostatic hyperplasia is the abnormal growth of prostate cells, but the condition is not cancerous.

### Signs and Symptoms

In benign prostate growth, the prostate undergoes abnormal growth and presses against the urethra and bladder, interfering with the normal flow of urine (Figure 2-10). As they age, most men will develop benign enlargement of the prostate, which may cause severe enough urinary dysfunction to warrant treatment.

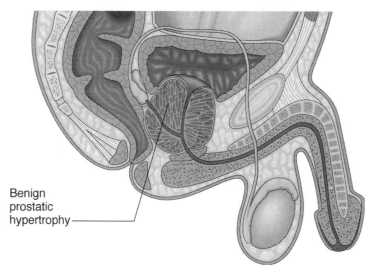

Benign
prostatic
hypertrophy

**Figure 2-10** Enlarged prostate

## Treatment

Several medications are available for the treatment of benign enlargement of the prostate (e.g., finasteride, doxazosin, prazosin, tamsulosin, and terazosin). Prostatits may be surgically treated.

## Testing

A rectal exam, during which a finger is inserted into the rectum to feel the size and shape of the prostate gland, is the most common test to detect prostate enlargement. Blood tests may also indicate prostatitis.

## BERIBERI

### Description

Beriberi is a disease caused by a deficiency in thiamine (vitamin $B_1$), which is essential in the digestion of carbohydrates. Thiamine is also necessary in the synthesis of acetylcholine, which functions in the nervous system. Cardiovascular disease, digestive disease, muscular diseases, and nervous system diseases can occur in relationship to beriberi. Beriberi of the cardiovascular system is known as wet beriberi, and beriberi of the nervous system is known as dry beriberi or Wernicke-Korsakoff syndrome. In the United States, the enrichment of foods with vitamins limits beriberi to a rare disease, and most cases occur among those who abuse alcohol and among breast-fed infants whose mothers have an inadequate intake of thiamine. Severe thiamine deficiencies have also been reported among HIV-positive patients. In the Far East, beriberi is primarily caused by consuming milled rice. Polishing the rice removes the outer coat that contains thiamine. Beriberi is endemic in Indonesia, and there are high morbidity rates among low-income families (Batres, 2003; Hart, 2004c).

### Signs and Symptoms

Symptoms of beriberi include pain, irritability, depression, tingling or loss of sensation in the hands and feet, atrophy of the lower extremities leading to paralysis, congestive heart failure, brain damage, and death.

### Treatment

Beriberi is treated with thiamine, which results in rapid improvement. Although nervous system damage may be reversible, cardiovascular disease can be fatal. Beriberi has a high mortality rate when left untreated.

### Testing

Both testing of urine and blood for levels of thiamine are conducted when diagnosing beriberi. In addition, the clinical response to administered thiamine is evaluated. Whole-blood and erythrocyte transketolase activity are also tested.

## BERYLLIOSIS

### Description

Berylliosis is a disorder of the lungs, known as a pneumoconiosis, caused by inhalation of beryllium dust. Beryllium is the second lightest of all metals and is, therefore, a useful component in nuclear, aerospace, and manufacturing industries. Beryllium is found in coal, oil, soil, volcanic ash, and in many rocks. Beryllium is used in the manufacture of golf clubs, dental applications, nonsparking tools, wheelchairs, and a variety of electronic instruments (Beryllium Network, 2004).

## Signs and Symptoms
Symptoms of berylliosis include cough, difficulty breathing, fatigue, fevers, skin rash, and night sweats. In the later stages, lung tissue becomes scarred. In severe cases, the right side of the heart may be strained due to increased pressure in the pulmonary artery from lung damage.

## Treatment
Berylliosis may be treated but not cured. Adrenocortical steroids can reduce inflammation of the lung tissue. Physicians most commonly prescribe the steroid prednisone to treat the disease. Other steroids such as dexamethasone or prednisolone may also be useful.

## Testing
The beryllium lymphocyte proliferation test (BeLPT) is a blood test that examines how lymphocytes react to beryllium. If they react strongly, then the BeLPT is abnormal and indicates beryllium sensitization.

## BLACK LUNG DISEASE

### Description
Coal worker's pneumoconiosis is also known as black lung disease or anthracosis. At one time, coal miners spent a lifetime underground with picks and shovels, breathing the contaminants of coal mining. Although coal is mostly comprised of carbon, coal dust contains all of the minerals in the rock that surrounds the coal, including crystalline silica. As the miners swung picks into the face of the rock, they created tremendous amounts of dust. Proper ventilation and the use of respirators was not a priority in the early days of mining. Modern mining operations are much safer than those of 50 years ago and earlier.

### Signs and Symptoms
Figure 2-11 depicts the lungs of a coal worker with pneumoconiosis. Note the excessive amount of coal dust lodged in the fine tissues of the lung, which causes them to harden, making breathing difficult. Symptoms include severe cough, airway obstruction, and difficulty breathing.

### Treatment
There is no cure of black lung disease, so the treatment is aimed at relieving the symptoms.

### Testing
The combination of a history of exposure to coal dust and X-rays of the chest revealing black spots is an initial indication of black lung disease.

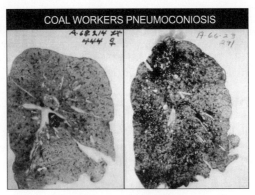

**Figure 2-11** Lungs of a coal worker with black lung disease. (Courtesy of the CDC)

## BLASTOCYSTOSIS

### Description
Blastocystosis is caused by *Blastocystis hominis,* which is a protozoan found commonly throughout the world. Although the method of transmission of *Blastocystis hominis* is unknown, the incidence of disease is higher in areas of the world with inadequate sanitation and poor personal hygiene.

### Signs and Symptoms
*Blastocystis hominis* is found in the intestine, where this microscopic parasite causes symptoms of watery or loose stools, diarrhea, abdominal pain, anal itching, weight loss, and excessive gas. It is not uncommon for people to be infected with *Blastocystis hominis* and have no symptoms of disease. *Blastocystis hominis* may remain in the intestine for weeks, months, or years. Because *Blastocystis hominis* is found in the feces of infected persons, handwashing is a strong deterrent to the spread of blastocystis.

### Treatment
Metronidazole and iodoquinol are used to treat bastocystosis.

### Testing
Diagnosis is based on finding the cystlike stage in feces. Permanently stained smears are preferred over wet mount preparations because fecal debris may be mistaken for the organisms in the latter. Specimens should not be washed in water during concentration procedures as this will lyse (disintegrate) the organisms.

## BLASTOMYCOSIS

### Description
Blastomycosis is a rare fungal infection caused by *Blastomyces dermatitidis,* which is a fungus found in wood and soil (Levy, 2004b). The disease

is spread through the inhalation of fungal spores, so individuals with exposure to soil (e.g., farmers, foresters, campers, hunters) are most at risk of contracting blastomycosis. Gilchrist's disease is another name for blastomycosis. The incidence of occurrence of blastomycosis is highest in the midwestern United States, the south-central United States, and Canada (*Blastomycosis*, 2004).

## Signs and Symptoms
The initial lung infection may cause no symptoms, but if the infection spreads throughout the body, skin lesions, bone lesions, and disorder of the urogenital system may occur. Symptoms of blastomycosis include cough with brown or bloody sputum, difficulty breathing, sweating, fever, fatigue, arthritis, muscle pain, rash, and chest pain.

## Treatment
Although individuals with limited skin lesions and mild lung involvement may recover completely after antibiotic treatment; if left untreated, more severe disease is progressive and potentially fatal.

## Testing
The diagnosis of blastomycosis is made by direct culture, KOH preparations, special stains, and measurement of complement fixing antibodies to various antigens.

## BLEPHARITIS

### Description
Blepharitis refers to a family of inflammatory disease processes of the eyelid (Lowery, 2004). Anterior blepharitis refers to inflammation mainly centered around the eyelashes and follicles; the posterior variant involves the meibomian gland orifices. Anterior blepharitis usually is subdivided further into staphylococcal and seborrheic variants. Frequently, a considerable overlap exists in these processes in individual patients. Blepharitis often is associated with systemic diseases, such as rosacea and seborrheic dermatitis, as well as ocular diseases, such as dry eye syndromes, chalazion, trichiasis, conjunctivitis, and keratitis.

### Signs and Symptoms
Blepharitis involves bacterial colonization of the eyelids. This results in direct microbial invasion of tissues and damage caused by the production of bacterial toxins, waste products, and enzymes. Symptoms of blepharitis may include burning, watery eyes, sensations of foreign material in the eye, crusting and mattering of the eyelashes, red eyelids, photophobia, pain, and decreased vision.

### Treatment
Treatment of blepharitis begins with the application of heat to warm the eyelid gland secretions and to promote cleansing of the secretory passages. The eyelid margins must be washed to remove any debris. Care should be

taken not to disturb the skin of the eyelids. Topical and oral antibiotics and corticosteroids are useful in the treatment of blepharitis.

## Testing

Diagnostic tests are not necessary in cases of blepharitis. However, testing for tear insufficiency or nasolacrimal drainage is necessary due to their likelihood of complicating the disease.

## BLIND LOOP SYNDROME

### Description

If the movement of food slows significantly or stops in the intestine causing it to become blocked, the amount of bacteria growing in the blocked section of the bowel increases. This condition is known as blind loop syndrome, stasis syndrome, or bacterial overgrowth syndrome. The body is unable to effectively absorb nutrients from the intestine, and bile salts that break down fats are unable to function properly. The increased level of bacterial activity consumes the available levels of vitamin $B_{12}$ in the food, resulting in vitamin $B_{12}$ deficiency in the body. Blind loop syndrome is associated with surgeries to remove part of the stomach or as complications associated with inflammatory bowel syndrome or scleroderma. Removal of part or all of the stomach and intestine is performed as part of various procedures to encourage weight loss among the morbidly obese (Stone, 2004b). The intestines may also stop normal muscular contraction for unknown reasons, or they may fail to function properly in cases of diabetic autonomic neuropathy, amyloidosis, or hypothyroidism.

### Signs and Symptoms

Blind loop syndrome is characterized by bloating, flatulence, loss of appetite, diarrhea, and unexplained weight loss. The primary complication of blind loop syndrome is the inability to properly absorb fats, carbohydrates, proteins, and vitamins from ingested food (Frye & Tamer, 2005).

### Treatment

Blind loop syndrome is treated with antibiotics, vitamin supplements, and possibly surgery to remove obstructions. Blind loop syndrome has a positive prognosis with treatment.

### Testing

Blind loop syndrome is diagnosed through imaging exams of the abdomen.

## BLOUNT'S DISEASE

### Description

Blount's disease, which is also known as tibia vara, is a disorder in which the tibia, which is the bone in the lower leg, is bent inward, resembling a bowleg (A. Chen, 2003a). Blount's disease is most common among blacks, due to their propensity to walk at an earlier age than other children and an increased elasticity of the ligaments in black children's knees and lower legs (Cheema & Harcke, 2003). The inner portion of the tibia, just below the knee, does not form properly for unknown reasons in all cases of Blount's disease. Obesity and early walking can be contributing causes to Blount's disease by placing stress on the already deformed tibia, causing it to bend further inward.

## Signs and Symptoms

Blount's disease is characterized by a marked inward bending of the tibia just below the knee. A bony protuberance can be felt along the inner aspect of the tibia near the knee. Patients may thrust the affected leg to the side while walking. Obesity is common in cases of Blount's disease.

## Treatment

Treatment for Blount's disease may include a brace or surgery to straighten the tibia by cutting the bone and securing it in place with pins. The prognosis is good with treatment.

## Testing

X-rays confirm diagnosis of Blount's disease.

## BOTULISM

### Description

Botulism is caused by an obligate anaerobic, gram-positive bacterial rod known as *Clostridium botulinum*. Botulin is the exotoxin produced by *C. botulinum* that causes food intoxication after ingesting the bacteria in contaminated foods such as home-canned vegetables, home-cured meats, and other preserved foods. The most common form of botulism in infants results from the ingestion of honey contaminated with *C. botulinum* spores. Only a small amount of botulin may block the release of the neurotransmitter acetylcholine from the end of nerves resulting in death (*Botulism*, 2001).

### Signs and Symptoms

Botulism is characterized by paralysis, cardiac failure, respiratory failure, nausea, double vision, blurred vision, and difficulty swallowing. Symptoms may appear as early as two hours or as late as three to eight days after ingestion of *C. botulinum*. Fever is not typically present in cases of botulism.

### Treatment

The respiratory failure and paralysis that occur with severe botulism may require a ventilator. After several weeks, the paralysis slowly improves. Botulism may be treated with an antitoxin, which blocks the action of toxin circulating in the blood. Removal of contaminated food from the gut by inducing vomiting or enemas may be necessary. Wound infections may require surgery to remove the source of the toxin-producing bacteria (see Color Plate 8).

### Testing

Tests for butulism may include a brain scan, spinal fluid examination, nerve conduction tests, and a tensilon test for myasthenia gravis. The most direct way to confirm the diagnosis is to demonstrate the botulinum toxin in the patient's serum or stool by injecting serum or stool into mice and looking for signs of botulism.

## BOUTONNEUSE FEVER

### Description

Boutonneuse fever, which is also known as Mediterranean spotted fever, is usually a mild rickettsial disease caused by *Rickettsia conorii;* however, severe complications can occur in some patients. Complications are more common in patients with underlying disease or in elderly persons. The brown-dog tick spreads Boutonneuse fever, which is endemic in the Mediterranean basin. *R conorii* invades and proliferates in the endothelial lining of small vessels, destroying them (Zalewska, 2003).

### Signs and Symptoms

In some patients, the only symptom is an isolated swelling of a lymph node. Other patients complain of a fever followed within a week by a rash with bumps on the lower legs. An area of dead tissue may be present at the site of the bite. Other symptoms may include stupor, pneumonia, lowered heart rate, jaundice, gastrointestinal bleeding, and coma, if the disease progresses.

### Treatment

Treatment of Boutonneuse fever includes antibiotics like tetracyclines with chloramphenicol and quinolones.

### Testing

Diagnosis is based on the presence of rashes with poxlike bumps, which are confirmed by using cultures. If the brain is involved, an MRI may be performed to identify white matter disturbances.

## BOWEL OBSTRUCTIONS

### Description

The small intestine and the large intestine are referred to as the bowel. When either becomes blocked, it is referred to as a bowel obstruction, which is depicted in Figure 2-12 and Figure 2-13. The leading cause of bowel obstruction is postoperative adhesions. If the intestine is cut during surgery, the two sides may grow together, affectively closing the lumen of the intestine. Other causes of bowel obstruction include cancer, Crohn's disease, bacterial infections, parasites, hernias, and paralysis of intestinal muscles. In children, bowel obstructions commonly result from congenital defects such as pyloric stenosis, volvulus, and intussusception of the intestines.

### Signs and Symptoms

Bowel obstructions are serious because the blood vessels may also become compressed within the occlusion, leading to a lack of blood flow to the bowel causing tissue death. Vomiting causes distention of the small

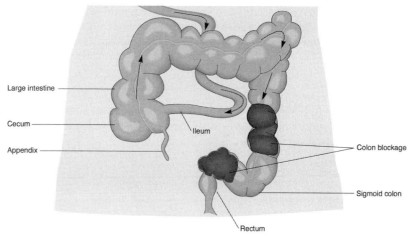

**Figure 2-12** Colon blockage

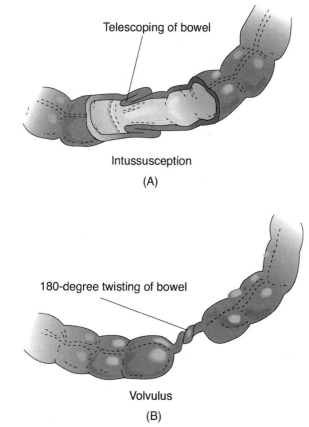

**Figure 2-13** Volvulus and intussusception

intestine, leading to increased pressure within the lumen of the intestines. The increased pressure compresses the lymphatic vessels in the mucosal layer of the intestines. The compression of the lymphatic vessels prevents them from removing excess fluid, and fluids cannot be resorbed. The fluid loss and dehydration that ensue are often a fatal combination.

## Treatment
The obstruction may be removed using a nasogastric tube in some cases. Surgery may be necessary. Complicating factors may include infection, gangrene, or bowel perforation.

## Testing
Tests for intestinal blockage may include barium enema, abdominal CT scan, upper GI and small bowel series, and abdominal X-rays.

## BRAINERD DIARRHEA

### Description
Brainerd diarrhea is an idiopathic disease characterized by the acute onset of watery diarrhea lasting four weeks or longer. Although its cause is unkown, it is believed to result from an infection. The disease is named after Brainerd, Minnesota, where the first outbreak occurred in 1983. Since that time, seven outbreaks have been reported. Six have occurred in the United States, and five of those were in rural settings. One outbreak occurred on a South American cruise ship based out of the Galapagos Islands. The original outbreak in Minnesota was attributed to drinking unpasteurized milk; however, contaminated water is believed to have been the cause in other outbreaks. Brainerd diarrhea does not appear to spread from person-to-person (*Brainerd Diarrhea*, 2003).

### Signs and Symptoms
Symptoms of Brainerd diarrhea include up to 20 episodes of explosive diarrhea per day, watery diarrhea, and diarrhea characterized by urgency and incontinence. Other symptoms include gas, abdominal cramping, and fatigue. More rare symptoms include nausea, vomiting, fever, and weight loss.

### Treatment
Brainerd diarrhea is self-limiting, although symptoms may last as much as three years. There have been no known cases of recurrence once the illness has completely resolved.

### Testing
There is no laboratory test that can confirm Brainerd diarrhea diagnosis.

## BREAST CANCER

### Description
The exact causes of breast cancer are not known, but the risk of developing breast cancer increases with age. Breast cancer is uncommon among

women under the age of 35, and most cases occur in women over the age of 50. Caucasian women develop breast cancer more frequently than African-American or Asian-American women (Donegan et al., 2002).

## Signs and Symptoms

Figure 2-14 is a photograph of a woman with breast cancer. In its early stages, breast cancer is painless and may present no signs or symptoms, but as the cancer grows, any or all of the following may be present:

- a lump or thickening in or near the breast or in the underarm area
- a change in the size or shape of the breast
- nipple discharge or tenderness
- nipple inverted into the breast
- ridges or pitting of the breast, which causes the breast to looks like the rind of an orange
- warm, swollen, red, or scaly breast, areola, or nipple

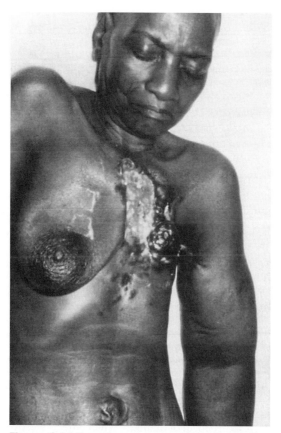

**Figure 2-14** Breast cancer complications after a mastectomy. (Courtesy of the CDC, Robert S. Craig)

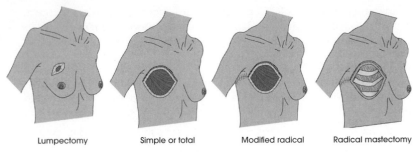

| Lumpectomy | Simple or total | Modified radical | Radical mastectomy |

**Figure 2-15** Types of mastectomy

## Treatment
Treatment for breast cancer may include chemotherapy, radiation therapy, and surgery (Figure 2-15).

## Testing
Breast cancer is diagnosed by biopsy.

# BRONCHITIS

## Description
Bronchitis is an inflammation of the bronchi, which are the main air passages to the lungs. The two forms of bronchitis are acute and chronic. To be classified as chronic bronchitis, there must be the presence of a cough with mucus most days of the month for at least three months per year (Blaivas, 2004a). Acute bronchitis usually is both bacterial and viral. Chronic bronchitis is almost always due to inflammation of the bronchi and not an infection.

## Signs and Symptoms
Bronchitis is characterized by a cough; coughing up blood; difficulty breathing; respiratory infections; wheezing; fatigue; headaches; and swelling of the ankles, feet, and legs.

## Treatment
There is no cure for chronic bronchitis. Respiratory irritants (e.g., tobacco smoke) should be avoided. Inhalants, antibiotics, and corticosteroids may be used in the treatment of bronchitis. In severe cases, oxygen therapy and even lung transplantation may be necessary.

## Testing
Diagnosis is based on pulmonary function tests, arterial blood gas, chest X-rays, pulse oximetry, CBC, exercise stress tests, and chest CT scans.

# BRONZE DIABETES

## Description
Bronze diabetes is a rare form of diabetes, which affects the liver's ability to metabolize iron, causing enlargement of the liver and a bronze discoloration

of the skin (Maxton, 2004). Bronze diabetes is also known as hemochromatosis. Primary hemochromatosis is an inherited disease. It is thought to be mainly caused by a mutation of a gene called HFE, which probably allows excess iron to be absorbed from the diet. This mutation is known as C282Y. Bronze diabetes is more common in men than in women, and it is more common among Caucasians. Bronze diabetes may lead to cardiac failure.

## Signs and Symptoms

Increasingly, people are being diagnosed with bronze diabetes without showing any symptoms. Symptoms can be difficult to spot, as they are often mild initially, with many potential causes. Fatigue, joint pain, impotence in men, and loss of menstruation in women are important early signs.

## Treatment

The main treatment for bronze diabetes is regular bloodletting known as therapeutic venesection. One unit of blood (approximately 500 ml) is taken at a time. The iron in the red blood cells is removed until body iron stores return to normal, which may require lifelong treatment.

## Testing

Blood tests (e.g., a transferrin saturation test or a serum ferritin test) can determine whether the amount of iron stored in the body is too high. It is also possible to test directly for the defective gene.

## BRUCELLOSIS

## Description

Brucellosis is a disease caused by human contact with animal products from animals infected by bacteria of the genus *Brucella*. These bacteria infect sheep, goats, cattle, deer, elk, pigs, dogs, and other animals. Humans can contract brucellosis by ingesting something contaminated with *Brucella*, inhalation of the bacteria, or through open wounds on the skin. Tourists are at a particular risk for infection if they eat village cheeses, which are unpasteurized cheeses in areas of the world where brucellosis is common. Although only about 100 to 200 cases of brucellosis occur in the United States annually, the disease is much more prevalent in certain parts of the world where animal control programs have not reduced the amount of disease among animals. These areas include Portugal, Spain, southern France, Italy, Greece, Turkey, Africa, South America, Central America, Eastern Europe, Asia, the Carribbean, and the Middle East (*Brucellosis*, 2004).

## Signs and Symptoms

Symptoms of brucellosis in humans are similar to the flu and include fever, sweats, headache, back pain, and weakness. The most common symptom of brucellosis is GI symptoms (e.g., loss of appetite, nausea, voming, abdominal pain, and diarrhea). Brucellosis may also lead to more severe infections of the central nervous system or lining of the heart. Chronic cases of brucellosis may include fevers, arthritis, and severe fatigue.

## Treatment

Treatment for brucellosis is based on a combination of doxycycline and either streptomycin or rifampin.

## Testing

Diagnosis of brucellosis is based on serum agglutination tests, positive blood or bone marrow aspirate culture, and the Western blot test.

## BUERGER DISEASE

### Description

Buerger disease, also known as thromboangiitis obliterans, is a disease of small arteries and veins in the arms and legs. Although the cause of Buerger disease is unknown, exposure to tobacco is strongly linked to the disease. Buerger disease is more common in countries with heavy use of tobacco and is perhaps most common among natives of Bangladesh who smoke a specific type of cigarettes, homemade from raw tobacco, called "bidi." Whereas the overwhelming majority of patients with Buerger disease smoke, a few cases have been reported in nonsmokers that have been attributed to the use of chewing tobacco. The use of tobacco results in blood vessel dysfunction and the formation of clots. Buerger disease is relatively less common in people of northern European descent. Natives of India, Korea, and Japan and Israeli Jews of Ashkenazi descent have the highest incidence of the disease.

### Signs and Symptoms

The signs of Buerger disease typically occur prior to age 45. Patients usually have a current history of tobacco use. They exhibit pain in the forearms, hands, legs, and feet due to diminished blood flow. The pain worsens during rest and may be accompanied by ulcers on the toes, feet, or fingers. The hands and feet of the patient are typically cold and slightly swollen. Most patients experience symptoms of numbness, tingling, and burning in three to four extremities.

### Treatment

Absolute discontinuation of tobacco use is the only strategy proven to prevent the progress of Buerger disease. Smoking as few as one cigarette daily, using chewing tobacco, or using nicotine replacements may keep the disease active. Except for absolute tobacco avoidance, there is no treatment for Buerger disease. Gene therapy is showing promise (Hanly, 2004).

### Testing

There is no specific laboratory test for Buerger disease. Angiography is used to identify the lesions in the arteries associated with Buerger disease.

## BULLOUS PEMPHIGOID

### Description

Bullous pemphigoid is a skin disorder characterized by large blisters that usually appear on the areas of the body that flex or move (Chan, 2003). Some people also develop blisters in the mouth. Bullous pemphigoid is an idiopathic disease, but it is believed to be related to immune system disorders. Bullous pemphigoid is more common among the elderly.

### Signs and Symptoms

Bullous pemphigoid may occur in various forms, from no symptoms, to mild redness and irritation, to multiple blisters. It is characterized by a pattern of exacerbations and remissions. The disease is noted by the presence of bullae, which are large blisters usually located on the arms, legs, or trunk. Bullae may also occur in the mouth. The bullae may weep and crust over through time. These blisters are often found deep below the surface of the skin, where they may cause erosion of the skin, causing ulcers. Symptoms include itching, rashes, bleeding gums, and sores in the mouth.

### Treatment

Treatment is focused on relief of symptoms and prevention of infection through corticosteroids and other medications, such as methotrexate, azathioprine, mycophenolate, or cyclophosphamide, and antibiotics in the tetracycline family. In most people, bullous pemphigoid is self-resolving within six years.

### Testing

Skin lesion biopsy indicates a characteristic blistering pattern. Blood tests may be ordered to rule out other diseases.

## BURKITT LYMPHOMA

### Description

Burkitt lymphoma is a high-grade B-cell cancer of the lymph tissues and has two major forms: the endemic (African) form and the nonendemic (sporadic) form (Huang, 2002). Burkitt lymphoma is a childhood tumor, but it is observed in adult patients. Burkitt lymphoma is one of the fastest growing malignancies in humans.

### Signs and Symptoms

Under the microscope, Burkitt lymphoma has a "starry sky" appearance. Symptoms of the African form of Burkitt lymphoma include swelling of the affected jaw, loosening of the teeth, and swelling of the lymph nodes of the neck or below the jaw. Symptoms of the sporadic form of Burkitt lymphoma include abdominal tumors causing swelling and pain in the affected area (see Color Plate 9).

## Treatment

Before aggressive chemotherapy, fatality rates for children with Burkitt lymphoma were quite high. With chemotherapy, the survival rate is now at least 60 percent. Patients with limited disease have a survival rate of 90 percent. Patients with bone marrow and brain involvement have a poor prognosis. In AIDS patients, Burkitt lymphoma usually is advanced and death often occurs shortly after diagnosis.

## Testing

Testing, which should be expedited due to the rapid growth of Burkitt tumors, includes biopsy of lymph nodes, biopsy of bone marrow, evaluation of cerebrospinal fluid, and examination of peritoneal and pleural fluids.

## BURSITIS

### Description

Bursitis is inflammation of the bursae in certain joints of the body. There are over 150 bursae in the body, and their job is to cushion pressure points between the bones and tendons as the muscles move near the joints. Bursae are small, fluid-filled sacs, and they become inflamed causing joint pain in cases of bursitis. Bursitis is typically due to overuse, stress or strain of a joint, or repeated bumping or pressure from kneeling. Less commonly, bursitis may be due to staphylococcal infections, arthritis, or even tuberculosis.

### Signs and Symptoms

Commonly affected joints include the shoulders, elbows, and hips. Less common sites of bursitis include the knees, heels, and the base of the big toes. Bursitis pain typically subsides within about a week with treatment, but recurrence is common. Symptoms of bursitis include a dull ache or stiffness in the affected joint, worsening pain upon movement of the affected joint, swelling of the affected joint, and heat and redness surrounding the inflamed joint.

### Treatment

Treatment for bursitis includes resting and immobilizing the affected area, applying ice and taking nonsteroidal anti-inflammatory drugs. Bursitis is self-resolving within two weeks.

### Testing

Testing includes a physical exam, blood tests, and examination of fluids from the bursae.

## CANAVAN DISEASE

### Description

Canavan disease, which is also known as spongy degeneration of the brain or aspartoacylase deficiency, is an inherited disorder that primarily affects Ashkenazi Jews and Saudi Arabians. The white matter in the brain becomes spongy due to the presence of multiple fluid-filled spaces.

Canavan disease is caused by a deficiency in the enzyme aspartoacylase, which causes the accumulation of N-acetylaspartic acid in the tissues of the brain.

## Signs and Symptoms

Symptoms of Canavan disease appear in infancy. Affected infants are usually quiet and apathetic, and they exhibit rapidly progressing disease characteristics including mental retardation, decline in previously acquired motor skills, poor neck muscle tone, lack of head control, increased head size, nasal regurgitation, vomiting, and feeding difficulties. Eventually children with Canavan disease become paralyzed and blind.

## Treatment

There is no specific treatment for Canavan disease except to treat symptoms. Canavan disease is generally fatal by the age of four, but some patients may live to the age of approximately twenty (NINDS Canavan Disease, 2005).

## Testing

Eye exams indicate optic atrophy in cases of Canavan disease. Imaging tests of the head are conducted to determine the extent of white matter deterioration. The blood, urine, and cerebrospinal fluid exhibit increased levels of N-acetylaspartic acid. Genetic tests indicate mutation of the aspartoacylase gene (Hart, 2004).

## CANCER OF THE BLADDER

### Description

Bladder cancer is typically caused by transitional cell carcinomas, which may appear in any part of the urinary tract including the renal pelvis, ureter, bladder, or urethra. Bladder cancer is categorized as low grade or high grade and as superficial or muscle invasive. Primary bladder tumors are rare but may include small-cell carcinoma, lymphoma, or sarcoma. Urinary bladder cancers may also include adenocarcinomas, squamous cell carcinomas, leiomyosarcomas, or rhabdomyosarcomas. It is believed that bladder cancer may be due to agents in cigarette smoke (i.e., nitrosamine, 2-naphthylamine, and 4-aminobiphenyl) and industrial exposure to aromatic amines in dyes, paints, solvents, leather dust, inks, combustion products, rubber, and textiles.

### Signs and Symptoms

One of the only initial signs of bladder cancer is painless, bloody urination.

### Treatment

Treatment of bladder cancer includes radiation therapy, chemotherapy, and surgery.

### Testing

Tests for bladder cancer may include CT scan, urinalysis, intravenous pyelogram (IVP), cytoscopy and biopsy, and urine cytology.

## CANCER OF THE PANCREAS

### Description
Most pancreatic cancers begin in the ducts that carry pancreatic fluids. When cancer of the pancreas metastasizes outside the pancreas, cancer cells are often found in nearby lymph nodes, the peritoneum, the liver, and the lungs (*Cancer of the Pancreas*, 2002).

### Signs and Symptoms
Pancreatic cancer is sometimes called a silent disease because early pancreatic cancer often does not cause symptoms. Later, pancreatic cancer is characterized by jaundice, dark urine, weakness, loss of appetite, nausea, vomiting, weight loss, and pain in the upper abdomen or upper back.

### Treatment
Treatment for pancreatic cancer includes radiation therapy, chemotherapy, and surgery. Cancer of the pancreas is extremely difficult to control with current treatments, and many patients' only option is medication that is still in the clinical trial stage. The mortality rate for pancreatic cancer is high.

### Testing
Tests for pancreatic cancer include a physical exam for jaundice and acities, lab tests for bilirubin, CT scan, ultrasonography, endoscopic retrograde cholangiopancreatography (ERCP), percutaneous transhepatic cholangiography (PTC), and biopsy.

## CANDIDIASIS

### Description
Candidiasis is a disease caused by the fungus *Candida albicans*. The normal microbes in the body's mucous membranes are generally sufficient to prevent the growth of *C. albicans*. Among infants who do not have a mature immune system, people with diseases that suppress the immune system, and when the normal microbes are removed from mucous membranes, however, the fungus is able to grow.

### Signs and Symptoms
Infants often develop a white overgrowth of the tongue called thrush (see Color Plate 10). People with AIDS can develop a systemic infection caused by *C. albicans* that can overgrow the esophagus or respiratory system causing death. *C. albicans* can cause yeast infections in women due to frequent douching, which kills the normal bacteria of the vagina that would otherwise retard the growth of *C. albicans*. Diabetics and the obese may develop candidiasis of the moist skin. Candidiasis can also infect the nails (see Color Plate 11).

### Treatment
Candidiasis is treated with topical and ingested antifungal medications. *C. albicans* is the fourth most common cause of nosocomial bloodstream

infections in the United States, and it is 40 percent fatal once it reaches the systemic level.

## Testing
Candidiasis can be diagnosed through cultures.

## CAPILLARIASIS

### Description
Capillariasis is an intestinal infection caused by the roundworm *Capillaria philippinensis*, that humans contract by eating raw or undercooked fish. Two other *Capillaria* species are also known to cause rare infections in humans: *C. hepatica* and *C. aerophila* cause hepatic capillariasis and pulmonary capillariasis, respectively. Intestinal capillariasis, hepatic capillariasis, and pulmonary capillariasis are all potentially fatal diseases. The most common areas of the world to contract capillariasis are the Philippines and Thailand, although cases have been reported worldwide (*Capillariasis*, 2004).

### Signs and Symptoms
Intestinal capillariasis is characterized by abdominal pain, diarrhea, and general wasting of the body. Hepatic capillariasis is an acute hepatitis accompanied by dissemination of the bacteria to other organs. Pulmonary capillariasis is characterized by fever, cough, asthma, and pneumonia.

### Treatment
Medications for capillariasis include mebendazole or albendazole.

### Testing
Cultures indicate the presence of *Capillaria philippinensis*.

## CAPUT SUCCEDANEUM

### Description
Caput succedaneum, or simply caput, occurs when pressure on the head during delivery of an infant causes the baby's scalp to swell. The pressure is exerted on the head by the uterus and vagina during contractions. Caput is caused when these pressures force the baby's head through the narrowed cervix (Blackman, 2004b).

### Signs and Symptoms
The swelling in the head may be on any part of the scalp in the newborn. The head may be discolored due to minor bruising.

### Treatment
No treatment is necessary, as caput heals spontaneously within a few days.

### Testing
No testing is necessary in cases of caput succedaneum.

## CARBON MONOXIDE POISONING

### Description
Carbon monoxide is a colorless, tasteless, odorless gas produced by burning material containing carbon. Carbon monoxide poisoning is sometimes referred to as a silent killer because carbon monoxide is nonirritating. The most common sources of carbon monoxide are motor vehicle exhaust, smoke from fires, engine fumes, and nonelectric heaters. Carbon monoxide poisoning is often associated with malfunctioning or obstructed exhaust systems and with suicide attempts (Cole, 2002).

### Signs and Symptoms
In a small, closed garage, the average car exhaust can induce a lethal coma within five minutes. Some of the signs and symptoms of carbon monoxide poisoning include headache, dizziness, nausea, drowsiness, difficulty breathing, chest pain, confusion, hallucination, agitation, vomiting, abdominal pain, visual impairment, and seizure. Among individuals who die from carbon monoxide poisoning, a characteristic cherry-red discoloration of the skin and mucous membranes is present due to carboxyhemoglobin in the blood. Swelling and hemorrhaging of the brain may also occur.

### Treatment
Carbon monoxide poisoning is treated by immediately removing the patient from the carbon monoxide source. Having the person remain still is important to conserve oxygen in the blood. Oxygen therapy, which may include artificial ventilation, may be required. Hemoglobin, which transports carbon dioxide and oxygen in red blood cells, has an affinity 200 times stronger for carbon monoxide than it does for oxygen. Once carbon monoxide bonds with hemoglobin, the mere introduction of oxygen is not sufficient to restore proper levels of oxygen in the blood.

### Testing
Blood gases indicate the presence of carbon monoxide.

## CARDIOMYOPATHY

### Description
Cardiomyopathy is a disease of the heart muscle due to a variety of causes. Alcoholic cardiomyopathy is due to excessive alcohol consumption. Hypertrophic cardiomyopathy is enlargement of the infant cardiac septum. Hypertrophic cardiomyopathy may lead to congestive heart failure but is often asymptomatic, with the exception of a heart murmur. Although hypertrophic cardiomyopathy may go unnoticed for a lifetime, it may also result in acute cardiac failure during exercise. Parasitic cardiomyopathy is an infection in the myocardium associated with parasitic organisms. Restrictive cardiomyopathy results from a lack of flexibility of the walls of the heart's chambers. Primary cardiomyopathy is idiopathic; secondary cardiomyopathy is caused by toxic chemicals, metabolic disorders such as diabetes mellitus, or inherited cardiac disorders.

## Signs and Symptoms

Cardiomyopathy may result in a blockage before any other symptoms appear.

## Treatment

Anticoagulant drug therapy may be needed, and arrhythmias may require antiarrhythmic drugs. More rarely, a pacemaker may be required.

## Testing

An EKG and an echocardiogram are common tests in the diagnosis of cardiomyopathy.

## CARPAL TUNNEL SYNDROME

### Description

Carpal tunnel syndrome is caused by compression of the median nerve at the wrist. The related numbness, tingling, pain, and weakness are thought to be caused by a lack of blood flow to the nerve rather than physical damage to the nerve itself. As the tissues of the wrist swell, the transverse carpal ligament holds the passageway, causing the swelling to compress the median nerve. Carpal tunnel syndrome is caused by repetitive motions of the hand and wrist such as typing, packing boxes in a factory, playing a musical instrument, or doing craftwork. Women are more prone to develop carpal tunnel syndrome due to swelling of the wrist related to pregnancy, premenstrual syndrome, and menopause.

### Signs and Symptoms

Carpal tunnel syndrome is characterized by weakness in the hand. Pain and numbness are also present in the thumb, ring finger, and middle finger. Symptoms are normally in both wrists and become progressively worse. The pain may eventually radiate into the forearm and elbow.

### Treatment

Treatment begins by wearing night splints and use of assistive devices to reduce stress on the wrist. Medications used in the treatment of carpal tunnel syndrome include anti-inflammatories and corticosteroids. Carpal tunnel release is a surgical procedure that cuts into the ligament to relieve pressure on the median nerve. Surgery is successful about 85 percent of the time.

### Testing

During a physical examination, tapping over the median nerve at the wrist may cause pain to shoot from the wrist to the hand, which is known as Tinel's sign. Bending the wrist forward all the way for 60 seconds will usually result in numbness, tingling, or weakness, which is known as Phalen's test. Opinions concerning the value of tests for Tinel's sign and Phalen's sign differ (Freedman, 2004; Steele, 2004). Electromyography and nerve conduction velocity may be performed.

## CATARACT

### Description

Cataract is a vision-impairing disease characterized by gradual, progressive thickening of the lens (Ocampo, 2004). It is one of the leading causes of blindness in the world today. As such, early detection, close monitoring, and timely surgical intervention must be observed in the management of senile cataracts.

### Signs and Symptoms

As the lens ages, its weight and thickness increase while its flexibility decreases. As new tissues are added in a concentric pattern, the central nucleus is compressed and hardened in a process called nuclear sclerosis. Symptoms include decreased visual acuity, increased glare, and nearsightedness.

### Treatment

The definitive management for senile cataract is surgical lens extraction.

### Testing

Diagnosis of cataract is made thorough a history and physical examination. Laboratory tests are requested to detect coexisting diseases (e.g., diabetes mellitus, hypertension, cardiac anomalies). An important test is the swinging flashlight test, which detects for a Marcus Gunn pupil or a relative afferent pupillary defect indicative of optic nerve lesions or macular involvement.

## CATSCRATCH DISEASE

### Description

Catscratch (also rendered cat-scratch or cat scratch) disease, which is also known as *Bartonella henselae* infection, is a bacterial disease spread by cat bites or scratches. Forty percent of cats are estimated to carry *Bartonella henselae* at some time in their lives, and kittens are more likely to be infected than adult cats. Many cats are asymptomatic but are still capable of spreading the infection to humans (Spoonemoore, 2002).

### Signs and Symptoms

Catscratch disease begins with a mild infection at the injury site. Later, the lymph nodes—primarily of the head, neck, and upper limbs—become swollen. Other symptoms include fever, headache, fatigue, and loss of appetite. Among persons with HIV, and rarely in others, catscratch disease can lead to bacillary angiomatosis.

### Treatment

Catscratch disease is normally self-limiting, but it may be treated with antibiotics.

### Testing

Diagnosis is based on the presence of *Bartonella henselae*.

## CELLULITIS

### Description

Cellulitis is an inflammation and infection of the superficial layers of the skin that can be fatal if bacteria spread in the body. Cellulitis can be caused by both *Streptococcus* and *Staphylococcus* bacteria, which may enter the skin through breaks, insect bites, puncture wounds, surgery, or other events that weaken the integrity of the skin (*Cellulitis*, 2004).

### Signs and Symptoms

Cellultis often appears as a slightly painful area of redness, swelling, and warmth without noticeable margins. Cellulitis may be accompanied by fever, malaise, rigors, headache, and an elevated white blood cell count. Although cellulitis can occur anywhere on the body, the skin of the ankles and shins are the most common sites of infection.

### Treatment

Cellulitis is treated with antibiotics.

### Testing

Diagnosis is based on the physical appearance of the skin, blood tests, and wound cultures.

## CEREBRAL PALSY

### Description

Cerebral palsy is a term used to describe a group of chronic disorders characterized by the impairment of control over movement. The impairment generally appears in the first few years of life and typically does not progress over time. It is believed that cerebral palsy is caused by developmental anomalies or damage to areas in the brain, disrupting its ability to control movement and posture. Some of the causes of cerebral palsy include head injury, jaundice, Rh incompatibility, and German measles (NINDS Cerebral Palsy, 2001).

### Signs and Symptoms

Individuals with cerebral palsy have difficulty with fine motor tasks, such as writing or using scissors. In addition, they struggle to maintain balance and walk. They may also lack full control of their voluntary movements. Symptoms may be as severe as having seizures or mental impairment, but symptoms differ between individuals and may change through time. Signs of cerebral palsy are typically apparent by the age of 3. Infants may develop normally, but they exhibit difficulty learning to roll over, sit, crawl, smile, or walk.

### Treatment

There is no cure for cerebral palsy, and treatment is aimed at improving motor skills and reducing muscle spasms. Treatment begins with physical therapy, the use of mechanical aids, and medications, like botox, that reduce spasms. A pump may also be inserted surgically that delivers baclofen to reduce spasms.

## Testing

Diagnosis of cerebral palsy normally occurs before the age of 3 and is based on tests of motor skills and medical history.

## CERVICAL CANCER

### Description

There are two primary categories of cervical cancer: The most common is squamous cell carcinoma, which develops from the flat cells covering the outer surface of the cervix at the top of the vagina; the other type is adenocarcinoma, which develops from the glandular cells lining the cervical canal.

### Signs and Symptoms

Cervical cancer is characterized by abnormal bleeding between periods or after sexual intercourse, a malodorous vaginal discharge, and discomfort during intercourse. Color Plate 12 highlights the erosion of the cervix that accompanies cervical cancer.

### Treatment

Treatment includes surgery, chemotherapy, and radiation therapy.

### Testing

Precancerous cells in the cervix are diagnosed through regular cervical smears. Although the smear test is designed to detect precancerous cells, it may also detect an existing cancer.

## CHAGAS DISEASE

### Description

Chagas disease, which is also known as American trypanosomiasis, is an infection caused by the protozoan parasite *Trypanosoma cruzi*. Approximately 16 million to 18 million people are infected with Chagas disease, and of those infected, 500,000 die annually (Lazdins, 2004). Chagas disease is spread by insects known as reduviid bugs, or "kissing bugs," which live in substandard housing and bite people, especially babies, on the lips. The insects become infected after biting an infected animal or person. The protozoa are spread to humans when an infected insect deposits feces on a person's skin, usually while sleeping. The person then rubs the infected feces into a bite wound, an open cut, the eyes, or the mouth. Chagas disease primarily occurs among low-income people living in rural areas of South America, especially during childhood. Those living in dwellings constructed from thatch, adobe, or mud are most at risk (*Chagas disease,* 2004).

### Signs and Symptoms

There are three stages of infection with Chagas disease. During the acute stage of infection, only about 1 percent of the people develop symptoms, but it can be fatal, particularly to infants due to swelling of the brain. The most recognized characteristic of acute Chagas infection is the Romana's sign, which is observable as swelling of the eye on one side of the face, usually at the bite wound or the site where the feces was rubbed into the eye. Other nonspecific symptoms may include fatigue, fever, enlarged spleen, swollen lymph glands, rash, loss of appetite, diarrhea, and vomiting. Illness lasts about a month during the acute stage and leaves without treatment. The next stage of Chagas disease is devoid of symptoms and is known as the indeterminate period. Finally, in some people, the chronic stage begins between 10 and 20 years after infection. During this severe stage, serious illness occurs, including cardiac disorders and enlargement of the digestive tract.

### Treatment
There is no vaccine to prevent Chagas disease, and although medications can be effective during the acute stage, they are less effective as the disease progresses.

### Testing
Diagnosis is based on the presence of *Trypanosoma cruzi*.

## CHANCROID

### Description
Chancroid is a sexually transmitted disease characterized by painful ulcers and painful regional enlargement of the lymph glands (see Color Plate 13). The disease is uncommon in industrialized nations, but it is a frequent cause of genital ulcer disease in developing countries. In some areas of the United States, chancroid is endemic, and it is known to occur in discrete outbreaks (Abbuhl, 2004). Chancroid is caused by the small gram-negative rod, *Haemophilus ducreyi*.

### Signs and Symptoms
The organism is transmitted by direct contact through the skin, presumably through minor abrasions. After an incubation period of about 10 days, a pustule erupts that erodes to form a painful ulcer with ragged margins. The ulcer may be quite deep, and more than one half of patients have multiple ulcers. Chancroid lesions occur on the penis of men, or on the labia, vagina, or cervix of women. Pus-filled, enlarged, draining, inguinal lymph nodes, which are known as buboes, are common in the majority of infected persons.

### Treatment
Antibiotics are indicated in all cases of chancroid. If chancroid is diagnosed and treated, the infection usually is cured. In HIV-positive patients, cure rates are lower.

### Testing
Gram stain has limited utility in diagnosing chancroid, and a definitive diagnosis requires culturing *H. ducreyi* on a special culture medium that is not always readily available. Even with the proper medium, the sensitivity

is not higher than 80 percent. New diagnostic techniques are evolving rapidly, and DNA probes and polymerase chain reaction (PCR) appear promising.

## CHEDIAK-HIGASHI SYNDROME

### Description

Chediak-Higashi syndrome is a rare genetic disorder of children in which the immune system is affected, resulting in chronic infections. The genetic mutation that causes Chediak-Higashi syndrome occurs in the CHS1 gene. These children may exhibit decreased pigmentation in their eyes and skin, and they suffer neurological diseases as well. They also bruise and bleed easily. During the accelerated stage of the disease, multiple organs become infiltrated with nonmalignant lymphomalike growths. During this stage, patients are more susceptible to infection from the Epstein-Barr virus. The lungs, skin, and respiratory tract may also become infected with bacteria (e.g., *Staphylococcus aureus*, *Streptococcus pyogenes*, and *Pneumococcus* species). Few patients with Chediak-Higashi syndrome will live to adulthood, and most die due to these infections (Newicki & Szarmach, 2003; Stewart, 2003c).

### Signs and Symptoms

Chediak-Higashi syndrome is characterized by small white ulcers of the mouth, decreased vision, sensitivity to light, various skin infections, albinism, muscle weakness, and mental retardation.

### Treatment

There is no specific treatment for Chediak-Higashi syndrome. Some treatments include bone transplants, surgical drainage of abscesses, antibiotics, and steroids.

### Testing

Chediak-Higashi syndrome is diagnosed by the presence of giant granules in blood smears and white blood cells that are positive with stains for peroxidases. Biopsies of skin, muscle, and nervous tissue indicate giant granules. Imaging tests may be performed to determine the degree of brain atrophy, and genetic tests indicate mutation of the CHS1 gene.

## CHICKENPOX

### Description

Chickenpox is an acute inflammatory disease caused by the varicella-zoster virus that also causes shingles. Chickenpox is a contagious disease spread by respiratory tract transmission (Varicella Disease, 2003).

### Signs and Symptoms

The primary symptom of chickenpox is the development of lesions on the skin (see Color Plate 14). The blisters last three to four days and fill with pus, causing crusting. Lesions are typically found on the face, neck, and lower back but can occur on the chest and shoulders. Chickenpox can be fatal from related encephalitis and viral pneumonia. Chickenpox is a childhood disease but can be contracted by adults. Adults are likely to develop more severe symptoms with a higher mortality rate than children who contract the disease.

## Treatment
Chickenpox is normally self-limiting, but acyclovir may be prescribed in severe cases.

## Testing
Diagnosis of chickenpox is based on the presence of the varicella virus.

## CHILDBIRTH FEVER

### Description
Puerperal sepsis, which was first known as childbed fever and is now also known as childbirth fever, is a septic disease mainly caused by *Streptococcus pyogenes*, although it may be caused by other bacteria. It is a nosocomial infection of the uterus resulting from childbirth or abortion. The *S. pyogenes* bacterium is spread to the uterus via contaminated surgical instruments or hands of medical workers. The infection spreads from the uterus to the abdominal cavity causing peritonitis. Modern disinfection techniques have reduced the occurrence of puerperal sepsis.

### Signs and Symptoms
The most common sign of puerperal sepsis is fever within two weeks after delivery, although fever may be due to other causes.

### Treatment
Puerperal sepsis is treated with antibiotics such as penicillin.

### Testing
Diagnosis is predicated on the presence of a bacterial infection.

## CHLAMYDIAL PNEUMONIA

### Description
The causative agent of chlamydial pneumonia is a recently recognized species of bacteria known as *Chlamydia pneumoniae*. This organism is an important respiratory pathogen, known to cause pneumonia, acute respiratory disease, and pharyngitis. Recently, *C. pneumoniae* has been believed to be a causative agent of otitis media, asthma, and cardiovascular disease. *C. pneumoniae* is the third most common cause of infectious respiratory diseases, accounting for about 10 percent of outpatient and hospitalized cases of pneumonia.

### Signs and Symptoms
About 90 percent of the infections show no symptoms and, therefore, go undiagnosed. It is still unknown how *C. pneumoniae* infections are spread.

**Treatment**

Chlamydial pneumonia is treated with antibiotics.

**Testing**

Diagnosis is based on the presence of *C. pneumoniae.*

## CHLONORCHIASIS

**Description**

Chlonorchiasis is caused by the trematode *Clonorchis sinensis,* which is also known as the Chinese or oriental liver fluke. Chlonorchiasis is contracted by ingestion of raw, undercooked, salted, pickled, or smoked freshwater fish. After ingestion, the organism ascends the biliary tract through the ampulla of Vater and matures, which takes about one month. Although most cases of clonorchiasis occur in Asia, cases have been reported in the United States.

**Signs and Symptoms**

Initial obstruction of the biliary ducts causes abdominal pain, nausea, and diarrhea. In chronic cases of chlonorchiasis, cholangitis, cholelithiasis, pancreatitis, and cholangiosarcoma can develop, which may be fatal.

**Treatment**

Chlonorchiasis may initially be treated with medications; however, the fluke may need to be surgically removed depending on the development of the organism.

**Testing**

Diagnosis of chlonorchiasis is based on the presence of *Clonorchis sinensis* in cultures.

## CHOLANGITIS

**Description**

Cholangitis is an acute infection of the bile duct, which is illustrated in Figure 2-16. The blockage of the flow of bile provides a breeding ground for the bacteria that cause the infection. Gallstones are the most common cause of obstruction, although strictures, stenosis, or tumors may also cause cholangitis. Bacteria are not normally present in bile, but they are common in gallstones. Mortality from cholangitis is high due to the underlying diseases and the spread of the infection throughout the blood. Historically, mortality was 100 percent; currently it ranges from 7 to 40 percent (Santen, 2001a).

**Signs and Symptoms**

Advanced cholangitis is characterized by pain in the upper right quadrant of the abdomen, fever, jaundice, blood poisoning, and mental status changes.

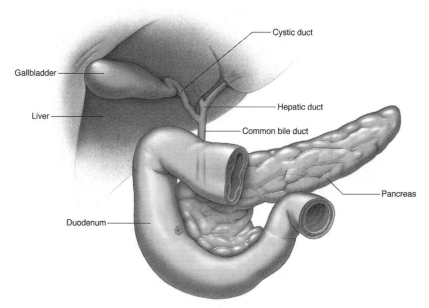

**Figure 2-16** Liver, gallbladder, and pancreas

## Treatment

The infection associated with cholangitis is treated with antibiotics. The obstruction may be drained by endoscopic retrograde cholangiopancreatography (ERCP) or percutaneous transhepatic cholangiogram (PTCA).

## Testing

Tests for cholangitis include magnetic resonance cholangiopancreatography (MRCP), endoscopic retrograde cholangiopancreatography (ERCP), percutaneous transhepatic cholangiogram (PTCA), and ultrasound, in addition to blood and stool cultures.

## CHOLECYSTITIS

## Description

Cholecystitis is an inflammation of the gallbladder, usually caused by obstruction of the bile duct by gallstones. There are three types of gallstones, the most common of which is composed of cholesterol. The other types include pigment gallstones and mixed gallstones. Each type is formed when bile becomes crystallized within the gallbladder or the bile duct, as shown in Figure 2-17. When the gallstones block the flow of bile, the gallbladder and the bile duct can become inflamed. Gallstones are more common in women because women have more estrogen. The estrogen causes increased cholesterol secretion; progesterone inhibits the flow of bile. Cholecystitis may also be caused by infections similar to that pictured in Color Plate 15, which is caused by a typhoid infection.

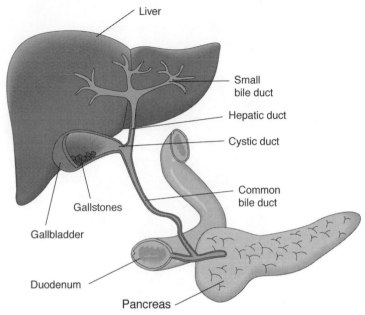

**Figure 2-17** Gallstones

## Signs and Symptoms

Most gallstones cause no significant signs or symptoms because they do not block the flow of bile. When the flow of bile is blocked, however, a common symptom is pain that radiates from the upper right quadrant of the abdomen to the shoulder. Other symptoms include indigestion, belching, bloating, and intolerance for fatty foods. The ingestion of fatty foods causes the release of bile for proper digestion, which causes pain because the bile duct is occluded.

## Treatment

The most common treatment for gallstones is a cholecystectomy.

## Testing

Gallstones are often detected during an abdominal X-ray, CT scan, or abdominal ultrasound.

## CHROMOBLASTOMYCOSIS

### Description

Chromoblastomycosis is a chronic fungal infection of the skin and the subcutaneous tissue caused by a specific group of fungi (usually *Fonsecaea pedrosoi, Phialophora verrucosa, Cladosporium carrionii,* or *Fonsecaea compacta*). Chromoblastomycosis occurs universally but is more prevalent in rural populations in countries with a tropical or subtropical climate.

The fungi often gain entry into the human body by contact with wood splinters or thorns (Castro, 2003).

## Signs and Symptoms

Patients usually do not complain of discomfort, and they tend to not seek medical care until secondary infection or elephantiasis ensues. After several years, a small, raised bump develops. Numerous black dots may occur at the site of the bumps. Secondary infection with bacteria is common, giving the lesion a characteristic ill odor. The sites most commonly affected are the lower extremities, especially the feet.

## Treatment

Surgical excision or electrodesiccation of lesions should be avoided because the infection might spread. Treatment with oral itraconazole and cryosurgery with liquid nitrogen are two common treatments.

## Testing

Diagnosis of chromoblastomycosis may include tests of lesion scrapings, which indicate the presence of thick-walled, cigar-colored, sclerotic cells known as Medlar bodies.

## CHRONIC FATIGUE SYNDROME

### Description

Chronic fatigue syndrome is a debilitating disorder characterized by profound fatigue that is not improved by bed rest and that worsens with physical or mental activity (*Chronic fatigue syndrome*, 2003).

### Signs and Symptoms

Nonspecific symptoms may include weakness, muscle pain, impaired memory and concentration, and insomnia.

### Treatment

Because the cause of chronic fatigue syndrome is unknown, treatment is aimed at relief of specific symptoms. Pharmaceutical treatment may include antidepressants, stimulants, anxiolytic agents, NSAIDS (e.g., aspirin and ibuprofen), and medications to affect sleep patterns.

### Testing

Currently, to be diagnosed with chronic fatigue syndrome, a person must (1) have severe chronic fatigue of at least six months' duration with other known medical conditions excluded by clinical diagnosis, and (2) concurrently have four or more of the following symptoms:

- substantial impairment in short-term memory or concentration
- sore throat
- tender lymph nodes
- muscle pain
- multijoint pain without swelling or redness

- headaches of a new type, pattern, or severity
- unrefreshing sleep
- postexertional fatigue lasting more than 24 hours

The symptoms must have persisted for six or more consecutive months of illness and must not have predated the fatigue.

## CHRONIC OBSTRUCTIVE PULMONARY DISEASE

### Description

Chronic obstructive pulmonary disease (COPD) is an umbrella term for a group of respiratory diseases in which the bronchioles become blocked and the alveolar sacs become deyhydrated (Blaivas, 2004b). Approximately 16 million Americans are believed to suffer from COPD (COPD International, 2005). Both emphysema, chronic bronchitis, and chronic asthma are the most common forms of COPD. In cases of COPD, the bronchioles become plugged with mucus, which promotes excessive growth of bacteria. The bacterial infection restricts the airflow through the lungs, which makes it difficult to inhale and to exhale.

### Signs and Symptoms

COPD is characterized by difficulty breathing and a persistent cough. Patients may flare their nostrils when inhaling, and they may purse their lips in an effort to inhale more air. The action of the intercostal muscles of the chest are more pronounced during inhalation as the patient struggles to inhale and exhale. Patients also often exhibit an increased respiratory rate, and a wheezing sound is heard during breathing.

### Treatment

COPD is treated with inhalers, theophyline, and steroids. Antibiotics may be used to treat infections. Surgery to reduce lung volume, lung transplants, and artificial ventilation may be options for treatment of severe cases of COPD.

### Testing

Imaging exams of the chest are used to diagnose COPD. Arterial blood gases indicate hypoxia and high levels of carbon dioxide causing respiratory acidosis. Pulmonary function tests are also performed.

## CIRRHOSIS

### Description

Cirrhosis is a chronic, degenerative disorder of the liver. Figure 2-18 identifies some of the most common characteristics of cirrhosis of the liver. In the United States, cirrhosis of the liver is mainly caused by long-term alcoholism, poisoning, or hepatitis. Cirrhosis of the liver is characterized by fatty and cellular infiltration and degeneration of liver cells, causing hardening of the liver (Stone, 2004c).

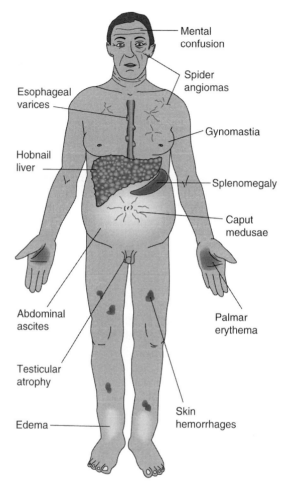

**Figure 2-18** Signs of cirrhosis of the liver

## Signs and Symptoms

As a result of loss of liver function, increased blood pressure in the hepatic portal system may develop, leading to ammonia toxicity in the body. Liver disorders may be characterized by fluid in the abdomen, dementia, jaundice, and blood clotting disorders. Cirrhosis is also characterized by swelling of the lower extremities; bloody vomit; weakness; impotence; bleeding hemorrhoids; and small, red, spiderlike blood vessels on the skin. Cirrhosis may also cause decreased urine output, pale or clay colored stools, nosebleed, bleeding gums, gynecomastia, abdominal pain, indigestion, and fever (Cirrhosis of the liver, 2002).

## Treatment

Patients must stop use of damaging medications and alcohol. Bleeding varices are treated with upper endoscopy. Ascites is treated with diuretics, fluid and salt restrictions, and paracentesis. Coagulopathy is treated with blood products or vitamin K. Encephalopathy is treated with medication lactulose, antibiotics, and the avoidance of protein in the diet. Liver transplant may be required.

## Testing

Physical examination may reveal enlarged liver or enlarged spleen, distended abdomen, jaundice, red spiderlike blood vessels on the skin, excess breast tissue, small testicles in men, reddened palms, contracted fingers, or dilated abdominal wall veins. Tests indicate anemia, coagulation abnormalities, elevated liver enzymes, elevated bilirubin, and low serum albumin. Liver biopsy indicates cirrhosis.

## CLEFT PALATE AND LIP

### Description

A cleft lip is a separation of the two sides of the lip, which may include the bones of the upper jaw (known as the maxillae). A cleft palate occurs when the two sides of the palate fail to fuse during fetal development. This results in an opening between the palatine bones that form the roof of the mouth. According to the Cleft Palate Foundation (2003), one of every 700 newborns is affected by cleft lip and/or cleft palate. Color Plate 16 pictures a child with a cleft lip, and Color Plate 17 pictures a cleft palate.

### Signs and Symptoms

A one-sided cleft is known as a unilateral cleft lip or a unilateral cleft palate. Clefts occurring on both sides are known as bilateral cleft lip or bilateral cleft palate. Because the lip and the palate develop separately, individuals may have a cleft lip, a cleft palate, or both cleft lip and cleft palate.

### Treatment

Treatment for cleft lip and cleft palate may include surgery, dental/orthodontic care, and speech therapy.

### Testing

Cleft palate and cleft lip are diagnosed based on physical appearance, and there is no test needed. Imaging exams are used in surgical procedures.

## COCCIDIOIDOMYCOSIS

### Description

Coccidioidomycosis is a respiratory disease caused by the fungus *Coccidioides immitis* (Levy, 2004m). Other names for this disease include Posada-Wernicke disease, coccidioidal granuloma, valley fever, desert rheumatism, valley bumps, and California disease. *C. immitis* spores are found in dry, alkaline soils in the American Southwest, Mexico, and parts of South America. *C. immitis* is one of the most virulent mycotic pathogens in humans—inhaling only a few organisms results in infection. The wind carries the spores, transmitting the infection. Simply passing through endemic areas can lead to infection (Coccidioidomycosis, 2002).

### Signs and Symptoms
Symptoms of the disease are chest pain, fever, coughing, loss of appetite, headache, and weight loss for six weeks or longer. If the disease progresses to a secondary stage, it is accompanied by nodule formation, progressive pulmonary disease, and brain involvement.

### Treatment
Most infections are subclinical, with less than 40 percent of those infected developing symptoms. Coccidioidomycosis can be fatal, however, and Filipinos and African Americans run the highest risk of the disease becoming systemic. Among HIV-positive populations, a severe pulmonary disease may occur. Bed rest and treatment of flulike symptoms until fever disappears may be recommended. Disseminated or severe disease is treated with amphotericin B, ketoconazole, fluconazole, or itraconazole.

### Testing
Tests for coccidioidomycosis include a Potassium hydroxide (KOH) test, sputum culture, serum coccidioides complement fixationtiter, CBC with differential indicating elevated eosinophils, chest X-rays, and coccidioidin or spherulin skin tests.

## COLD SORES

### Description
The herpes simplex 1 virus is transmitted by oral or respiratory routes. Almost everyone has been infected with the herpes simplex 1 virus during infancy. Cold sores may appear due to excessive exposure to ultraviolet (UV) rays from the sun, emotional upsets, or hormonal changes during menstruation. Herpes labialis is an infection caused by the herpes simplex virus, characterized by cold sores on the skin of the lips, mouth, gums or the skin around the mouth. During latency, the herpes simplex 1 virus remains dormant in the trigeminal nerve ganglia of the brain (McKinley Health Center, 2002).

### Signs and Symptoms
Symptoms begin with itching, burning, increased sensitivity, or tingling sensations about two days before cold sores appear. The blisters appear on the lips, mouth, and gums, and they are filled with a clear to yellowish fluid (see Color Plate 18). They are red and painful, and they break, ooze, and crust before sloughing off to reveal the underlying healing skin. Mild fever may also occur.

### Treatment
Cold sores are usually self-resolving within two weeks. Antiviral medication may be given to shorten the course of symptoms and decrease pain.

Blisters should be gently washed with antiseptic soap and water to minimize spread. Ice or warmth may be applied to reduce inflammation.

### Testing

Diagnosis is made on the basis of the appearance of the lesion. Viral culture or Tzanck test of the skin lesion may reveal the herpes simplex virus.

## COLITIS

### Description

Colitis is an inflammation of the large intestine. There are a variety of types of colitis including pseudomembranous colitis, Crohn's disease, ulcerative colitis, ischemic colitis, irritable bowel syndrome, necrotizing enterocolitis, cryptosporidium enterocolitis, and cytomegalovirus colitis. Colitis may be caused by both acute and chronic infections disorders like ulcerative colitis and Crohn's disease. A lack of blood flow to the large intestine may cause ischemic colitis. A history of radiation to the large intestine has been known to cause colitis (Lehrer, 2003; Ulcerative Colitis, 2003).

### Signs and Symptoms

Symptoms of colitis include abdominal pain, diarrhea, dehydration, abdominal bloating, intestinal gas, and bloody feces.

### Treatment

Treatment is directed at the cause of the disease, which may be infection, inflammation, ischemia, or other cause.

### Testing

Diagnosis of colitis is based on flexible sigmoidoscopy or colonoscopy. Biopsies, barium enemas, abdominal CT scan, abdominal MRI, and abdominal X-rays may also be used.

## COLOR BLINDNESS

### Description

The term *color-blind* is misleading because color-blind people are not blind at all; instead, they cannot distinguish between some colors, and some may not see colors at all. Color blindness is due to defects in specialized cells in the retina of the eye called cones that enable humans to see in color, as opposed to many nonhuman animals that have no color perception. Although color blindness can be acquired, most cases are inherited, and it affects males almost exclusively (Steefel, 1999).

### Signs and Symptoms

There are three basic types of color blindness, and they are described in Table 2-2.

### Treatment

There is no treatment or cure for congenital color blindness, but acquired color blindness may be temporary.

**Table 2-2** Types of Color Blindness

| | |
|---|---|
| Red/green color blindness | People with red/green color blindness can distinguish between red and green when comparing the two side-by-side. However, they cannot determine whether a color is red or green when shown only one of the two colors. |
| Blue color blindness | Individuals with blue color blindness cannot distinguish between blue and yellow; they, instead, see only white or grey. Blue color blindness usually occurs due to physical disorders, such as liver disease or diabetes mellitus. |
| Achromatopsia | Total color blindness is known as achromatopsia, which is an extremely rare, hereditary disorder. These individuals cannot see any colors, and their vision is limited to black, white, and shades of gray. Achromatopsia results in poor visual acuity and extreme sensitivity to light. |

## COLORECTAL CANCER

### Description

Cancer that begins in the colon is called colon cancer, and cancer that begins in the rectum is called rectal cancer. When cancer affects either of these portions of the large intestine, it may be called colorectal cancer (Stone, 2004c).

### Signs and Symptoms

Colorectal cancer is characterized by changes in bowel habits, diarrhea, constipation, bloody feces, gas, bloating, abdominal cramps, unexplained weight loss, and vomiting. Most colorectal cancer develops gradually from benign polyps. So, the early detection and removal of polyps may help prevent colorectal cancer.

### Treatment

The majority of colon cancer cases are asymptomatic, so regular screening for colon cancer before symptoms occur is essential for treatment. Based on the stage of the tumor, colon cancer is treated with surgery, chemotherapy, and radiation.

### Testing

Tests for diagnosing colon cancer may include colonoscopy, sigmoidoscopy, imaging tests, and blood tests such as a fecal occult blood test.

## COMMON COLD

### Description

Over 1 billion colds occur in the United States each year (*Health Matters*, 2001). Symptoms and signs generally last only two weeks, but the common cold is one of the leading causes of health care visits and school or job absences. In 1996, colds caused 45 million days of restricted activity and 22 million days lost from school in the United States. There are more than 200 different viruses known to cause the symptoms of the common cold. Rhinoviruses and coronaviruses are two of the most common causes of colds. The common cold is age dependent, with children having between 6 and 10 colds per year due to their relative lack of resistance to infection, whereas people over age 60 have 1 or less colds per year. Children in school or day care, and adults who work with children are more likely to get a cold. Because colds are spread through both direct and indirect contact, hand-washing is one of the best ways to reduce the spread of the common cold.

### Signs and Symptoms

Symptoms of the common cold usually begin about two or three days after infection and often include nasal discharge, obstructed nasal breathing, swelling of the sinuses, sneezing, sore throat, cough, and headache. Occasionally, colds lead to secondary bacterial infections of the middle ear or sinuses.

### Treatment

Chicken soup has been used for treating common colds at least since the twelfth century (Greene, 2004a). The heat, fluid, and salt may actually help fight the infection. Over-the-counter medications may relieve symtpoms, but they do not shorten the length of a cold. Rest and fluids are the best treatment for a cold. Children should not be forced to eat, and antibiotics should not be taken, because they are not effective in the treatment of viral infections.

### Testing

There is no specific test for the common cold.

## CONCUSSION

### Description

A concussion is a traumatic injury to the head resulting in temporary loss of consciousness, paralysis, vomiting, and seizures. It is believed that microscopic shearing of nerve fibers in the brain from sudden deceleration may result from head injury.

### Signs and Symptoms

Figure 2-19 illustrates damage to the brain resulting from concussion. Immediate symptoms may include altered level of consciousness, coma, confusion, repeated vomiting, unequal pupils, unusual eye movements, gait abnormalities, and muscle weakness on one or both sides.

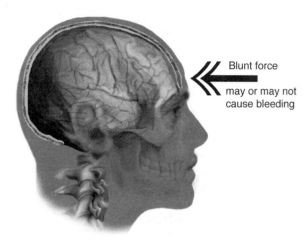

Blunt force may or may not cause bleeding

**Figure 2-19** Concussion

## Treatment

Recovery occurs in hours or days, without permanent injury, with the exception of memory loss surrounding the traumatic event. It is important to rest, prevent re-injury, limit exposure to drugs, and be observed by a responsible adult. Severe concussion requires immobilization.

## Testing

Testing includes a neurological exam and head imaging, such as X-rays, MRI, or CT scan.

## CONGESTIVE HEART FAILURE

### Description

Congestive heart failure is a disorder affecting multiple body systems, in which the heart is unable to pump as much blood as the venous system supplies. Instead of pumping out all of the blood from the ventricles when the heart pumps, some amount of blood remains in the lower chambers of the heart. Blood, therefore, becomes congested throughout the venous system. At the same time, an insufficient amount of blood enters the arterial system. Fluids accumulate in the venous system, and associated tissues become swollen. Congestive heart failure may result in cardiac failure and involve either the left side, the right side, or the entire heart.

### Signs and Symptoms

Figure 2-20 illustrates some of the most common signs of congestive heart failure. Right-sided heart failure leads to anasarca, which is severe generalized swelling, especially in the hands, feet, and abdomen. Chronic right-sided heart failure also leads to enlargement of abdominal organs such as the liver. Congestive heart failure on the left side of the heart causes the development of pulmonary edema in the chest because the heart cannot

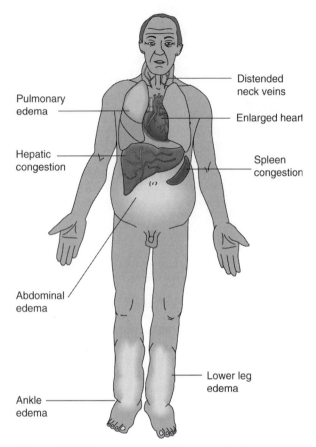

Pulmonary
edema

Distended
neck veins

Enlarged heart

Hepatic
congestion

Spleen
congestion

Abdominal
edema

Lower leg
edema

Ankle
edema

**Figure 2-20** Signs of congestive heart failure

remove the excess fluid from the lungs as part of pulmonary circulation, which is illustrated in Figure 2-21. Individuals with left-sided heart failure commonly experience shortness of breath. Decreased left-sided cardiac output eventually results in less blood entering the kidneys. The kidneys respond by reabsorbing more sodium and water into the blood vascular system, resulting in an increase in blood volume, which adds to the congestion and causes the heart to work that much harder. Congested blood quickly becomes clotted and can result in embolisms that can cause stroke or blockage of the coronary artery. Congestive heart failure eventually leads to failure of the heart to beat properly, resulting in sudden death.

## Treatment
Common medications used in the treatment of congestive heart failure include ACE inhibitiors (e.g., Captopril and enalapril), diuretics (e.g., thiazide, loop diuretics, potassium-sparing diuretics), digitalis glycosides, angiotensin receptor blockers (e.g., losartan and candesartan), and beta-

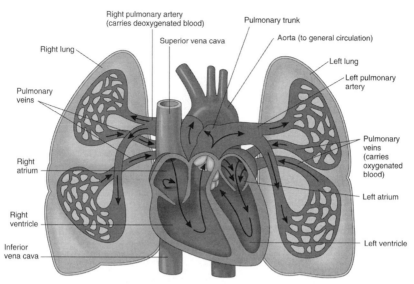

**Figure 2-21** Cardiopulmonary circulation

blockers. Hospitalization may be required to receive oxygen therapy and intravenous vasodilators, diuretics, and inotropic agents (e.g., dobutamine and milrinone). Unstable patients may require hemodynamic monitoring with Swan-Ganz catheterization. Severe cases may require dialysis, intra-aortic balloon pumps, left ventricular assist devices, or a heart transplant.

## Testing
Diagnosis of congestive heart failure may include echocardiogram, heart catheterization, chest X-ray (see Color Plate 19), chest CT scan, cardiac MRI, nuclear heart scans, and electrocardiogram.

## CONTUSION OF THE BRAIN

### Description
A contusion is a head injury of sufficient force to bruise the brain, causing blood to pool between the brain and the membranes that surround it. Contusions are more serious than concussions because contusions include hemorrhaging into the brain tissue (see Figure 2-22).

### Signs and Symptoms
Contusions may occur at any point at which the brain is in contact with the skull, but are most common in the frontal, temporal, and occipital lobes of the brain. Although the skull is often intact, it may contain fractures. Interestingly, the site of contusion does not indicate the point of blunt force trauma. For example, during a falling accident on the back of the head, a contusion may occur on the front of the brain as it is jarred

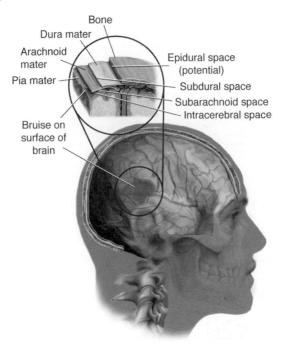

**Figure 2-22** Contusion

against the forehead, with no contusion present in the back of the brain where the impact occurred.

### Treatment

Treatment for contusion is typically centered around close observation for changes in levels of consciousness. Headache and dizziness are common, but if they persist or become severe, medical attention may be required. Surgery may be required in severe cases to relieve intracranial pressure or stop hemorrhaging. Improvement after brain injury may be slow, and changes may only be noticed by health-care providers during periodic visits.

### Testing

Testing includes a neurological exam and head imaging, such as X-rays, MRI, or CT scan.

## CORONARY ARTERY DISEASE

### Description

Coronary artery disease, which is also known as ischemic heart disease or coronary heart disease, is the most common cause of death in economically developed countries, including the United States. The coronary artery supplies blood to the heart, as illustrated in Figure 2-23. Coronary artery

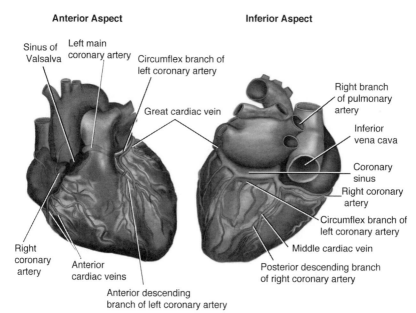

**Figure 2-23** Arteries and veins of the heart

disease is characterized by the narrowing of the lumen of the coronary arteries due to atherosclerosis, as represented in Figure 2-24. There are three changes that can contribute to the severity of coronary artery disease, including acute plaque changes, blood clots in the coronary artery, and spasms of the coronary artery.

## Signs and Symptoms

A waxy substance called plaque—which is made of cholesterol, fatty compounds, calcium, and a blood-clotting material called fibrin—reduces the flow of blood in the coronary artery. The presence of plaque may result in blood clot formation within the coronary artery. Thickening of the arterial walls may also lead to spasms in the muscular layer of the coronary artery. The coronary artery then cannot supply blood to the heart. The loss of oxygen-rich blood starves the heart muscle and leads to its death, which is referred to as myocardial infarction.

## Treatment

Treatment of coronary artery disease may include weight loss, reducing cholesterol levels, reducing sodium, regular exercise, and quitting smoking. Medications may include antiplatelet agents (e.g., aspirin, ticlopidine, clopidogrel), glycoprotein IIb-IIa inhibitors (e.g., abciximab, eptifibatide, tirofiban), antithrombin drugs (e.g., heparin), beta-blockers, nitrates, calcium-channel blockers, ACE inhibitors, and diuretics (Amaldo, 2004a and 2004b). Procedures may include coronary angioplasty, coronary

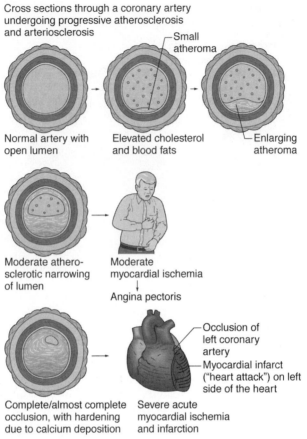

Cross sections through a coronary artery undergoing progressive atherosclerosis and arteriosclerosis

Small atheroma

Normal artery with open lumen

Elevated cholesterol and blood fats

Enlarging atheroma

Moderate athero-sclerotic narrowing of lumen

Moderate myocardial ischemia
↓
Angina pectoris

Complete/almost complete occlusion, with hardening due to calcium deposition

Severe acute myocardial ischemia and infarction

Occlusion of left coronary artery

Myocardial infarct ("heart attack") on left side of the heart

**Figure 2-24** Coronary artery disease

atheroctomy, ablative laser-assisted angioplasty, catheter-based thrombolysis and mechanical thrombectomy, coronary stenting, and coronary radiation inplant or coronary brachytherapy. Surgical intervention may include coronary artery bypass surgery.

## Testing
Tests for coronary artery disease may include electrocardiogram, exercise stress test, echocardiogram, nuclear scan, coronary angiography/arteriography, and electron-beam computed tomography.

## CRANIOTABES

### Description
Craniotabes, which is also known as congenital cranial osteoporosis, is a softening of the skull. Craniotabes can be a normal finding in infants, especially premature infants. Studies suggest that it is present in one third

of newborns. Craniotabes is harmless although it may indicate rickets and osteogenesis imperfecta (Graham, 2003; Van Rijn & McHugh, 2004).

## Signs and Symptoms
Craniotabes is characterized by soft areas of the skull, especially along the suture line, which pop in and out like a squeezed Ping-Pong ball. Bones may feel soft, flexible, and thin along the suture lines.

## Treatment
Craniotabes is self-resolving and is, therefore, not treated.

## Testing
No testing is done unless osteogenesis imperfecta or rickets is suspected.

## CRETINISM

### Description
Cretinism is a hypothyroid condition of infants and children in which the thyroid gland does not secrete sufficient quantities of thyroid hormones. Among children who were not born with the disorder, it is largely the result of an iodine deficiency in the diet.

### Signs and Symptoms
Cretinism is characterized by arrested physical and mental development, dystrophy of the bones, and lowered basal metabolism. Signs in infants may include a thick, protruding tongue, poor feeding, choking episodes, constipation, prolonged jaundice, and short stature. Infants may also have a widely separated and large fontanelle, dry hair, low hairline, thick neck, shortened extremities, myxedema, broad hands with short fingers, hypotonia, and a hoarse-sounding cry or voice.

### Treatment
Cretinism is treated with the hormone thyroxine.

### Testing
Tests may include X-rays of long bones, free T4 thyroxine levels, serum thyroid stimulating hormone (TSH) levels, serum thyroxine binding globulin (TBG) levels, and a thyroid scan.

## CREUTZFELDT-JAKOB DISEASE

### Description
Creutzfeldt-Jakob disease (CJD) is thought to be caused by a prion, which is a particle of protein that acts in a way similar to disease-causing microorganisms. CJD is a progressive disease that causes spongiform— porous, like a sponge—degeneration of the brain. There is a long incubation period measuring between months, years, and decades associated with Creutzfeldt-Jakob disease. CJD has been transmitted to a pathologist via a scalpel nick during an autopsy, it has been experimentally transmitted

to chimpanzees, it has been transmitted via cornea donation, and it is believed to be inherited. CJD is an extremely rare disease, with approximately one case appearing per million population worldwide (New Variant CJD, 2003; NINDS Creutzfeldt-Jakob, 2001).

## Signs and Symptoms

Symptoms include failing memory, behavioral changes, and visual disturbances. Later, the individual experiences mental deterioration, involuntary movements, blindness, and coma.

## Treatment

Creutzfeldt-Jakob disease has no known cure. It is fatal in 90 percent of the cases within one year, and there is no treatment to control its progress.

## Testing

There is no diagnostic test for CJD, which is categorized as either sporadic CJD, hereditary CJD, or acquired CJD. The only way to confirm a diagnosis of CJD is by biopsy of the brain during an autopsy. A confirmed diagnosis of CJD while the person is still alive does not help the patient, so a brain biopsy of a living patient is rarely performed, unless it is used to confirm a treatable nervous system disorder.

## CRI DU CHAT SYNDROME

### Description

Cri du chat syndrome, which is also known as chromosome 5p deletion syndrome or 5p minus syndrome, is caused by the absence of a portion of the short arm of chromosome 5. The disease receives its name from the infant's cry, which is similar to the high-pitched mewing of kittens. The cry is due to dysfunction of the central nervous system and structural abnormalities of the larynx. Between 1 and 20,000 and 1 in 50,000 babies are affected by cri du chat syndrome, which is believed to occur from the spontaneous loss of a piece of chromosome 5 during development of an egg or sperm. Multiple genes are involved in this disease, including the telomerase reverse transcriptase (*TERI*) gene (H. Chen, 2005; Stewart, 2003d).

### Signs and Symptoms

Cri du chat syndrome is characterized by its distinctive cry, slowed development, hyperactivity, small head, low-set eyes, downward slant to the eyes, small jaw, low-set ears, and mental retardation. These children also exhibit a simian crease in their palms, and they may have partial webbing of the fingers or toes.

### Treatment

No specific treatment is available for cri du chat syndrome. Death occurs in approximately 8 percent of the cases. Most deaths result from pneumonia, aspiration pneumonia, heart defects, and respiratory distress syndrome.

## Testing

Parents should have genetic karyotype tests to make sure that they do not have rearranged chromosomes that predispose for children missing part of chromosome 5.

## CROHN'S DISEASE

### Description

Crohn's disease is an inflammatory bowel disease, which is the general name for diseases that cause inflammation in the intestines. It also may be called ileitis or enteritis, and its cause is unknown. Crohn's may occur at any age, but adolescence and early adulthood are the periods of highest risk. Other risk factors include a family history of Crohn's disease and Jewish ancestry. About 7 out of every 100,000 people will develop Crohn's disease (Stone, 2004e).

### Signs and Symptoms

The most common complication is blockage of the intestine, which occurs due to swelling and scar tissue formation in the intestinal wall. Ulcers that tunnel through the affected area into surrounding tissues such as the bladder, vagina, or skin may also be present. The tunnels, which are known as fistulas, are common and often become infected. Other complications associated with Crohn's disease include arthritis, skin problems, inflammation in the eyes or mouth, kidney stones, gallstones, and diseases of the liver and biliary system. Crohn's disease is characterized by abdominal pain in the lower right quadrant, diarrhea, rectal bleeding, weight loss, fever, and ulcers in the intestines. It is also characterized by clubbing of the fingers and toes, and foul smelling stools (Nachimuthu & Piccione, 2004).

### Treatment

Medications such as 5-aminosalicylate, corticosteroids, and immunomodulators such as azathioprine or 6-mercaptopurine may be used to control inflammation. Infliximab may be prescribed to control infections related to the abscesses and fistulas sometimes present in cases of Crohn's disease. Surgical removal of diseased or strictured segments of the bowel may also be required, although this does not cure the condition. Changes in diet are also recommended.

### Testing

Diagnosis of Crohn's disease may include endoscopy, colonoscopy, sigmoidoscopy, biopsies, barium enema, upper GI series, and stool guaiac.

## CROUP

### Description

Croup is an acute viral infection characterized by a barking cough, hoarseness, inspiratory stridor, and varying degrees of respiratory distress (Muniz, 2004). Symptoms can range from mild to severe with respiratory failure secondary to airway obstruction. This infection primarily involves the larynx and may extend into the trachea and bronchi. The causative virus is transmitted via the respiratory route. Parainfluenza types II, III, and IV; influenza A and B; adenovirus; respiratory syncytial virus; herpes simplex virus; measles; rhinovirus; coxsackievirus A and B; and echovirus all can cause mild sporadic croup.

### Signs and Symptoms
Croup begins with a few days of mild upper respiratory infection with nasal congestion, sore throat, and cough. Fever, hoarse voice, and a harsh, brassy, barklike cough follow. These conditions worsen at night. Croup usually peaks over three to five days and resolves within a week.

### Treatment
Treatment may include humidification, vasoconstrictors, and glucocorticoids. Severe croup that is unresponsive to therapy may require intubation. Some physicians have used a helium-oxygen (helium 60 to 80 percent) mixture in order to prevent intubation. Helium decreases the force necessary to move the gas through the airways and decreases the mechanical work of the respiratory muscles. Cases of severe croup may require frequent suctioning to prevent airway obstruction. Croup may lead to severe airway obstruction and death.

### Testing
The most direct test for croup is laryngoscopy, which usually reveals a pale and boggy laryngeal mucosa. This may be accompanied by abundant pus-filled fluids, mucus, and pseudomembranes.

## CRYPTORCHIDISM

### Description
Cryptorchidism, which is also known as cryptorchism, is defined as failure of the testicle to descend from its intra-abdominal location into the scrotum (Figure 2-25). A normal testicle descends at approximately 36 weeks of age, but for unknown reasons, cryptorchidism occurs in some male infants.

### Signs and Symptoms
There are usually no symptoms other than inability to find the testicle within the scrotum.

### Treatment
In most cases, cryptorchidism is self-resolving. In other cases, cryptorchidism is treated by orchiopexy, in which the testicle is sutured into place in the scrotum.

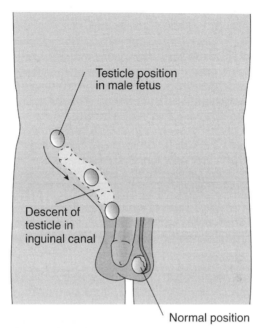

**Figure 2-25** Cryptorchidism

## CRYPTOSPORIDIOSIS

### Description

Over 403,000 people were involved in one waterborne outbreak of cryptosporidiosis, which is a protozoan disease caused by *Cryptosporidium parvum*. Many cases of traveler's diarrhea are caused by *C. parvum*, and it may be spread through contaminated food and water as well as the fecal-oral route. Epidemics have arisen from drinking water, swimming pools, a water slide, a zoo fountain, day-care centers, unpasteurized apple juice, and miscellaneous foods. The protozoa may be spread in the feces of infected humans and domestic animals such as dogs, pigs, and cattle. *C. parvum* is even more resistant to chlorine than *Giardia lamblia* (Cryptosporidiosis, 2003).

### Signs and Symptoms

The incubation period is approximately 4 to 12 days for this disease, with the symptoms lasting 10 to 14 days in most people. Cryptosporidiosis causes fever, loss of appetite, nausea, cramping abdominal pain, and profuse watery diarrhea. The disease is often fatal for individuals with suppressed immune systems.

### Treatment

In otherwise healthy people, cryptosporidiosis is self-resolving. There is no reliable treatment for cryptosporidiosis. Paromomycin, atovaquone, nitazoxanide, and azithromycin are sometimes prescribed, but they usually have temporary effects.

### Testing

A stool ova and parasite exam is used to diagnose cryptosporidiosis.

## CUSHING'S SYNDROME

### Description

Cushing's syndrome is an iatrogenic disorder of the adrenal glands due to chronic glucocorticoid hormone therapy. Prednisone is a commonly prescribed steroid for the management of chronic diseases, and its long-term use can cause Cushing's syndrome. Unlike Addison's disease, which results from a deficiency in cortisol from the adrenal cortex, Cushing's syndrome results from excesses of the hormone cortisol. Cushing's may also result from tumors of the adrenal glands or the pituitary gland (Corrigan, 1997).

### Signs and Symptoms

Color Plate 20 pictures a woman with a characteristic moon face resulting from steroid therapy. Cushing's syndrome is characterized by a rounded face due to excess fat deposits (moon face), obesity in the upper body, and obesity in children. Cushing's syndrome also includes purple stretch marks on the skin, thin skin, muscle weakness, easy bruising, hypertension, and destruction of bone tissue. Patients may also experience diabetes mellitus, impaired immune function, excessive facial hair, balding in women, kidney stones, perforations of the viscera, and fungal infections.

### Treatment

Cessation of the use of medications causing Cushing's syndrome is required for treatment; however, such changes should occur slowly. Surgical removal of tumors may be required if Cushing's is not due to the use of steroids.

### Testing

Diagnosis of Cushing's syndrome is based on cortisol levels in the urine, dexamethasone suppression tests, serum cortisol levels, ACTH, and MRI and CT scans for pituitary tumors or an adrenal mass.

## CUTANEOUS ANTHRAX

### Description

The overwhelming majority of anthrax cases in the world are cutaneous anthrax. When wounds such as skin cuts, abrasions, or insect bites become contaminated with anthrax spores, a small lesion appears about two to three days later. This lesion develops into a ring of small blisters that surround a dark center that eventually ulcerates and dries. This area of dead tissue is known as an eschar, which does not form pus or cause pain (see Color Plate 21 and Color Plate 22). Within two to three weeks, the eschar dries, separates from the skin, and falls off, leaving a scar (Dixon, 1999).

## Signs and Symptoms

Cutaneous anthrax lesions usually remain localized, but they may spread to the lymph glands. If a septic infection occurs, its symptoms are fever, malaise, and headache; although in normal cases of cutaneous anthrax, septic infection does not develop.

## Treatment

Several antibiotics are effective in the treatment of cutaneous anthrax, including penicillin, doxycycline, and ciprofloxacin (Cipro). The length of treatment is usually 60 days because spores may take up to 60 days to germinate.

## Testing

Cutaneous anthrax is diagnosed through a culture of the skin lesion.

## CYCLOSPORIASIS

## Description

Cyclosporiasis is a disease caused by the protozoon *Cyclospora cayetanensis*. This parasite was first described as the causative agent of cyclosporiasis after an outbreak in 1979 in Papua, New Guinea. Outbreaks have also been reported in the United States and Canada. *Cyclospora* is spread by ingestion of contaminated food or water. *Cyclospora* requires days or weeks to become infective after being passed in human feces, so it is not believed to be passed through direct contact with infected hosts. It is unknown whether animals can spread cyclosporiasis (Upton, 2001).

## Signs and Symptoms

*Cyclospora* infects the small intestine, and although some infected persons are asymptomatic, others experience watery diarrhea, frequent and explosive diarrhea, loss of appetite, weight loss, bloating, gas, abdominal cramps, nausea, vomiting, muscle pain, low-grade fever, and fatigue. The time between infection and illness is about one week. Cyclosporiasis can last up to a month or longer if untreated, and it can be a recurrent disorder.

## Treatment

The recommended treatment for *Cyclospora* infection is trimethoprim-sulfamethoxazole, which is also known as Bactrim, Septra, or Cotrim.

## Testing

Diagnosis is based on stool sample testing for the presence of *Cyclospora*.

## CYSTIC FIBROSIS

## Description

Cystic fibrosis (CF) is the most common, fatal genetic disease in the United States. According to the National Human Genome Research Institute (2003), about 30,000 people in the United States have the disease. Cystic fibrosis is caused by mutations in the cystic fibrosis transmembrane regulator gene. The protein associated with this gene should allow cells to release chloride and other ions, but in cystic fibrosis, the cells are defective and do not release the chloride. The lack of chloride results in a salt imbalance in the cells. The defective cells produce a thick, sticky mucus that clogs the lungs, leads to infection, and blocks the pancreas. In addition, the presence of this thick mucus stops digestive enzymes from reaching the intestine where they are required for proper digestion. Diabetes mellitus is frequently found in cases of cystic fibrosis. CF is a terminal disease in most cases at an average age of 20.

## Signs and Symptoms

CF is characterized by a lack of bowel movements in the first two days of life, pale or clay colored stool, foul smelling stool that floats, salty skin, recurrent persistent respiratory infections, coughing, weight loss, delayed growth, and fatigue.

## Treatment

Medications include antibiotics for respiratory infections and replacement of pancreatic enzymes. Inhaled bronchodilators are used to relieve chronic obstruction of the airways. Ibuprofen may slow lung deterioration, primarily in children ages 5 to 13 (Hait, 2002). Other treatments include postural drainage and chest percussion. Lung transplant may be required in some cases. Dornase (Pulmozyme) may be used to replace DNase enzymes (Cystic Fibrosis Research, 1997).

## Testing

Diagnosis of CF is based on sweat chloride tests, DNA testing, fecal fat tests, upper GI, and measurement of pancreatic function.

## CYSTICERCOSIS

### Description

Cysticercosis is an infection caused by a tapeworm found primarily in pigs, known as *Taenia solium*. Infection occurs most frequently in areas with poor sanitation and hygiene. The tapeworm is spread when pigs ingest contaminated human feces. Ingestion of contaminated pork products, water, or food or direct contact with contaminated surfaces allows the completion of the tapeworm life cycle. The larvae of the tapeworm form cysts throughout the body (*Cysticercosis*, 2003).

### Signs and Symptoms

Infection in the brain is known as neurocysticercosis, and it causes seizures, headaches, confusion, lack of attention to people and surroundings, difficulty with balance, swelling of the brain, and potentially death. Infection of the muscles is often asymptomatic, with the exception of lumps under the skin. Rarely, cysts may develop in the eyes, causing disturbances in vision, swelling of the eye, and possible detachment of the retina.

### Treatment

Cysticercosis is treated with antiparasitic drugs, steroids, and surgery to remove the affected area.

## Testing

Diagnosis may be predicated on antibody tests and the identification of lesions with X-rays, CT scans, MRI, and biopsy of the affected area.

## DACRYOADENITIS

### Description

Dacryoadenitis is an inflammatory enlargement of the lacrimal gland, which is the gland in the eye that produces tears (Singh, 2001). It is believed that infectious dacryoadenitis is caused by an agent that travels from the eye through the lacrimal ducts into the lacrimal gland. Common causes may include viruses, bacteria, and fungi. The disease may also be associated with sarcoidosis, Graves' disease, Sjögren's syndrome, orbital inflammatory syndrome, or benign lymphoepithelial lesions.

### Signs and Symptoms

Dacryoadenitis is characterized by rapid onset of severe pain, redness, and pressure in the orbit of the eye. The palpebral lobe of the lacrimal gland often is involved and is seen easily by everting the upper lid. Other associated physical signs of dacryoadenitis include swelling of the conjunctiva, pustular discharge, inflammation of the eyelids, inflammation of the submandibular lymph tissues, displacement of the eyeball inferiorly and medially, parotid salivary gland enlargement, and fever.

### Treatment

Viral forms of dacryoadenitis are usually self-limiting, and treatment may include warm compresses and nonsteroidal anti-inflammatories. Bacterial forms of dacryoadenitis should be treated with cephalosporins (e.g., Keflex) until culture results are obtained. If the patient needs to be hospitalized due to the severity of illness, IV cefazolin (Ancef) may be administered.

### Testing

Diagnostic tests may include smear and culture of pus, if it is present. Blood cultures should rule out *N. gonorrhoeae* infections, and CT scans of the orbits with contrast may be utilized.

## DENGUE

### Description

Dengue, which can progress into dengue hemorrhagic fever, is caused by one of four closely related viruses of the genus *Flavivirus* (Levy, 2003a). Dengue hemorrhagic fever has been a serious global problem since an outbreak in Southeast Asia at the end of World War II. In endemic areas of the world, it is a leading cause of hospitalization and death of children. Since the 1980s, dengue fever has also been a serious cause of disease throughout Africa. Since 1997, dengue has been the most reported mosquito-borne viral disease in the world, with tens of millions of cases annually. Recovering from dengue hemorrhagic fever does not provide immunity against the other serotypes of *Flavivirus*, so it is possible to contract dengue hemorrhagic fever four times. The virus is spread primarily in the tropics by the *Aedes aegypti* mosquito (*Dengue fever*, 2003).

## Signs and Symptoms

Dengue begins with flulike symptoms characterized by fever, and it progresses into dengue hemorrhagic fever, which can result in circulatory failure and death, especially in children. Symptoms include fever, rashes, muscle pain, arthralgia, headache, nausea, vomiting, and enlarged lymph nodes.

## Treatment

Treatment includes reducing fever and rehydration.

## Testing

Diagnosis is based on a CBC indicating increased leukocytes, decreased platelets, and increased hematocrit. Tests also indicate an increase in antibody titer for dengue virus types.

## DEQUERVAIN'S DISEASE

### Description

DeQuervain disease, which is also known as deQuervain tenosynovitis, is caused by narrowing of the tendons of the wrist, which includes the tendons of the abductor pollicis longus and the extensor pollicis brevis. DeQuervain disease commonly is seen in patients who use their hands and thumbs in a repetitive fashion (Foye, 2004).

### Signs and Symptoms

Patients with deQuervain disease usually report pain in the wrist with referral of pain toward the thumb and forearm. Swelling of the affected wrist is also common.

### Treatment

Various forms of physical therapy or occupational therapy may be used in treatment of patients with deQuervain tenosynovitis.

### Testing

The most classic finding in deQuervain tenosynovitis is a positive Finkelstein test. This test is performed by having the patient make a fist with the thumb inside the fingers. The wrist is then moved, which causes the symptomatic wrist pain. The Finkelstein test is performed on both wrists to compare with the uninvolved side.

## DIABETES INSIPIDUS

### Description

Diabetes insipidus and diabetes mellitus are different diseases. Diabetes mellitus is caused by a disorder of the pancreas, whereas diabetes insipidus is caused by a disorder between the pituitary gland and the kidneys. Diabetes insipidus is an uncommon condition resulting from the inability of the kidneys to conserve water. This function of the kidney is controlled by the release of antidiuretic hormone (ADH) from the pituitary gland in the brain. Diabetes insipidus is either caused by damage to the hypothalamus or pituitary gland as a result of surgery, infection, tumors, or head injury. Diabetes insipidus may also be caused by defects in the kidney that may be inherited in male children from their mothers (Brown, 2003b). Other diseases, like polycystic kidney disease, and the effects of drugs like lithium and amphotericin B may cause diabetes insipidus as well. There are four types of diabetes insipidus. Pituitary diabetes insipidus, which is also known as neurogenic, hypothalamic, or neurohypophyseal diabetes insipidus, is caused by a lack of vasopressin, which is an antiduretic hormone that controls urine output. Nephrogenic diabetes insipidus, which is also known as vasopressin-resistant diabetes insipidus, is caused by a lack of response by the kidneys to the effects of vasopressin. Gestagenic diabetes insipidus, which is also known as gesta-tional diabetes insipidus, is also caused by a deficiency in vasopressin, but it only occurs during pregnancy. Dipsogenic diabetes insipidus, which is also known as primary polydipsia, results from abnormal thirst and excessive consumption of liquids (Robertson, 2003).

### Signs and Symptoms
The most pronounced symptoms of diabetes insipidus are extreme thirst and excessive urination. The loss of water can result in fatal dehydration.

### Treatment
Diabetes insipidus is treated by focusing on the underlying cause when possible. Medications used in the treatment of diabetes insipidus may include vasopressin, indomethacin, and the diuretics hydrochlorothiazide and amiloride.

### Testing
Diagnosis of diabetes insipidus may include urinalysis and an MRI of the head. The effect of ADH on urine output may also be used to distinguish between central diabetes insipidus and nephrogenic diabetes insipidus. In central diabetes insipidus, a dose of ADH suppresses urinary output, and in cases of nephrogenic diabetes insipidus, a dose of ADH does not sup-press urinary output.

## DIABETES MELLITUS

### Description
Diabetes mellitus is categorized into two types: Type I (insulin-dependent diabetes) and Type II (non–insulin-dependent diabetes). Diabetes mellitus is a metabolic disorder, in which carbohydrates, which break down into sugars in the digestive system, are not digested effectively by the body due to a lack of appropriate insulin production in the pancreatic islets, which are also known as the islets of Langerhans. When left untreated, diabetes

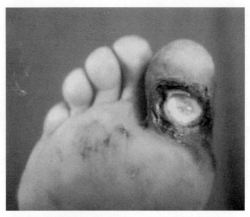

**Figure 2-26** Perforating ulcer of the big toe (Courtesy of the CDC)

mellitus can lead to coma and death (Brown, 2003a). Diabetes may cause blindness, carbuncles of the legs and feet, and ulcers of the feet, as indicated in Figure 2-26. Amputation of parts of the lower extremities is not uncommon, and diabetes mellitus can also cause renal failure and cardiac disorders. Diabetes mellitus can cause a variety of complications, including elevated blood sugar levels, polyuria, excessive thirst, and increased appetite (American Diabetes Association, 2005).

## Signs and Symptoms

Diabetics may have a sweet smell to their breath due to the presence of acetone in the body. Symptoms of Type I diabetes may include increased thirst, increased urination, weight loss, loss of appetite, fatigue, nausea, and vomiting. Type II diabetes is characterized by increased thirst, increased urination, increased appetite, fatigue, blurred vision, slow-healing infections, and impotence in men.

## Treatment

Diet, exercise, and proper medication are essential aspects of the treatment of diabetes. There is no cure for diabetes, and the immediate concern is to stabilize blood sugar and eliminate the symptoms of hyperglycemia. Medications to treat diabetes may include insulin and hypoglycemic agents. Some patients use an insulin pump, which delivers a steady flow of insulin throughout the day. Medications that increase insulin production by the pancrease include Amaryl, Gucotrol, Micronase, DiaBeta, Glynase, Prandin, and Starlix. Medications that increase sensitivity to insulin include Glucophage, Avandia, and Actos. Medications that delay absorption of glucose include Precose and Glyset.

## Testing

Tests for diabetes may include a urinalysis to look for glucose and ketones from the breakdown of fats, fasting blood glucose levels, random blood glucose levels, and oral glucose tolerance tests.

## DIABETIC RETINOPATHY

### Description

Diabetes mellitus causes an array of long-term systemic complications, of which the most common and potentially most blinding is diabetic retinopathy. The exact mechanism by which diabetes causes retinopathy remains unclear, but growth hormone appears to play a causative role in the development and progression of diabetic retinopathy. In addition, several blood abnormalities related to diabetes lead to loss of blood flow to the retina of the eye. Approximately 8,000 eyes become blind each year due to diabetes (Valero, 2004).

### Signs and Symptoms

In the initial stages, patients are generally asymptomatic. Later, patients experience vision loss and floaters, which are translucent specks that move across the eye. Hemorrhage into the vitreous humor may cause a haze as blood clots within the gel. Swelling and thickening of the eye may also occur.

### Treatment

The treatment of diabetic retinopathy may include laser photocoagulation, glucose control, and laser burns over the retina.

### Testing

Fluorescein angiography is used to diagnose diabetic retinopathy.

## DIENTAMOEBA FRAGILIS INFECTION

### Description

*Dientamoeba fragilis* infection causes gastrointestinal illness in humans. *Dientamoeba fragilis* is a parasitic protozoan that is found worldwide and is a commonly diagnosed cause of illness in the United States (Mack, 2003).

### Signs and Symptoms

Symptoms of *Dientamoeba fragilis* infection include diarrhea, stomach pain, loss of appetite, nausea, and fatigue, although many cases are asymptomatic. *Dientamoeba fragilis* is transmitted through the fecal-oral route. Those at highest risk for infection live in institutions that have poor sanitary conditions, travelers who visit developing countries, and the immunosuppressed (*Dientamoeba fragilis infection*, 2004).

### Treatment

*Dientamoeba fragilis* infection is treated with iodoquinol. Paromomycin, tetracycline, or metronidazole may also be used.

### Testing

*Dientamoeba fragilis* infection is diagnosed through stained fecal smears to detect trophozoites, which are not detectable by stool concentration methods. *Dientamoeba fragilis* can be easily overlooked because they are pale-staining and their nuclei may resemble those of *Endolimax nana* or *Entamoeba hartmanni*.

## DIGEORGE SYNDROME

### Description

DiGeorge syndrome is a genetic disorder causing specific cardiac malformations, a subset of facial attributes, hormone, and immune anomalies. The cause of DiGeorge syndrome has been identified as a deletion of chromosome 22 in the DiGeorge chromosomal region (*DiGeorge syndrome* NCBI, 2004; *DiGeorge syndrome* NPIRC, 2004; *DiGeorge syndrome*, 2002).

### Signs and Symptoms

Persons with DiGeorge syndrome may have tetralogy of Fallot, interrupted aortic arch type B, truncus arteriosus, aberrant left subclavian artery, right infundibular stenosis, or ventricular septal defect. Some of the facial characteristics of DiGeorge syndrome are a divided uvula, high-arched palate, small mouth and wide-set eyes, down-slanting eyes, hooded eyes, long face, cupped low-set ears, bulbous nasal tip, and a dimpled or bifurcated nasal tip. They may also exhibit immune deficiency of varying severity. The thymus gland and parathyroid glands are malformed and dysfunctional. Learning disorders are common.

### Treatment

The initial treatment is to control hypoparathyroidism. Intravenous calcium gluconate is administered to stop and prevent hypocalcemic seizures, followed by a low phosphorus diet, calcium supplements, and vitamin D. Transplant with fetal thymus from a stillborn fetus, thymic factor replacement, and bone marrow transplantation have been tried with varying results. Correction of congenital heart defects is usually needed. Patients require prompt treatment of infection, may benefit from *Pneumocystitis carinii* antibiotic prophylaxis, and must avoid live virus vaccinations (Fratterelli, 2002).

### Testing

The presence of prolonged hypocalcemia, congenital hypoparathyroidism, and elevated serum phosphorus in a child with congenital heart disease is suggestive of DiGeorge syndrome. X-ray examination of the chest may reveal congenital malformation of the heart and vessels and absence of the thymus gland. Genetic studies using chromosomal markers to study chromosome 22 are usually performed.

## DIPHTHERIA

### Description

Diphtheria occurs in two forms: respiratory and cutaneous. The pathogen that causes diphtheria is *Corynebacterium diphtheriae*. Until 1935, diphtheria was the leading infectious killer of children in the United States (Levy, 2004c). Now, however, it is considered uncommon in North America and

Western Europe. Due to immunization programs in the United States, in particular the DTaP vaccine, the number of cases of diphtheria reported annually has fallen to five or fewer. Although *C. diphtheriae* is readily killed by heat and most disinfectants, it is resistant to drying and remains viable in the environment for weeks. The diphtheria toxin is extremely potent and is lethal for humans in small amounts because it is able to block the production of proteins in human cells. Humans are the only natural host for *C. diphtheriae*, which is spread through airborne droplet transmission or hand-to-mouth contact (NFID, 2003).

### Signs and Symptoms
Diphtheria is characterized by sore throat, red abdominal rash, fever, fatigue, swelling of the neck, bleeding in the throat, and paralysis. Color Plate 23 pictures a skin lesion caused by diphtheria infection. As the disease advances, a grayish-white pseudomembrane forms in the throat. The membrane contains dead tissue, fibrin, and bacterial cells. If the infection reaches the kidneys or heart, it can cause sudden death.

### Treatment
Diphtheria is treated by the administration of antitoxins commercially produced in horses. The infection is then treated with antibiotics, such as penicillin or erythromycin.

### Testing
Tests for diphtheria include Gram stain or throat culture and an electrocardiogram for individuals in which myocarditis is suspected.

## DIPHYLLOBOTHRIASIS

### Description
Diphyllobothriasis is a gastrointestinal disease caused by the largest human tapeworm, *Diphyllobothrium latum*. This tapeworm is spread by ingesting contaminated fish. Diphyllobothriasis occurs in areas where lakes and rivers coexist with human consumption of raw or undercooked freshwater fish, primarily in Eastern Europe, Asia, North America, Uganda, and Chile (Smith, 2003a).

### Signs and Symptoms
Symptoms of diphyllobothriasis include diarrhea, stomach pain, loss of appetite, nausea, and fatigue, although many cases are asymptomatic.

### Treatment
Treatment for diphyllobothriasis may include niclosamide or paraziquantel to treat the tapeworm infection. In addition, vitamin $B_{12}$ may be needed for megaloblastic anemia (Rai & Weisse, 2002).

### Testing
Visible segments of worms may be present in the stool, and a CBC may reveal macrocytic anemia. Stool smears may also be conducted for the presence of tapeworm eggs.

## DIVERTICULITIS

### Description

Diverticulosis is the development of small sacs in the wall of the colon, without inflammation or symptoms (Stone, 2004f). These saculations are asymptomatic unless they become inflamed. Inflammation of diverticula occurs when feces are trapped inside these abnormal sacs. This causes the feces to stagnate in the colon and turn to gangrene with the possibility of perforation of the bowel (Sherif & Perez, 2004).

### Signs and Symptoms

Diverticulitis is characterized by chronic constipation, chills and fever, nausea, vomiting, mucus in the stool, and a gripping abdominal pain.

### Treatment

Diverticulitis requires antibiotic therapy; perforations, fistulas, or abscesses may require surgery. Chronic diverticulitis is treated by increasing high-fiber foods and additives such as psyllium in the diet.

### Testing

In cases of diverticulitis, a CT scan may reveal thickening of the inflamed area, a mass in the lower left quadrant, and an elevated white blood cell count.

## DOWN SYNDROME

### Description

Down syndrome is named after J. Langdon Down, a nineteenth-century British physician. It also goes by the name of trisomy 21. It receives its alternate name because people with Down syndrome have an extra chromosome, usually number 21 or 22. Mental retardation occurs in Down syndrome to varying degrees. According to the National Institute of Child Health and Development (2003), mothers who become pregnant by the age of 30 have less than a 1 in 1,000 chance of having a baby with Down syndrome, in comparison to mothers over the age of 49, who have a 1 in 12 chance (Facts about Down Syndrome, 2003).

### Signs and Symptoms

The signs of Down syndrome are observable in the child in Color Plate 24. Down syndrome is characterized by an enlarged tongue, sloped forehead, small ear canals, low-set ears, a dwarfed physical appearance, and a flattened nose or absent nasal bridge. Persons with Down syndrome also are noted for the presence of short, broad hands with a single palmar crease, and they may have gray or light yellow spots on the iris of their eyes (Stewart, 2003e).

### Treatment

There is no specific treatment for Down syndrome.

## Testing

A heart murmur may be present, and early and massive vomiting may indicate obstruction of the upper digestive tract. Tests may include a chromosome study, imaging tests for the presence of cardiac abnormalities, and gastrointestinal imaging to show obstructions.

## EBOLA HEMORRHAGIC FEVER

### Description

The Ebola virus causes a severe hemorrhagic fever with a high mortality rate (88 percent) that has appeared sporadically since it was initially discovered in 1976 in Zaire, Africa (now known as the Democratic Republic of the Congo). The Ebola virus is named after the river where it was first identified. The Ebola virus is an RNA virus that infects both human and nonhuman primates. Ebola virus was isolated from African imported monkeys in the United States. There have been no cases of Ebola hemorrhagic fever in the United States; however, several American research scientists were infected with the virus but did not become ill. The disease can spread between people by way of nosocomial routes, needle-stick injury, or contact with infected bodily fluids. It is not known why some individuals recover from the disease and others do not (Wener, 2004c).

### Signs and Symptoms

Ebola hemorrhagic fever is characterized by fever, headache, arthritis, muscle pain, sore throat, diarrhea, vomiting, rash, red eyes, hiccups, and internal and external hemorrhaging (Ebola hemorrhagic fever, 2002).

### Treatment

There is no known cure for Ebola hemorrhagic fever. Hospitalization and intensive care will likely be needed. In addition, supportive measures for shock will be used, and transfusions of platelets or fresh blood may be needed to correct bleeding abnormalities.

### Testing

Tests for Ebola hemorrhagic fever include coagulation studies to determine blood clotting ability, serologic studies for exposure to Ebola virus, and a CBC demonstrating leukopenia and thrombocytopenia.

## ECLAMPSIA AND PRE-ECLAMPSIA

### Description

Pre-eclampsia is a serious condition that occurs during pregnancy. It is characterized by high blood pressure, weight gain, and protein in the urine. Pre-eclampsia may progress into eclampsia, which is the occurrence of seizures during pregnancy that cannot be attributed to another cause after the 20th week of gestation. The causes of both pre-eclampsia and eclamspia are unknown. There is an increased risk for pre-eclampsia with first-time pregnancies; with teenage pregnancies; among mothers over the

**Table 2-3** Characteristics of Pre-Eclampsia and Eclampsia

| Pre-Eclampsia | Eclampsia |
|---|---|
| swelling of hands and face upon arising | seizures |
| sudden weight gain over one or two days | severe agitation |
| persistent headache | periods of unconsciousness |
| upper abdominal pain | aches and pains after seizures |

age of 40; among African-American women; in multiple pregnancies; and among women with a history of diabetes, hypertension, or renal diseases (Brooks, 2001; Pre-eclampsia [n/d]).

### Signs and Symptoms

Table 2-3 compares the characteristics of pre-eclampsia and eclampsia.

### Treatment

The treatment for eclampsia is to deliver as soon as it is safe for the fetus because prolonging such pregnancies may result in fetal death and complications for the mother. Treatment includes medications to control elevated blood pressure and seizures.

## ECTOPIC PREGNANCY

### Description

Ectopic pregnancy is the implantation of the fertilized ovum somewhere other than the normal site in the uterine cavity (Marchiano, 2004). It is a condition in which the fertilized egg fails to implant itself in the uterine wall and implants outside the uterus, where the fetus begins to develop. In most cases, the egg implants within the fallopian tube, although it may implant in the ovary, abdomen, or cervix (Figure 2-27). Ectopic pregnancies rarely progress to full term (Bourgon & Outwater, 2004).

Ectopic pregnancies occur when an obstruction blocks the fertilized egg from passing through the uterine tube to the uterus. Possible causes of ectopic pregnancy include physical blockage in the tube or failure of the tubal epithelium to move the fertilized egg down the tube and into the uterus. Previous tubal infection or surgery might also have caused scarring of the lining of the tube, which can inhibit the passage of the fertilized egg toward the uterus. Many women who experience tubal pregnancies also have a history of salpingitis or pelvic inflammatory disease. Occasionally, ectopic pregnancies are due to unknown causes.

### Signs and Symptoms

Ectopic pregnancy is characterized by lower abdominal or pelvic pain, mild cramping on one side of the pelvis, abnormal vaginal bleeding (e.g., spotting), breast tenderness, nausea, and low back pain. If rupture

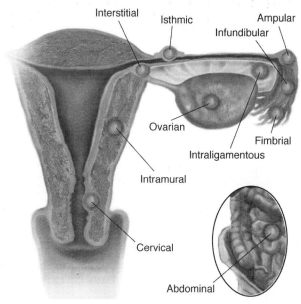

**Figure 2-27** Possible sites of implantation in ectopic pregnancy

and hemorrhaging occur before successfully treating the pregnancy, symptoms may worsen and include sharp and sudden pain in the lower abdominal area and referred pain to the shoulder area.

## Treatment

The first symptom of nearly 20 percent of ectopic pregnancies is pelvic organ rupture leading to hemorrhage and shock (Marchiano, 2004). Surgical laparotomy is performed to stop the immediate loss of blood, to confirm the diagnosis of ectopic pregnancy, to remove the products of conception, and to repair surrounding tissue damage. In some cases, removal of the involved fallopian tube may be necessary. In nonemergency cases, minilaparotomy or laparoscopy are the most common surgical treatments. In nonsurgical management for ectopic pregnancies without suspected immediate danger of rupture, methotrexate is administered with serial human chorionic gonadotropin (hCG), CBC, and liver function tests. Ectopic pregnancies cannot continue to term, so removal of the developing cells is necessary to save the life of the mother.

## Testing

Diagnosis is based on blood work indicating a pregnancy combined with imaging exams indicating an empty uterus. A culdocentesis, a laparoscopy, or a laparotomy may be necessary.

## ECZEMA

### Description

Eczema is a general term for a variety of inflammatory skin conditions (Kantor, 2004a). Among infants, eczema occurs on the forehead, cheeks, forearms, legs, scalp, and neck. In children and adults, eczema occurs on the face, neck, and the insides of the elbows, knees, and ankles. Skin affected by eczema may become easily infected (Mishky, 2004).

### Signs and Symptoms

Eczema is characterized by dry, red, extremely itchy patches on the skin that may ooze an inflammatory fluid (see Color Plate 25). Ear discharges and bleeding may also be present.

### Treatment

Contact with water should be brief, and soap should be used sparingly. After bathing, it is important to trap the moisture in the skin by applying lubricating cream on the skin while it is damp. Temperature changes and stress may cause sweating and aggravate the condition. Chronic areas may be treated with ointments containing tar compounds, corticosteroids, and skin humectants and emollients. Topical immunomodulators, which are steroid-free, including tacrolimus (Protopic) and pimecrolimus (Elidel), are also used in the treatment of eczema.

### Testing

Diagnosis is based on the appearance of the skin, biopsy, and personal and family history.

## EHLERS-DANLOS SYNDROME

### Description

Ehlers-Danlos syndrome is a group of inherited disorders characterized by excessive looseness of the joints, hyperelastic skin that is fragile and bruises easily, and easily damaged blood vessels. The syndrome also may involve rupture of internal organs (Schaefer, 2002; Stewart, 2003f).

### Signs and Symptoms

Ehlers-Danlos syndrome is characterized by joint dislocation, arthritis, flat feet, soft and velvity skin, easy scarring, poor wound healing, and joint hypermobility and laxity. In addition, patients may exhibit mitral valve prolapse; periodontitis; platelet aggregation failure; rupture of intestines or uterus; visual impairment; and soft, thin, or hyperextensible skin.

### Treatment

There is no specific cure for Ehlers-Danlos syndrome, except to treat symptoms.

### Testing

Tests associated with Ehlers-Danlos syndrome may include collagen typing, collagen gene mutation testing, lysyl hydroxylase or oxidase activity, and an echocardiogram.

## EHRLICHIOSIS

### Description

Ehrlichiosis is caused by several bacterial species in the genus *Ehrlichia*, which are known to cause disease in dogs, cattle, sheep, goats, and horses (Wener, 2004d). Currently, there are three species of *Ehrlichia* in the United States and one in Japan known to cause disease in humans. In the United States, ehrlichiosis occurs primarily in the southeastern and south central regions of the country and is primarily transmitted by the lone star tick (*Amblyomma americanum*), the black-legged tick (*Ixodes scapularis*), and the western black-legged tick (*Ixodes pacificus*) (*Human ehrlichiosis*, 2000).

### Signs and Symptoms

Initial symptoms of ehrlichiosis include fever, headache, muscle pain, fatigue, nausea, vomiting, diarrhea, cough, arthritis, confusion. Rash may also be present among infected children.

### Treatment

Ehrlichiosis is usually treated effectively with tetracycline or doxycycline.

### Testing

Diagnositic tests indicate leukopenia, thrombocytopenia, elevated liver transaminase, and a fluorescent antibody test may turn positive for *E. chaffeensis* or granulocytic *Ehrlichia*.

## EIKENELLA INFECTION

### Description

*Eikenella corrodens* is part of the normal bacteria found in the mouth and digestive tract in humans. Most infections occur as a result of traumatic events such as human bites. Infections are typically mixed with other bacteria.

### Signs and Symptoms

*Eikenella* infections have been known to cause meningitis, empyema, pneumonia, osteomyelitis, arthritis, and cellulitis in intravenous drug abusers as a result of direct inoculation after licking the needle clean instead of sterilizing it.

### Treatment

*Eikenella* infection is treated with antibiotics. These infections are characteristically resistant to clindamycin and the aminoglycosides. In vitro isolates demonstrate sensitivity to penicillin, ampicillin, cefoxitin, chloramphenicol, carbenicillin, and imipenem.

### Testing

Cultures indicate the presence of *E. corrodens*.

## EMBOLISM

### Description

An embolism is the sudden obstruction of a vessel by debris. An embolism is caused by an embolus, which is a free floating object in the bloodstream. Some of the most common emboli are blood clots, cholesterol-containing plaques, bacteria, cancer cells, amniotic fluid, fat from the marrow of broken bones, and injected substances such as air bubbles. Embolisms can be life-threatening conditions. Emboli that block the flow of blood to the heart or brain can result in sudden death.

### Signs and Symptoms

Embolisms cause sudden shortness of breath, unequal breathing sounds in the lungs, low blood pressure, weak pulse, elevated blood pressure in the veins, cyanosis, sharp chest pain, coughing up blood, and loss of consciousness. Table 2-4 lists and describes some of the more common forms of emboli.

### Treatment

Emboli require prompt hospitalization to control symptoms and to improve interrupted blood flow. Intravenous analgesics are administered for pain control, and clots are broken down by thrombolytics such as streptokinase. The development of new clots is prevented with anticoagulants (e.g., warfarin, heparin) or antiplatelet medications (e.g., aspirin, ticlopidine, clopidogrel). Surgical procedures may include thromboaspiration, embolectomy, or angioplasty.

### Testing

Tests to diagnose arterial embolism or reveal the source of emboli may include a Doppler ultrasound exam of an extermity, a transcranial Doppler, echocardiography, transesophageal echocardiography, myocardial contrast echocardiography, MRI, angiography, arteriography, or plethysmography.

## EMPHYSEMA

### Description

Emphysema is a chronic inflammatory disease of the respiratory system, characterized by the presence of air pockets at the terminal ends of the bronchioles. The walls of the alveolar sacs become desiccated and tear. Because the individual is able to inhale, but is unable to properly exhale, a characteristic barrel chest develops, as illustrated in Figure 2-28. Individuals with emphysema may also purse their lips when exhaling in an effort to expelled trapped air from the alveoli. Emphysema is often a secondary disease brought on by infections, long-term smoking, or pneumoconiosis.

### Signs and Symptoms

Emphysema is characterized by shortness of breath, cough, wheezing, anxiety, weight loss, fatigue, and swelling in the lower extremities.

**Table 2-4** Common Emboli

| Type | Description |
|------|-------------|
| Fragments of thrombi | One of the most common forms of embolism occurs when a blood clot (thrombus) breaks apart, fragmenting small pieces of the clot throughout the bloodstream where they may become lodged in smaller vessels blocking the flow of blood. |
| Microorganisms | Many microorganisms spread throughout the body by multiplying in the blood, which is known as septicemia. For example, bacteremia, which occurs when bacteria multiply in the blood, can cause congestion of the tissues and death due to blood poisoning. |
| Tumor cells | Metastasis is the process in which cancer cells spread throughout the body. For example, a single tumor cell may break off of a larger tumor in the lung and spread through the blood to the liver, where a new, secondary tumor grows. It is also possible for tumor cell emboli to block blood vessels, preventing the flow of blood. |
| Animal parasites | A variety of animal parasites are capable of spreading through the blood, and certain of those require this stage in their life cycle to grow and replicate. |
| Fat | During crushing injuries, fat globules in the tissues may enter damaged blood vessels. This is particularly common in fractures of bone, where fat globules from the yellow bone marrow are able to enter the blood vessels. If a fat embolus occludes an artery of the heart or brain, it can cause sudden death. |
| Gas | Bubbles may enter the blood during chest injuries, during surgery, or during a simple inoculation (a shot). In another example, divers may experience a condition known as the bends, in which nitrogen that is dissolved in the blood forms nitrogen bubbles causing serious illness or death. |
| Foreign bodies | Emboli can be formed of any free-floating object in the blood; therefore, any foreign object small enough may become an embolus. Examples of foreign body emboli include bullet fragments, microscopic glass shards, grains of sand, or any other object small enough to float in the blood after trauma. |

## Treatment

Smoking cessation is the most important and effective treatment. Medications used to improve breathing include bronchodilators, diuretics, and corticosteroids. Antibiotics may be prescribed when respiratory infections

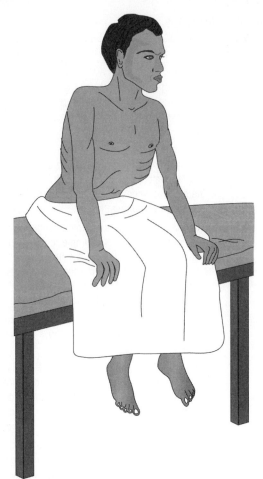

**Figure 2-28** Pursed lips and barrel chest of emphysema

occur. Low-flow oxygen and pulmonary rehabilitation may improve quality of life. Lung transplantation may be required.

### Testing

Tests used in the diagnosis of emphysema may include pulmonary function tests, chest X-rays, arterial blood gases, perfusion scans, and chest CT.

## ENCEPHALITIS

### Description

Encephalitis is inflammation of the brain, typically caused by an infection of the brain caused by a virus (Campellone, 2004b). Although rare, encephalitis can be a severe and potentially fatal disease. The two forms of encephalitis are primary encephalitis and secondary encephalitis. Primary encephalitis occurs when a virus directly invades the brain and spinal cord. In cases of secondary encephalitis, which is also known as postinfectious encephalitis, the virus first infects another part of the body and then spreads to the brain (Edwards, 2003).

Encephalitis is caused by three broad categories of viruses: herpes virus, childhood infections, and arboviruses. Both herpes simplex virus types 1 and 2 are the most common causes of encephalitis, with herpes simplex virus 1 causing more cases than herpes simplex virus 2. Another potential cause of encephalitis is the varicella-zoster virus, which causes chickenpox and shingles. Finally, the Epstein-Barr virus, which causes infectious mononucleosis, can cause a form of encephalitis that results in death about 8 percent of the time.

### Signs and Symptoms
Although most people with encephalitis have little or no symptoms, more severe cases can include drowsiness, confusion, seizures, fever, headache, nausea, vomiting, convulsions, or tremors.

### Treatment
Treatment of encephalitis may include antiviral medications for viral infections; however, specific antiviral drugs are often unavailable to combat the infection. Antibiotics, antiseizure medications such a phenytoin, and steroids such as dexamethasone may also be used to treat encephalitis.

### Testing
Diagnosis of encephalitis may include viral cultures of cerebrospinal fluid obtained through lumbar puncture, serology tests, EEG, brain MRI, and CAT scans of the head.

## ENDOCARDITIS

### Description
An inflammation of the endocardium of the heart, which may include the heart valves or the cardiac septum, is known as endocarditis (Wener, 2004e). Endocarditis may occur when the surface of the lining of the heart is damaged due to blood clots that traumatize the tissues. Bacteria may then infect the damaged tissue (see Color Plate 26). In this form of endocarditis, the heart valves may become involved. Damaged heart valves may disrupt the flow of blood through the heart because the heart valves are unable to properly function. Endocarditis may also result from an infection after the implantation of artificial heart valves, and endocarditis is commonly associated with the use of intravenous drugs. The infections associated with endocarditis may spread to the kidneys, inflaming the lining of the renal blood vessels (Marill, 2001; Ryan, 2004).

### Signs and Symptoms
Endocarditis may cause symptoms of fatigue, weakness, fever, chills, severe night sweats, weight loss, heart murmur, difficulty breathing,

bloody urine, swelling of the lower extremities, hemorrhages under the nails, paleness, and abnormal urine color. Patients may also present with red, painless skin spots, located on the palms and soles, called Janeway lesions. Endocarditis may also cause red, painful nodes in the pads of the fingers and toes called Osler's nodes.

## Treatment

Endocarditis is treated with antibiotics. If heart failure develops as a result of damaged heart valves, or if the bacterial colonies fragment causing stroke or vascular occlusions, surgery may be needed to replace the affected heart valve.

## Testing

Diagnosis of endocarditis is based on blood cultures, serology specific bacteria, erythrocyte sedimentation rate (ESR), CBC, ECG, echocardiogram, transesophageal echocardiogram, and chest X-rays.

## ENDOMETRIOSIS

### Description

Endometriosis is a condition in which the lining of the uterus (i.e., endometrium) grows in other areas of the body, such as the pelvic area, the surface of the uterus, the ovaries, the intestines, the rectum, or the bladder (Figure 2-29). Endometriosis is an idiopathic disorder, which can cause pain, irregular bleeding, and infertility as the disease progressess (P. Chen, 2004b).

### Signs and Symptoms

Although some women are asymptomatic, endometriosis can cause abdominopelvic pain lasting for approximately a week surrounding menstruation, pain during or following sexual intercourse, painful bowel movements, premenstrual spotting of blood, and infertility.

### Treatment

Treatment of endometriosis depends on the degree of symptoms and the extent of the disease. The woman's desire for future childbearing and the woman's age are also factors to consider. Analgesic therapy may be indicated for women with mild to moderate premenstrual pain, with no pelvic examination abnormalities, and with no immediate desire to become pregnant. Treatment may also include progesterone, amen, cycrin, provera, megace, zoladex, danazol, and antigonadotropin drugs such as Synarel and Depo-Lupron. Surgery may be indicated for severe cases of endometriosis (Kapoor & Davila, 2004).

### Testing

Diagnosis of endometriosis may include a pelvic examination, a pelvic ultrasound, and laparoscopy.

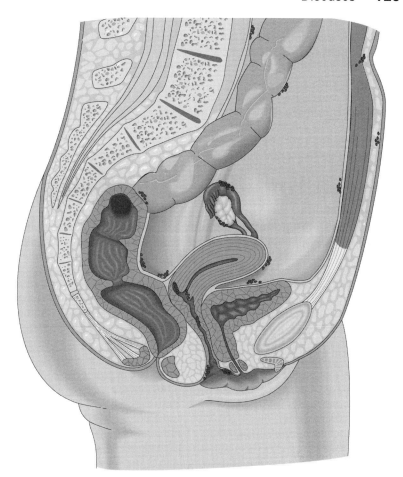

**Figure 2-29** Endometriosis

## ENTERITIS

### Description

Enteritis is an inflammation of the intestine caused by an infection. Micro-organisms are usually ingested in contaminated food or water. There are a variety of microorganisms that can cause enteritis, but some of the more common include S*taphylococcus, Salmonella, Shigella, Campylobacter,* and *E. coli.* Enteritis is most common after traveling to areas with untreated or contaminated water.

### Signs and Symptoms

Symptoms of enteritis may include abdominal pain, cramping, diarrhea, fever, and dehydration. Vomiting is rarely associated with enteritis

(Stone, 2003a). These symptoms may appear soon after exposure, or they may take several days to manifest. Enteritis is most dangerous to infants and the elderly.

### Treatment

Symptoms usually resolve in one to five days without treatment. The goal of treatment is to control symptoms and prevent dehydration due to diarrhea.

### Testing

Diagnosis of enteritis may include a stool culture and an upper endoscopy.

## EPIDURAL HEMATOMA

### Description

Epidural hematoma is a traumatic accumulation of blood between the skull and the dural membrane, which is most frequently due to rupture of a meningeal artery. The inciting event often is a focused blow to the head, such as that produced by a hammer, baseball bat, or windshield. The middle meningeal artery is firmly attached to the skull at the squamous portion of the temporal bone, so injury to the temple region of the head frequently results in its rupture. In most cases this trauma results in an overlying fracture (Price & Wilson, 2001).

### Signs and Symptoms

The typical symptom pattern of loss of consciousness, followed by alertness, then loss of consciousness again may not appear in all people, but is highly indicative of an extradural hemorrhage (Jasmin, 2004). Other characteristics of extradural hemorrhage include severe headache, drowsiness, confusion, nausea, vomiting, dizziness, unilateral pupil enlargement, and weakness of part of the body on the opposite side of the enlarged pupil. Symptoms may occur within minutes to hours after a head injury. Notice in Figure 2-30 how the brain tissue is compressed by the hematoma.

### Treatment

An extradural hematoma is an emergency condition that may require life support to prevent permanent damage to the brain. Emergency surgery, which may include drilling a hole in the skull to relieve pressure and allow drainage of blood from the brain, is almost always necessary to reduce intracranial pressure. Large hematomas need to be removed through a craniotomy. Medications may include anticonvulsants and hyperosmotic agents like mannitol, glycerol, and hypertonic saline to reduce brain swelling. Epidural hematoma can have an excellent prognosis if the bleeding can be controlled, but epidural hemorrhage has a high fatality rate.

### Testing

Diagnosis of epidural hematoma is based on imaging tests such as a head CT scan to pinpoint the location of the hematoma and associated skull fractures.

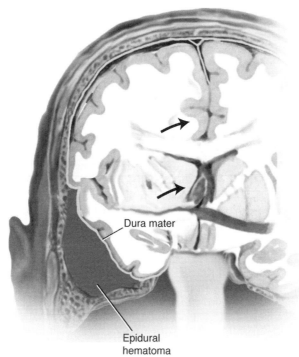

Dura mater

Epidural
hematoma

**Figure 2-30** Epidural hematoma. The arrows indicate a
shift in the position of the brain

## EPIGLOTTITIS

### Description

Epiglottitis is an inflammation of the cartilage that covers the trachea,
and it is usually caused by the bacterium *Haemophilus influenzae* (Felter,
2001). There are fewer cases of epiglottitis since the introduction of the
*H. influenzae* group b (Hib) vaccine in the late 1980s. Epiglottitis is a life-
threatening disease in which the epiglottis becomes inflamed, obstructing
the airway. Respiratory distress increases rapidly as the epiglottis swells.
Spasm may cause the airway to close abruptly. Death may follow within
minutes of airway obstruction.

### Signs and Symptoms

Epiglottitis is characterized by drooling, sore throat, difficulty swallowing,
difficulty breathing, stridor, hoarseness, chills, fever, and cyanosis.

### Treatment

Epiglottitis is a medical emergency requiring intensive care, which may
include humidified oxygen, intubation, IV fluids, antibiotics, and

corticosteroids. Although life-threatening, with proper treatment, many patients respond positively.

### Testing
Diagnostic tests for epiglottitis may include laryngoscopy, blood culture, throat culture, CBC, and X-rays of the neck to identify epiglottis enlargement.

## EPILEPSY

### Description
Epilepsy is a recurrent degenerative disorder of the nervous system marked by repetitive abnormal electrical discharges within the brain known as seizures (Campellone, 2004c). Epilepsy is characterized by sudden convulsions and seizures or altered consciousness, depending on the type of attack. There are two basic types of seizures associated with epilepsy: grand mal and petite mal.

Grand mal seizures are characterized by fecal and urinary incontinence, uncontrolled contraction of the muscles of the extremities, loss of consciousness, and a cry caused by contraction of the respiratory muscles forcing exhalation. Petite mal seizures differ from grand mal seizures in that the individual ceases activity for a few seconds. Petite mal seizures are more common in children, who often outgrow the disorder (Types of Seizures, 2003).

### Signs and Symptoms
The severity of symptoms can vary greatly from simple staring spells to loss of consciousness and violent convulsions. For many patients, the event is stereotyped (the same event over and over), but some patients have many different types of seizures that cause different symptoms each time. The type of seizure a person experiences depends on a variety of factors, such as the part of the brain affected, the cause, and individual response. An aura consisting of a strange sensation, such as tingling, smell, or emotional changes, signals a seizure in some people.

### Treatment
Treatment may include surgical repair of tumors or brain lesions. Anticonvulsants may reduce the number of seizures. Another treatment for epilepsy is the implantation of a vagal nerve stimulator in the chest, which can help reduce the number of seizures.

### Testing
Tests used in the diagnosis of epilepsy may include an EEG, blood tests, cerebrospinal fluid analysis, and head CT or MRI scan.

## EPISCLERITIS

### Description
Episcleritis is inflammation of the episclera that occurs in the absence of an infection. The episclera is a membrane that covers the sclera of the eye.

Episcleritis is usually mild and rarely progresses to scleritis. Episcleritis may be idiopathic, but it may be associated with certain diseases (e.g., rheumatoid arthritis, Sjögren's syndrome, syphilis, herpes zoster, tuberculosis) (Feinberg, 2004a; Roy, 2004).

## Signs and Symptoms
Episcleritis is characterized by a pink or purple discoloration of the white part of the eye, eye pain, sensitivity to light, eye tenderness, and tearing of the eye.

## Treatment
Episcleritis is typically self-resolving in one to two weeks. Treatment with corticosteroid eyedrops may shorten the course of the symptoms.

## Testing
Eye examination is usually sufficient to diagnose the disorder. No special tests are usually necessary.

## ERYSIPELAS

### Description
Erysipelas is a type of skin infection that is generally caused by group A streptococci (Lehrer, 2003a). Erysipelas is more likely to occur after local trauma to the skin, if ulcers are present, or in cases of venous or lymphatic drainage disruption. Erysipelas occurs most frequently on the lower extremities, but may also occur on the face, primarily occurring on the cheeks and bridge of the nose (Levy, 2004e).

### Signs and Symptoms
Erysipelas skin lesions typically have a raised, sharply demarcated border (see Color Plate 27). The underlying skin is painful, intensely red, hardened, swollen, and warm. Fever and shaking chills may also occur. Streaking of the affected skin and necrosis of the tissue may occur (Davis & Benbensity, 2003).

### Treatment
Erysipelas is treated with antibiotics such as penicillin. If appropriate antibiotic therapy is given early, the outcome is favorable. Skin changes may take up to a few weeks to normalize, and peeling is common.

### Testing
The diagnosis of erysipelas is based on the characteristic appearance of the skin lesion. Skin biopsies are usually not needed.

## ERYSIPELOID

### Description
*Erysipelothrix rhusiopathiae* is a nonsporulating, gram-positive, rod-shaped bacterium that has a tendency to form long filaments (Farrar, 1989). It was identified more than 100 years ago as the etiologic agent of swine

erysipelas, and it is still commonly found in domestic swine. Humans become infected through exposure to infected or contaminated animals or animal products. This occupational disease is most significant to persons whose work involves handling fish and animal products.

## Signs and Symptoms

Erysipeloid lesions are typically present on the hands or fingers at the site of original infection. The incubation period is one to four days. Erysipeloids are sharply defined, slightly elevated, purplish areas that spread peripherally as the discoloration in the central area of the erysipeloid fades. Low-grade fever, joint pain, and inflammation of the lymph glands may also occur. These symptoms may last up to several months.

## Treatment

Erysipeloid is a self-limiting infection that normally heals within a month. The problem is that second attacks can occur, and relapses are common. The infection is susceptible to penicillins, cephalosporins, erythromycin, and clindamycin, but it is often resistant to many other antibiotics, including vancomycin, which is frequently used in infections due to gram-positive bacteria.

## Testing

The organism may be isolated from biopsy or blood specimens on standard culture media. It is identified by morphology, lack of motility, and biochemical characteristics. Identification may be confirmed by the mouse protection test.

## ERYTHRASMA

### Description

Erythrasma is a chronic bacterial infection usually seen in skin folds caused by *Corynebacterium minutissimum* (Crawford, 2003; Kibbi, 2002). The typical appearance is a reddish-brown, slightly scaly patch with sharp borders. The lesions occur in moist areas such as the groin, axilla, and skin folds. Erythrasma is most prevalent among obese persons, diabetics, and among persons living in warm climates.

### Signs and Symptoms

The symptoms of erythrasma are itchy, scaly, reddish-brown lesions found in the axilla, groin, between the toes, and in skin folds.

### Treatment

Gently washing the lesions with antibacterial soap and applying topical erythromycin gel typically clear cases of erythrasma.

### Testing

Tests used in the diagnosis of erythrasma may include cultures of the skin and a Wood's lamp test, during which the lesions glow a coral-red color.

## ESCHERICHIA COLI INFECTIONS

### Description

The most significant opportunistic pathogen of all the enterics is *E. coli,* which is normally found in the human intestine. *E. coli* may cause several types of diarrheal illnesses, meningitis in newborns, urinary tract infections, and infections of wounds. The spread of the infection has been identified through processed meats, such as undercooked hamburgers from fast food restaurants, unpasteurized milk, and apple cider. When individuals travel from industrialized countries to developing countries, they may acquire this illness due to inadequate sources of drinking water and a lack of proper sanitation. Two strains of *E. coli* cause severe diarrheal illnesses. Enteroinvasive *E. coli* and enterohemorrhagic *E. coli* cause damage to the intestines that penetrates the intestinal wall (Levy, 2004d).

### Signs and Symptoms

Mild *E. coli* infection is characterized by low-grade fever, watery diarrhea, nausea, and abdominal cramps. Enteroinvasive *E. coli* is transmitted from person to person through the fecal-oral route and results in fever, severe abdominal cramps, malaise, and watery diarrhea with pus, mucus, and blood. In cases of hemorrhagic diarrhea and colitis caused by *E. coli,* the classic progression is from watery diarrhea to a bloody diarrhea with cramps that may or may not present with a low-grade fever. The infection is fatal because it is accompanied by low platelet count, hemolytic anemia, and kidney failure (Hiong & Cunha, 2004).

### Treatment

*E. coli* infections usually are self-resolving within three days. Antidiarrheal medication may delay the elimination of the organism from the digestive tract, and therefore may not be recommended.

### Testing

The primary test for *E. coli* infection is a stool culture.

## ESOPHAGITIS

### Description

Esophagitis is inflammation of the esophagus, and it is caused by backflow of acid-containing fluid from the stomach to the esophagus (Stone, 2004g). It can also be caused by vomiting, surgery, medications, or hernias. Esophagitis may also be caused by an infection (e.g., herpes, cytomegalovirus, Candida) among the immunocompromised. Esophagitis results in ulcers of the esophagus (Tsoi, 2002).

### Signs and Symptoms

Esophagitis is characterized by difficulty swallowing, painful swallowing, and heartburn (acid reflux).

## Treatment

Esophagitis is treated with antibiotics and medications to control acid production.

## Testing

Tests involved in the diagnosis of esophagitis may include endoscopy, barium swallow, biopsy, and cultures.

## ESSENTIAL TREMOR

## Description

Essential tremor is a nerve disorder in which a person shakes while moving or trying to move (Campellone, 2004d). Essential tremor is an idiopathic disorder that is sometimes genetic. Essential tremor is worsened by stressful circumstances, such as fatigue, anger, fear, or using certain substances (e.g., coffee or cigarettes). New research indicates that the cerebellum does not appear to function properly in persons who have essential tremor, although no evident brain lesions have been identified. Over time, the tremors may affect the hands, arms, head, larynx, eyelids, or other muscles. An essential tremor rarely involves the legs or feet.

## Signs and Symptoms

Essential tremors may be occasional, temporary, or intermittent, and they occur at the rate of approximately 6 to 10 per second. Essential tremors may not affect both sides of the body equally, they worsen with voluntary movement, and they disappear during sleep. For unknown reasons, essential tremor typically improves with alcohol (Burke & Hauser, 2001).

## Treatment

Essential tremors may not be treated, if they do not interfere with the ability to perform daily activities. Medications do not benefit 25 percent of patients with essential tremors. Propranolol and primidone block neurotransmitters containing compounds related to adrenaline. Other medications used in the treatment of tremors include antiseizure drugs (gabapentin), mild tranquilizers (alprazolam or clonazepam), and calcium-channel blockers (flunarizine and nimodipine). Intramuscular injections of botulinum toxin or surgical implantation of a deep brain stimulator in the basal ganglia of the brain may also alleviate severe essential tremors.

## Testing

There is no diagnostic laboratory test for essential tremor, although tests may be conducted to rule out other tremor-inducing disorders.

## EWING'S SARCOMA

## Description

Ewing's sarcoma is a malignant bone tumor that affects children, most commonly occurring during puberty during accelerated bone growth. It is uncommon in African-American, African, and Chinese children. The tumor usually develops in long bones, the pelvis, or the chest, but may arise at any point in the body. Metastasis is present in approximately one third of children with this condition at the time of diagnosis (Blackman, 2004c; Strauss, 2002).

## Signs and Symptoms

Ewing's sarcoma is characterized by pain and swelling at the site of the tumor. Fever may also occur, and pathological fracture of affected bones may occur.

## Treatment

Treatment of Ewing's sarcoma includes chemotherapy, radiation therapy, and surgery.

## Testing

Diagnostic testing includes imaging tests and tissue biopsy.

## FANCONI'S ANEMIA

### Description

Fanconi's anemia results from the decreased production of all types of blood cells due to bone marrow dysfunction. This inherited disease prevents cells from fixing damaged DNA or removing toxic oxygen free radicals that damage cells. The deficiency in blood cells causes numerous problems including susceptibility to infections and a variety of blood disorders. Fanconi's anemia should not be confused with Fanconi's syndrome, which is a rare disorder of the kidneys. There have been 1,200 reported cases of Fanconi's anemia since 1927. This genetic disease results from mutations in eight genes ranging from *FANCA* through *FANCG*. Fanconi's anemia is more common among Ashkenazi Jews and Afrikaners in South Africa (Alter & Lipton, 2004).

### Signs and Symptoms

Fanconi's anemia is characterized by café-au-lait spots, vitiligo, and dark areas of the trunk, neck, and areas of skin that experience increased friction (e.g., between the scrotum and leg, between the breast and chest). Patients may exhibit short stature, underdeveloped forearms, and deformities of the thumbs. Underdevelopment of the genitals and skeletal deformities may also be present.

### Treatment

Fanconi's anemia is treated with growth factors (e.g., erythropoietin, G-CSF, GM-CSF), bone marrow transplant, and androgen therapy (e.g., oxymetholone, nandrolone decanoate) combined with low-dose steroids (e.g., hydrocortisone and prednisone). Fifty to seventy-five percent of patients respond to androgen therapy, but they rapidly relapse when the drugs are stopped. Faconi's anemia is typically fatal by the age of 30.

## Testing

Tests used in the diagnosis of Fanconi's anemia include CBC, imaging exams, bone marrow biopsy, human leukocyte antigen (HLA) tissue typing, and hearing tests. Clastogenic stress-induced chromosomal breakage analysis on blood cells of patients and their siblings is also conducted. Fanconi's anemia can be identified prenatally through amniocentesis or chorionic villous sampling (Cohen, 2003b).

## FASCIOLIASIS

### Description

Fascioliasis is a rare infection caused by parasites known as liver flukes (*Fasciola hepatica*) that live in plant-eating animals. Liver flukes can be found in areas where sheep and cattle are raised, and where humans consume raw watercress, including Europe, the Middle East, and Asia (*Fascioliasis*, 2004).

### Signs and Symptoms

Symptoms of fascioliasis begin during the acute phase, which is caused by migration of the immature fluke through the liver, and include abdominal pain, enlarged liver, fever, vomiting, diarrhea, and hives. These symptoms may last for several months. During the chronic phase, which occurs when the liver fluke migrates into the bile ducts, intermittent biliary obstruction and inflammation occur. The liver flukes may also be located occasionally in the intestinal wall, lungs, subcutaneous tissues, or mucous lining of the throat. Infection in the pharynx is called Halzoun syndrome.

### Treatment

Unlike infections with other flukes, *Fasciola hepatica* infections may not respond to praziquantel. The drug of choice is triclabendazole with bithionol as an alternative.

### Testing

Microscopic identification of eggs is useful in the chronic (adult) stage. Eggs can be recovered in the stools or in material obtained by duodenal or biliary drainage. They are morphologically indistinguishable from those of *Fasciolopsis buski*. Antibody detection tests are useful in the early invasive stages, when the eggs are not yet apparent in the stools, or in ectopic fascioliasis.

## FATAL FAMILIAL INSOMNIA

### Description

Fatal familial insomnia is a genetic disorder within families that results from a mutation of the normal protein in the brain. The specific portion of the brain affected in this disease is the thalamus, which is the sleep control center for the body. The presence of the waxlike buildup of amyloid tissues in the brain is a common aspect of fatal familial insomnia (Akroush, 1997).

## Signs and Symptoms

As its name indicates, the disease ends in death, but first the following complications occur from sleep deprivation: hallucinations, inefficient core body temperature regulation, blood pressure irregularities, abnormal heart rate, dementia, poor reflexes, inability to produce tears, and failure to feel pain.

## Treatment

There is no cure for fatal familial insomnia, but research is focused on gene therapy.

## Testing

Techniques such as DNA sequencing or molecular hybridization with a probe that seeks to detect the defective gene may be used for early diagnosis.

## FIBROMYALGIA

### Description

Fibromyalgia is an idiopathic condition characterized by widespread, long-standing pain with defined tender points (Peng, 2004a). Fibromyalgia can develop secondary rheumatoid arthritis or systemic lupus. The significant swelling, destruction, and deformity of joints seen in diseases such as rheumatoid arthritis does not occur with fibromyalgia syndrome alone. The cause of this disorder is unknown. Physical or emotional trauma may play a role in development of the syndrome. Evidence suggests that fibromyalgia may be associated with abnormal pain transmission responses. Fibromyalgia is most frequent among women 20 to 50 years old.

### Signs and Symptoms

Fibromyalgia is characterized by fatigue, morning stiffness, sleep problems, headaches, numbness in hands and feet, depression, and anxiety. Other disease characteristics include multiple tender areas on the back of the neck, shoulders, sternum, lower back, hips, shins, elbows, and knees (Giardino & Giardino, 2004).

### Treatment

In mild cases, symptoms may go away when stress is decreased or lifestyle changes are implemented. Treatment for fibromyalgia may also include antidepressant medications that can decrease depression, relax muscles, improve sleep, and reduce pain. Anti-inflammatory pain medications and medications that work on pain transmission pathways, such as gabapentin, may also be prescribed.

### Testing

Laboratory and imaging tests are done to confirm diagnosis based on physical examination and to rule out other diseases.

## FIFTH DISEASE

### Description

Fifth disease is a mild rash illness in children caused by parvovirus B19, which is not the same type of virus that affects animals. Fifth disease spreads from contact with contaminated respiratory secretions (e.g., saliva, sputum, nasal mucus).

### Signs and Symptoms

Children with fifth disease have a characteristic slapped-cheek rash on their face and a red rash on their trunk and limbs. The rash is self-resolving within 7 to 10 days. Patients are contagious during the early part of the illness, prior to the appearance of the rash, after which the patient is no longer contagious. Adults contract fifth disease at a much lower rate than do children. Lasting immunity results from fifth disease (*Parvovirus B19*, 2003).

### Treatment

No treatment is usually required for fifth disease (Banerjee, 2004a).

### Testing

Blood tests for antibodies against parvovirus B19, which may indicate infection, are available, although they are not commonly necessary, unless there is a question of exposure in a pregnant mother whose immune status is not known.

## FILARIASIS

### Description

Filariasis is an infection caused by eight species of roundworms that inhabit the lymphatics and subcutaneous tissues of humans. The three species responsible for most cases of filariasis are *Wuchereria bancrofti*, *Brugia malayi*, and *Onchocerca volvulus*, which causes onchocerciasis, which is also known as river blindness. Filariasis is spread by biting arthropods such as mosquitoes, midges, deerflies, and blackflies. The roundworms infest the blood vessels and lymphatic vessels, where they cause lymphatic disorders leading to swelling. Filariasis occurs globally (*Filariasis*, 2004).

### Signs and Symptoms

The disease characteristics of filariasis are dependent upon the species of roundworm, but generally include inflammation of the lymph glands, swelling of the scrotum, and elephantiasis. In Asia, a specific type of filariasis, known as pulmonary tropical eosinophilia syndrome, may cause cough, wheezing, fever, and red blood cell disorders. River blindness, another type of filariasis, may be accompanied by generalized itching, inflammation of the skin, nodules under the skin, and inflammation of the lymph glands.

### Treatment

Diethylcarbamazine, ivermectin, and albendazole have all been used in the treatment of filariasis.

## Testing

Tests used in the diagnosis of filariasis may include identification of microfilariae by microscopic examination, blood sample, or tissue biopsy.

## FLAIL CHEST

### Description

The arched design of the rib cage allows it to absorb blunt force due to its flexibility, and the intercostal muscles and fascia offer further strength and stability. Crushing injuries associated with heavy objects or sudden deceleration injuries may break a rib in one position, but only a significant impact breaks a rib in two or more positions. It is not the flail chest itself that is most significant, however, it is the amount of injury to the respiratory system and heart that typically causes fatality. A flail chest can be caused by such trauma as motor vehicle accidents, falls, and physical assault; although, it may also result from minor trauma in persons with an underlying disease such as osteoporosis, which weakens the ribs (Bjerke, 2002).

### Signs and Symptoms

A flail chest is the paradoxical movement of a segment of chest wall caused by three or more ribs broken in two or more places (Figure 2-31).

### Treatment

Overall, patients with flail chest do better with medical management of their pulmonary insufficiency and do not require prolonged mechanical ventilation or surgery.

### Testing

Chest radiography is the easiest test to perform to delineate the number of fractured ribs. Three-dimensional reformation of a thoracic helical CT scan also identifies rib fractures.

## FOLLICULAR LYMPHOMA

### Description

Follicular lymphomas usually arise or are present in lymphoid tissues, such as lymph nodes, spleen, and bone marrow, although lymphomas can arise in any organ (Freytes, 2002). Most lymphomas originate from lymph node tissue and frequently metastasize to other organs, where they cause detrimental effects by organ invasion and obstruction of anatomical structures.

### Signs and Symptoms

Follicular lymphomas are characterized by fever, night sweats, weight loss, or weakness. Involved nodes typically are nontender, firm, and rubbery in consistency.

### Treatment

Defining a standard treatment for follicular lymphomas is difficult. Because many patients are asymptomatic at the time of diagnosis and are

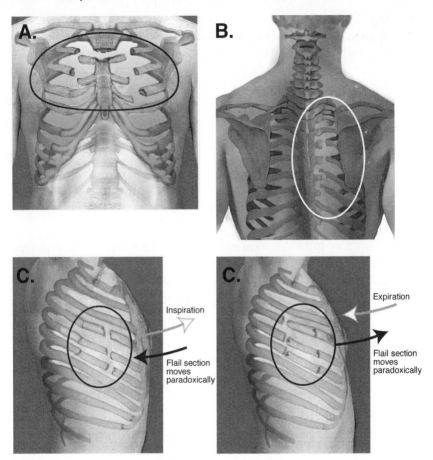

**Figure 2-31** Flail chest. (A) front, (B) back, (C) side

incurable with conventional chemotherapy, many experts recommend a watch-and-wait approach. Medications may include antineoplastic agents, corticosteroids, monoclonal antibodies, and antimetabolites.

### Testing
Tests involved in the diagnosis of follicular lymphoma may include blood tests, imaging tests, and biopsies.

## FOLLICULITIS

### Description
Folliculitis, which is also known as pseudofolliculitis barbae, tinea barbae, or barber's itch, is an infection of the hair follicles. The most common cause of folliculitis is the bacteria *Staphylococcus aureus*, although it may

be caused by *Pseudomonas aeruginosa*. Folliculitis has been known to spread from contaminated swimming pools or hot tubs.

## Signs and Symptoms

Folliculitis is characterized by the presence of small, red bumps that progress into pustules with a whitish or yellowish central zone. Lesions are most common at sites of friction such as the hips, buttocks, underarm, and scalp.

## Treatment

Treatment of folliculitis involves avoiding shaving of the affected area, minimizing friction from clothing, and the use of antibiotics such as Bactroban and dicloxacillin.

## Testing

Folliculitis is diagnose through cultures of the lesions.

## FOOD POISONING CAUSED BY STAPHYLOCOCCUS

### Description

Staphylococcal food intoxication is a gastrointestinal disorder caused by the poisons produced by the *Staphylococcus aureus* bacterium. The normal processes through which food intoxication takes place are common at many social events. During the preparation of food, the *S. aureus* bacteria are usually killed through the process of cooking. After the food is cooked, however, it is easily contaminated by food handlers who have bacteria on their hands. Food may also become contaminated by flies or ants, which may spread bacteria on their legs. If the food is then allowed to stand at room temperature to cool, or if it is cooked slowly in large masses, or if it is kept warm for any length of time at low temperatures, the bacteria have an opportunity to form poisons (i.e., enterotoxins). Reheating the food will kill the bacteria but not the toxin.

### Signs and Symptoms

One to 6 hours after ingesting contaminated food, the signs of food poisoning typically occur. Recovery is usually within 24 hours. Fever is not associated with food poisoning; however, the toxins may cause headaches, vomiting, abdominal cramps, and diarrhea. The mortality rate of staphylococcal food poisoning is quite low for healthy adults; however, it is significant in the elderly and children.

### Treatment

The objective of treatment is to replace fluids and electrolytes lost by vomiting or diarrhea.

### Testing

Tests for bacteria in vomit, blood, stool, and any leftover food may be used in the diagnosis of food poisoning.

## FUCHS HETEROCHROMIC UVEITIS

### Description

Fuchs heterochromic uveitis is a chronic, infection of the eye (Wong, 2002). The uveal tract structures of the eye include the iris, ciliary body, and choroids. The uveitis typically occurs in the lighter colored eye of a young adult with minimal symptoms and no related disease. Gradual progression of the disease is associated with cataract formation, glaucoma, and clouding of the vitreous fluids. The cause of the inflammation of the iris and the ciliary body is unknown.

### Signs and Symptoms

Small, clear lesions with fine filament projections are numerous on the cornea in cases of Fuchs heterochromic uveitis. A distinctive feature is scattering of the lesions over the entire surface of the back of the cornea. The eyes are different colors in most patients. Normally, a lighter colored eye becomes darker.

### Treatment

Fuchs heterochromic uveitis is not treated.

### Testing

There is no specific test for Fuchs heterochromic uveitis.

## FUNGAL MENINGITIS

### Description

*Cryptococcus neoformans* is the most common causative agent of a rare form of meningitis known as fungal meningitis, cryptococcal meningitis, or cryptococcosis. In cases of fungal meningitis caused by *C. neoformans*, a secondary fungal meningitis may also appear resulting from *Histoplasma capsulatum* infection, *Coccidioides immitis* infection, or *Aspergillus* species infection. Cryptococcosis may also infect the lung, as pictured in Figure 2-32. Even though fungi are widespread in the environment, fungal infections of the central nervous system in humans are rare.

### Signs and Symptoms

Fungal meningitis is usually a chronic form of meningitis. However, it may appear acutely, mimicking bacterial meningitis. Fungal meningitis is characterized by headache, low-grade fever, respiratory failure, deteriorating mental status, and stiff neck. *C. neoformans* is an encapsulate yeast cell present in the cerebrospinal fluid of infected persons. At autopsy, a mucus-like covering appears on the surface of the brain due to the capsule on these fungi. Microscopic flask-shaped cavities are also present in the brain tissue causing progressive dementia.

### Treatment

Fungal meningitis is fatal about 12 percent of the time. Antifungal medications are and IV therapy with amphotericin B are used to treat fungal meningitis. Injection of medication into the spinal cord may be required.

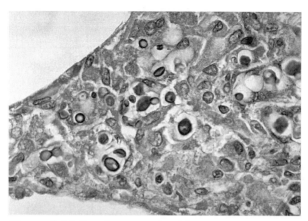

**Figure 2-32** Cryptococcosis of the lung in a patient with AIDS

High doses of fluconazole may also be an effective treatment for fungal meningitis.

## Testing

Diagnosis of cryptococcal meningitis requires a spinal tap. Tests on the cerebrospinal fluid allowing the diagnosis of cryptococcal meningitis include CSF stains indicating the presence of the yeast, CSF culture, and CSF cryptococcus antigen tests (Levy, 2004l, 2004m, 2004n).

## GALACTOSEMIA

### Description

Galactosemia is the inability of the body to metabolize the sugar galactose, which makes up half of lactose, the sugar found in milk (Stewart, 2004b). Galactosemia causes liver damage and central nervous system damage, and it is inherited as an autosomal recessive trait. Consumption of milk causes derivatives of galactose to build up in the person's system, causing damage to the liver, brain, kidneys, and eyes. Individuals with galactosemia cannot tolerate either human milk or animal milk. Exposure to milk products may result in liver damage, mental retardation, cataract formation, and kidney failure (Anadiotis, 2003).

### Signs and Symptoms

After drinking milk for a few days, a newborn with galactosemia will develop intolerance of feeding, jaundice, vomiting, tiredness, irritability, and convulsions. The liver will be enlarged, and the blood sugar may be low. Continued feeding of milk products to the infant leads to cirrhosis of the liver, cataract formation in the eye, and mental retardation.

### Treatment

Galactosemia is chronic and requires abstinence from milk and milk products for life. Infants can be fed with lactose-free formula.

## Testing

Tests used in the diagnosis of galactosemia include urinalysis for the presence of reducing substances and ketones. Blood tests for hypoglycemia and the measurement of enzyme activity levels in red blood cells may also be conducted.

## GANGRENE

### Description

Gangrene is an infection of dead tissue. Wet, or moist gangrene, is a form of liquefactive necrosis that results from bacterial or fungal infections that develop in areas of dead tissue. Ischemic gangrene, which is also known as dry gangrene, occurs when tissues become dehydrated if the blood supply is reduced. This may occur, for example, in the leg if calcification of the arteries is present in the form of arteriosclerosis. The tissues become black, dry, wrinkled, and greasy to the touch. There is also a clearly defined line of separation between the dead and healthy tissue, and there is no infection present (Hart, 2004d).

### Signs and Symptoms

The tissues become swollen, discolored, and blistered. Gangrene may exhibit a crackling sound known as crepitation when it is touched. Symptoms may include discoloration (blue or black, if skin is affected; red or bronze, if the affected area is beneath the skin), loss of sensation (which may occur after severe pain in the area), and a foul-smelling discharge. If the affected area is internal (such as gangrene of the gallbladder), the symptoms may include severe pain, fever, gas in tissues beneath the skin, and septic shock.

### Treatment

Gangrene is a medical emergency. Treatment may include surgical removal of dead tissue, amputation of the affected body part, repeated debridement, antibiotics, and surgery to restore blood supply to the affected area. Gangrene can be fatal.

### Testing

Diagnosis of gangrene may include blood tests, CT scan for internal conditions, surgical exploration, tissue biopsy, and tissue culture to identify bacterial infections (Hart, 2004a).

## GAS GANGRENE

### Description

Gas gangrene is a severe form of tissue death caused by *Clostridium perfringens* or Group A Streptococcus (Wener, 2004f). *Clostridium perfringens* is a gram-positive, endospore-forming bacterium. *Staphlococcus aureus* and *Vibrio vulnificus* can also cause similar infections. The bacteria cause the fermentation of carbohydrates in the tissues releasing carbon dioxide and hydrogen gases. The toxins move through the tissue causing further necrosis. Gas gangrene is often fatal, spreading throughout the body via the blood (see Color Plate 28). About 1,000 to 3,000 cases of gas gangrene occur in the United States annually. About one-third of cases occur spontaneously in patients who often have underlying vascular disease, diabetes, or colon cancer.

## Signs and Symptoms
The onset of gas gangrene is sudden and dramatic with inflammation beginning at the site of infection as a pale brownish-red and extremely painful tissue swelling. Gas may be felt in the tissue as a crackly sensation when the swollen area is pressed with the fingers. The gas spreads so rapidly that changes in the margins of the affected area are visible in only a few minutes. The involved tissue is completely destroyed, and the toxins cause rupture of red blood cells, decrease in circulation, and increased vascular permeability. Systemic symptoms develop early in the infection and consist of sweating, fever, and anxiety. If untreated, the individual develops a shocklike syndrome with hypotension, renal failure, coma, and death.

## Treatment
Prompt surgical debridement and potential amputation are necessary in cases of gas gangrene. Intravenous administration of penicillin-type antibiotics is a preferred method of treating gas gangrene.

## Testing
Gas gangrene is diagnosed initially through physical examination. Diagnosis is confirmed by blood tests, imaging tests, surgical exploration, tissue biopsy, and tissue culture to identify bacteria.

## GASTRITIS

### Description
Gastritis is inflammation of the stomach lining, and it can be caused by excessive alcohol consumption, prolonged use of nonsteroidal anti-inflammatory drugs, pernicious anemia, autoimmune disorders, or by the bacteria that cause ulcers. It may develop after major surgery, traumatic injury, burns, or severe infections (Muir, 2003a).

### Signs and Symptoms
Gastritis is characterized by abdominal pain, belching, bloating, nausea, vomiting, bloody vomit, hiccups, and bloody stool.

### Treatment
Gastritis is treated by avoiding inflammatory agents, acid-reducing medications, and antibiotics, if appropriate.

### Testing
Imaging exams, blood tests, and stool cultures are used to diagnose gastritis.

## GASTROENTERITIS

### Description
Gastroenteritis is a form of food intoxication caused by improper handling of meat during the slaughtering of animals. Intestinal contents are allowed to contaminate meat as it is slaughtered. Cooking the meat lowers the oxygen level and provides obligate anaerobes like *C. perfringens* the opportunity to grow. Keeping foods warm for over 20 minutes and inadequate refrigeration are two main causes of the growth of *C. perfringens* colonies.

### Signs and Symptoms
Most cases of food poisoning are mild, with symptoms appearing 8 to 12 hours after ingestion of the bacteria.

### Treatment
Treatment includes replacement of fluids and electrolytes. Antidiarrheal medications and antimicrobial therapy are not needed (Stone, 2003a).

### Testing
Tests used in the diagnosis of gastroenteritis include imaging exams, blood tests, examination of food for toxins and bacteria, stool Gram stains, and fecal smears.

## GASTROSCHISIS

### Description
Gastroschisis occurs when a hernia is present in the umbilical cord (Goldenring, 2004b).

### Signs and Symptoms
In cases of gastroschisis, the intestine protrudes through the abdominal wall near the umbilical cord. The unprotected intestine is exposed to irritating amniotic fluid, and as a result, gut motility and absorption may be affected.

### Treatment
Gastroschisis is treated with surgery, temperature regulation, and antibiotics.

### Testing
Prenatal ultrasonography and physical examination are used to diagnose gastroschisis.

## GAUCHER DISEASE

### Description
Gaucher disease is a disease that results in the buildup of glucosylceramide in parts of the body such as the spleen, liver, and bones (McGovern, 2003). Gaucher disease is a rare, inherited, potentially fatal disorder. Deficiency of the enzyme glucocerebrosidase leads to an accumulation of glucosylceramide in the lysosomes of certain cells. Deficiency of this enzyme causes the lysosomes to become congested with

glucosylceramide, which leads to decreased production of red blood cells and thinning of the bones.

## Signs and Symptoms

Gaucher disease is characterized by bone pain, fractures, easy bruising, fatigue, seizures, enlarged spleen, enlarged liver, anemia, low platelet counts, dysfunctional eye movement, and disorders of muscle control.

## Treatment

Previously, the only treatment for Gaucher disease was removal of the spleen, but now both gene therapy and injections of a replacement synthetic enzyme, known as Cerezyme/Ceredase, are available. Another treatment for Gaucher disease is a drug known as *N*-butyldeoxynojirimycin (OGT 918), which works by inhibiting the formation of glucocerebroside. Gaucher disease is usually fatal in children by the age of five, however treatment of the adult-chronic form results in near-normal life expectancy.

## Testing

Tests used in the diagnosis of Gaucher disease may include blood cell examination for decreased enzyme activity, white blood cell cultures for beta-glucosidase, bone marrow aspiration, spleen biopsy, and imaging tests. Genetic tests are designed to assess enzyme functional activity and to examine DNA for sequence mutations. Testing is complicated by the fact that the disease expression is extremely variable, and patients who test positive may be asymptomatic.

## GEOGRAPHIC TONGUE

### Description

Geographic tongue, which is also known as benign migratory glossitis, describes a maplike appearance of the tongue. This idiopathic disorder results from irregular patches on the surface of the tongue. Causes may include allergies and irritation from hot or spicy foods, alcohol, or tobacco. The pattern may change rapidly and is caused by the loss of papillae, which are fingerlike projections on the surface of the tongue. This gives areas of the tongue flat spots, and thus a geographic appearance (Newman, 2003a).

### Signs and Symptoms

Geographic tongue is characterized by a maplike appearance on the tongue. The lesions are smooth, red patches that change location from day to day. Tongue soreness and burning pain may occur in some cases. The patches are surrounded by yellow-white borders. The condition is more frequent in persons with psoriasis (Kelsch, 2003).

### Treatment

There is no cure for geographic tongue, and the condition is otherwise harmless. However, it can be persistent and uncomfortable.

### Testing

Diagnosis is based on physical exam, and tests are usually not necessary.

## GERMAN MEASLES

### Description

German measles, or rubella, is a contagious viral infection with mild symptoms associated with a rash (Ratner, 2003). German measles is caused by the rubella virus (which is pictured in Figure 2-33), which is spread via the respiratory route. The incubation period of German measles is approximately two to three weeks.

The most severe effects of the rubella virus are found among pregnant women. Congenital rubella syndrome is a form of birth defect that occurs when the mother becomes infected with the rubella virus in her first trimester. In 1964 and 1965, a rubella epidemic in the United States caused thousands of infants to be born with congenital rubella syndrome. Fifteen percent of babies born with congenital rubella syndrome die within their first year. The others suffer from stunted growth, disfigurement, deafness, cataracts, heart defects, and mental retardation. A vaccine has been developed to control the spread of rubella, and women who have been inoculated with the vaccine are protected 90 percent of the time for at least 15 years.

### Signs and Symptoms

German measles is a more mild form of measles than rubeola, and often its symptoms are subclinical. German measles are characterized by a rash of red spots and fever (see Color Plate 29). Encephalitis may occur in adults who have contracted German measles. Children generally have few symptoms, but adults may experience fever, headache, malaise, and a runny nose before the rash appears. A person is contagious from one week before the rash until two weeks after the rash. Lifelong immunity to German measles follows infection.

### Treatment

There is no treatment for German measles, but a safe and effective vaccine is available.

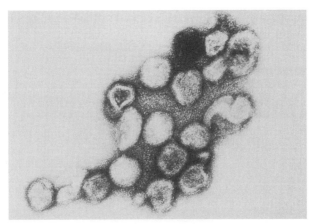

**Figure 2-33** Rubella virus causes German measles
(Courtesy of the CDC)

## Testing

Tests used in the diagnosis of German measles include a rubella serology and a nasal or throat swab for viral culture.

## GERSTMANN-STRÄUSSLER-SCHEINKER SYNDROME

### Description

Gerstmann-Sträussler-Scheinker syndrome is a rare central nervous system disorder of families that belongs to a family of human and animal diseases known as the *transmissible spongiform encephalopathies* (e.g., Creutzfeldt-Jakob disease, kuru, fatal familial insomnia). Onset of Gerstmann-Sträussler-Scheinker syndrome usually occurs between the ages of 35 and 55. Gerstmann-Sträussler-Scheinker syndrome is a slowly progressive condition usually lasting from 2 to 10 years. The disease ultimately causes severe disability and finally death, often after the patient goes into a coma or has a secondary infection such as aspiration pneumonia due to an impaired ability to swallow (*Gerstmann-Straussler-Scheinker disease*, 2003).

### Signs and Symptoms

Gerstmann-Sträussler-Scheinker syndrome is characterized by loss of reflexes in the legs and the development of dementia. Gerstmann-Sträussler-Scheinker is noted for spongiform degeneration of the brain and spinal cord with the presence of amyloid plaque. In the early stages, patients may experience varying levels of ataxia (lack of muscle coordination), including clumsiness, unsteadiness, and difficulty walking. As the disease progresses, the ataxia becomes more pronounced and most patients develop dementia. Other symptoms may include slurred speech, involuntary movements of the eyes, muscle spasms, and visual disturbances, sometimes leading to blindness. Deafness also can occur. In some families, Parkinsonian features are present.

### Treatment

There is no cure or treatment for Gerstmann-Sträussler-Scheinker syndrome.

### Testing

Diagnosis is based on physical examination of the brain at autopsy.

## GIANTISM

### Description

Giantism, a rare disease also known as gigantism, is excessive growth of the long bones resulting in an abnormally tall stature. Gigantism is caused by an excessive secretion of growth hormone during childhood prior to the closure of the bone growth plates. The most common cause of the excess growth hormone secretion is a pituitary gland tumor, which is never malignant. Giantism may also be caused by an underlying medical condition such as multiple endocrine neoplasia (MEN) type-1, McCune-Albright syndrome (MAS), neurofibromatosis, or Carney complex (Crawford, 2002; Sidhaye, 2004a; Stewart, 2004c).

## Signs and Symptoms
The abnormal height associated with giantism is accompanied by delayed puberty, and growth in muscles and organs that makes affected children extremely large for their age. Persons with giantism may exhibit a protruding forehead and a prominent jaw, thickening of the facial features, disproportionately large hands and feet with thick fingers and toes, increased perspiration, weakness, and irregular menstruation. They may also experience vision problems.

## Treatment
Treatment of giantism may include surgical removal of the pituitary tumor, followed by medication. The most effective medications are somatostatin analogs (e.g., octreotide or long-acting lanreotide), dopamine agonists (e.g., bromocriptine mesylate, cabergoline), and pegvisomant, which all reduce growth hormone secretion. If surgery and medications fail, radiation therapy may be used to treat giantism.

## Testing
Tests used to diagnose giantism may include examination of insulin growth factor-I (IGF-I) levels, serum GH levels after an oral glucose challenge, imaging tests of the head for pituitary tumors, hormone level tests (e.g., thyroid hormone, testosterone, estradiol, cortisol), and tests for the presence of elevated prolactin levels.

## GIARDIASIS

### Description
The most commonly identified waterborne illness in the United States is giardiasis (Smith, 2003b). It is caused by the protozoan *Giardia lamblia*, which is found in both clear mountain streams and the chlorinated water supplies of the largest cities. The life cycle of *G. lamblia* is illustrated in Figure 2-34. It also can be spread through the fecal-oral route. Contamination after diaper changing in day-care centers spreads the disease from the hands of the caregiver to the children. Giardiasis may also be spread sexually through anal intercourse. A single human stool can contain 300 million *G. lamblia* cysts, and the establishment of infection only requires 10 cysts. In cold water, the cysts can remain viable for up to two months, and chlorination of municipal water supplies is ineffective against these cysts (Giardiasis, 2001).

### Signs and Symptoms
About two-thirds of exposed individuals develop symptoms approximately 6 to 20 days after infection. Symptoms include loss of appetite, nausea, vomiting, explosive diarrhea, abdominal pain, fatigue, and weight loss.

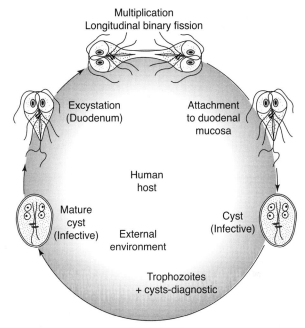

**Figure 2-34** Life cycle of *Giardia lamblia*

## Treatment

Giardiasis is normally self-resolving within about four weeks. Some cases, however, become chronic. Anti-infective agents such as metronidazole or quinacrine may be used for adults, and furazolidone is generally used to treat children. Cure rates are greater than 80 percent, but drug resistance may be a factor in treatment failures, requiring a change in antibiotic therapy.

## Testing

Tests used in diagnosing giardiasis include stool ova and parasite tests, a positive *Giardia* enzyme immunoassay (EIA) antibody test, a small bowel biopsy, and an immunofluorescence test (see Color Plate 30).

## GILBERT'S SYNDROME

## Description

Gilbert's syndrome is an inherited disorder affecting the way bilirubin is processed by the liver (Mukherjee, 2001). Other names for Gilbert's syndrome include icterus intermittens juvenilis, low-grade chronic hyper-bilirubinemia, familial non-hemolytic-non-obstructive jaundice, constitutional liver dysfunction, and unconjugated benign bilirubinemia. Gilbert's syndrome is relatively common among Caucasians.

## Signs and Symptoms

The most significant symptom of Gilbert's syndrome is jaundice. Affected individuals experience jaundice under conditions of exertion, stress, fasting, and infection. There may be no disease characteristics associated with Gilbert's syndrome in many people.

## Treatment

Usually no treatment is necessary because the jaundice associated with Gilbert's syndrome typically causes no health problems.

## Testing

A serial serum indirect bilirubin indicates changes consistent with Gilbert's syndrome.

# GINGIVITIS

## Description

Gingivitis is a disease of the gums, which are also known as the gingiva, involving an infection that can result in tissue destruction (Kapner, 2003). As it progresses, gingivitis may involve the tooth sockets. Gingivitis is caused by the long-term effects of plaque. Plaque may consist of bacteria, mucus, or particles of food. In time, plaque mineralizes into a hard deposit known as tartar. Gingivitis is more common in cases of uncontrolled diabetes, due to hormonal changes associated with pregnancy, and among those with poor dental hygiene.

## Signs and Symptoms

Gingivitis is characterized by mouth sores, inflammation of the gums, bleeding gums, and painful gums when touched.

## Treatment

Treatment begins by cleaning the teeth with instruments to loosen and remove deposits from the teeth by a dentist or dental hygienist. Meticulous oral hygiene is necessary after professional tooth cleaning.

## Testing

No testing is necessary, although dental X-rays and measuring the amount of bone loss may be performed to determine whether infection has spread to surrounding structures causing periodontitis.

# GINGIVOSTOMATITIS

## Description

Gingivostomatitis is a condition among children caused by a viral infection that results in sores on the mouth and gums (Newman, 2003b). Common viruses that cause gingivostomatitis include herpes viruses and coxsackieviruses.

## Signs and Symptoms

Gingivostomatitis is characterized by shallow ulcers with a grayish or yellowish base and a slightly red margin on the tissues of the gums or the lining of the cheeks. Gingivostomatitis infections range from mild and slightly uncomfortable to severe and painful.

## Treatment

Salt water or over-the-counter mouthwashes like hydrogen peroxide or Xylocaine may be used to treat gingivostomatitis. The sores generally resolve in three weeks with or without treatment.

## Testing

Normally, no special tests are required for the diagnosis of gingivostomatitis; however, tests may be conducted to rule out more serious infections.

## GLAUCOMA

### Description

Glaucoma is a disease of the eye in which increased fluid pressure inside the eye damages the optic nerve and causes partial vision loss and eventual blindness (Feinberg, 2004b; Noecker, 2003). Glaucoma is the third most common cause of blindness in the Unites States. Increased pressure occurs when the aqueous humor does not drain properly, creating pressure on the junction of the optic nerve and the retina, which reduces blood flow to the optic nerve. As the optic nerve deteriorates, blind spots develop in the field of vision, affecting peripheral vision and eventually central vision.

### Signs and Symptoms

Acute glaucoma is characterized by severe eye pain, facial pain, loss of vision, cloudy vision with halos appearing around lights, red eye, fixed and nonreactive pupils, nausea, and vomiting. Chronic glaucoma is characterized by gradual loss of peripheral vision, blurred or foggy vision, chronic headaches, and the presence of rainbow-colored halos around lights.

### Treatment

Acute glaucoma is a medical emergency necessitating the immediate reduction of intraocular pressure. Beta-adrenergic blocking agents (e.g., timolol, Betagan, OptiPranolol) are effective for treatment of glaucoma. Epinephrine drops are sometimes used in combination with other medications. Other medications may include Xalatan, Daranide, Diamox, and Neptazane. A surgical treatment for glaucoma, known as an iridotomy, involves the creation of a drainage hole in the iris to relieve pressure.

### Testing

Tests used to diagnose glaucoma may include a retinal exam, measurement of intraocular pressure by tonometry, visual field measurement, visual acuity, refraction, papillary reflex response, and a slit lamp exam.

## GLIOMAS

### Description

Gliomas are malignant tumors of glial cells, which provide supporting structure to the neurons of the brain (Cohen, 2002). Malignancies of the glial cells tend not to metastasize outside of the skull. Gliomas are extremely difficult to remove from the brain surgically because they do not encapsulate; instead, they grow into the surrounding brain tissue, making it difficult to know the extent of brain tissue to remove. Gliomas are fast growing tumors resulting in high mortality. There are three types of glioma named after the cells from which they originate: astrocytomas, ependymomas, and oligodendrogliomas, all of which occur in the frontal and temporal lobes of the cerebrum of the brain and spread through the cerebrospinal fluid to the spinal cord (Mixed Gliomas, 2001).

### Signs and Symptoms

Gliomas are characterized by headaches, vomiting, visual impairment, paralysis, lack of coordination, speech disorders, memory loss, and changes in mood, behavior, and personality. The symptoms of gliomas are caused by the blockage of the ventricles of the brain, leading to increased intracranial pressure due to the buildup of cerebrospinal fluid and the swelling of brain tissue.

### Treatment

Treatment for brain cancers includes surgery, radiation therapy, and chemotherapy. Depending on the location and extent of the glioma, it may be inoperable. Mortality for gliomas is high, and for unknown reasons, gliomas are more common in men than women.

### Testing

Examination often shows focal or general neurologic changes that are specific to the location of the tumor. Diagnosis may be confirmed, and the tumor localized, by imaging tests of the head (e.g., CT, MRI, angiography), EEG, cerebrospinal fluid examination, and tissue biopsy.

## GLOMERULONEPHRITIS

### Description

Glomerulonephritis is the most serious and potentially devastating form of renal disorders. Acute glomerulonephritis is characterized by the sudden onset of blood and protein in the urine accompanied by salt and water retention. There are both structural and functional changes associated with acute glomerulonephritis (Agha, 2003b).

### Signs and Symptoms

At the cellular level, there is an increase in the number of epithelial and endothelial cells in the glomerulus. Immune system cells known as neutrophils and monocytes are also present in large numbers in the glomerulus. The capillary walls within the glomerulus also thicken. As a result of these anatomical changes, the glomerulus undergoes physiological changes such as the excess secretion of proteins in the urine, blood in the urine, swelling, and high blood pressure. Acute glomerulonephritis may be accompanied by loss of appetite, itching, nausea, bruising, nosebleed, swelling of the face or legs, difficulty breathing, fluid in the abdomen, skin rash, skin pallor, and arthritis.

Acute glomerulonephritis may progress into chronic glomerulonephritis. In cases of chronic glomerulonephritis, the glomerulus becomes fibrous. Symptoms of chronic glomerulonephritis include weakness, loss of appetite, weight loss, pus in the urine, early morning nausea and vomiting, change in taste sensation, sleeping during the day and wakefulness at night, seizures, and tremors.

## Treatment

Acute glomerulonephritis may be caused by streptococcal throat infection, skin infection, hepatitis, diabetes, or intravenous drug use. Depending on etiology, acute glomerulonephritis is treated with antibiotics. Corticosteroids, immunosuppressives, or other medications may be used to treat some of the causes of chronic glomerulonephritis. Dietary restrictions on salt, fluids, protein, and other substances may be recommended to aid control of hypertension or renal failure. Dialysis or kidney transplantation may be necessary.

## Testing

Laboratory tests may reveal anemia or indicate reduced kidney functioning, including uremia. Urinalysis may indicate blood, casts, protein, or other abnormality. Findings are nonspecific for ultrasounds, abdominal CT scans, and IVP. Other tests for glomerulonephritis may include chest X-ray and kidney biopsy.

## GNATHOSTOMIASIS

### Description

Gnathostomiasis is caused by the roundworms *Gnathostoma spinigerum* and *Gnathostoma hispidum*, which infect vertebrate animals. The roundworms induce tumors in the gastric wall of the animals they infect (e.g., pigs, cats, dogs, wild animals). Humans become infected by eating undercooked fish or poultry containing the roundworm larvae or by drinking contaminated water. Gnathostomiasis is most common in Asia, especially Thailand and Japan, although it has recently emerged as an important human parasite in Mexico (*Gnathostomiasis*, 2004).

### Signs and Symptoms

As the organisms migrate through the subcutaneous tissues of the body, infected individuals experience intermittent, migratory, painful, itchy swellings. Migration to other tissues can result in cough, bloody urine, vision loss, meningitis, and myeloencephalitis.

## Treatment

Treatment for gnathostomiasis may include surgical removal of the worms and/or treatment with albendazole or ivermectin.

## Testing

Removal and identification of the worm is both diagnostic and therapeutic.

## GOITER

### Description

A goiter is an enlargement of the thyroid gland that is not associated with inflammation or cancer (Jain, 2003). A simple goiter occurs when the thyroid gland enlarges to overcome deficiencies in the production of thyroid hormone. The two forms of simple goiters are endemic goiters and sporadic goiters (Mulinda, 2004).

Endemic goiters are also known as colloid goiters, and they are generally the result of a lack of iodine in the diet. Iodine is essential in the production of thyroid hormone, and people residing in geographic areas away from the sea coast are unable to ingest sufficient quantities of iodine in their diets because the soil in these regions of the world is deficient in iodine. Endemic goiters are more common in central Asia and central Africa. They are rare in the United States due to the use of iodized table salt. In contrast to endemic goiters, sporadic goiters, which are also known as nontoxic goiters, have an unknown cause, but they may result from the use of certain medications like lithium and aminoglutethimide.

### Signs and Symptoms

Goiters are characterized by thyroid enlargement varying from a single small nodule to massive enlargement, difficulty breathing, cough, difficulty swallowing, neck vein distention, and dizziness when the arms are raised above the head.

### Treatment

A goiter is harmless and only needs to be treated if it is causing other symptoms. The enlarged thyroid can be treated with radioactive iodine to shrink the gland or with surgical removal known as a thyroidectomy.

### Testing

Tests used in the diagnosis of goiters include measurement of thyroid stimulating hormone and free thyroxine (T4) in the blood, thyroid scan and uptake, thyroid biopsy, and ultrasound of the thyroid.

## GONORRHEA

### Description

Gonorrhea is one of the most reported sexually transmitted bacterial diseases in the United States (Levy, 2004f). Gonorrhea is caused by the *Neisseria gonorrhoeae* bacterium, and it is spread through vaginal, oral, or anal sexual contact. Humans are the only natural host for *N. gonorrhoea*, which is an aerobic, gram-negative diplococcus. *N. gonorrhoea* is uniquely virulent due to its capsule, pili, cell-wall proteins, endotoxin, and enzymes. The majority of reported cases of gonorrhea in the United States are among African Americans. A condom can help protect both partners from gonorrhea. Condoms do not provide complete protection from sexually transmitted diseases, however, because bacteria and lesions may be present in areas not covered by the condom, resulting in transmission of infection to another person (Gonorrhea, 2001).

### Signs and Symptoms

Gonococcus is extremely virulent in the body and attaches to tissues via its pili. Its most common symptom is a pustular discharge from the genitalia and painful urination (see Color Plate 31). Symptoms of rectal infection include discharge, anal itching, soreness, bleeding, and sometimes painful bowel movements. The symptoms appear a few days after infection. Sterility is a complication of gonorrhea. Gonorrheal infections may also be transferred from the hands to the eyes, leading to possible blindness (see Color Plate 32). The heart, joints, meninges, and pharynx may also become involved in the infection. Color Plate 33 is a photograph of the feet of a person exhibiting gonococcal lesions.

### Treatment

Antibiotics can successfully cure gonorrhea. Penicillin is no longer used to treat gonorrhea because many strains of the gonorrhea bacterium have become resistant to penicillin. Because many people with gonorrhea also have chlamydia, antibiotics for both infections are usually given together. Some of the medications used to treat gonorrhea include ceftriaxone, cefixime, ciprofloxacin, ofloxacin, spectinomycin, cefuroxime axotal, cefpodoxime proxetil, enoxacin, and erythromycin.

### Testing

Tests used in the diagnosis of gonorrhea include a cervical Gram stain, endocervical culture, throat swab culture, skin lesion aspiration, and rectal culture.

## GOODPASTURE'S SYNDROME

### Description

Goodpasture's syndrome is a disorder in which antibodies collect in both the kidneys and the lungs, causing both glomerulonephritis and bleeding in the lungs (Koren, 2003a). Although Goodpasture's syndrome is an idiopathic disorder, it is believed to be an inherited autoimmune disease (Valentini, 2004).

### Signs and Symptoms

Antibody deposits in the lungs cause bleeding, resulting in bloody sputum. Other symptoms include protein and blood in the urine, kidney failure, and iron deficiency anemia. Other disease characteristics of Goodpasture's syndrome may include dark colored urine, decreased urine output, foamy urine, difficulty breathing, weakness, nausea, vomiting, chest pain, and skin pallor.

## Treatment

Treatment is most effective when begun early, before kidney function has deteriorated to the point of requiring dialysis. Corticosteroids or other anti-inflammatory agents and immunosuppressants, such as cyclophosphamide, may be used aggressively to treat Goodpasture's syndrome. Plasmapheresis, a procedure by which blood plasma is removed from the body and replaced with fluids or donated plasma, may be performed repeatedly to remove circulating antibodies. Dialysis and or kidney transplant may be required.

## Testing

Tests used to diagnose Goodpasture's syndrome may include blood tests for anemia, serum iron and ferritin levels, and increased BUN and creatinine levels. Urinalysis tests indicate the presence of proteins, blood, or casts. Serum antibody to normal human glomerular basement membrane is positive. Sputum stain may indicate macrophages containing iron pigments. Chest X-ray shows fluid in the lung tissues. A lung needle biopsy shows immune system deposits. Kidney biopsy shows immune system deposits with crescent shapes.

## GOUT

### Description

Gout is a common form of arthritis (Peng, 2003a). In particular, gout affects the joint at the base of the big toe, but it also affects other joints of the feet and ankle, as well as other parts of the body. Gout is a disorder caused by the accumulation of uric acid in the tissues. The body breaks down foods and builds up tissues in a process (i.e., purine metabolism) that naturally produces uric acid. When excess levels of uric acid are found in the blood, the condition is referred to as hyperuricemia. Excess uric acid leads to the formation of microscopic crystals (i.e., monosodium urate crystals) that infiltrate the tissues of the joints, which causes inflammation. Gout may be an inherited condition, but certain foods result in higher levels of uric acid through purine metabolism. These foods include, but are not limited to, beans, red meat, shellfish, organ meats (e.g., liver, kidneys, tongue), peas, and lentils.

### Signs and Symptoms

The cardinal sign of gout is pain at the base of the big toe. Other joints may exhibit pain, redness, swelling, and loss of function. Gout often appears suddenly, and it may become chronic, in which case joint deformity is not uncommon. In chronic cases of gout, larger crystals known as tophi may appear in the joints, and they are sometimes present in the ears.

## Treatment

Chronic gouty arthritis is treated with drugs like probenecid or sulfin-pyrazone, which reduce uric acid levels. Allopurinol is used to block the enzyme that produces uric acid. Colchicine may prevent acute attacks.

## Testing

Tests used to diagnose gout include synovial fluid analysis, blood tests for uric acid levels, and imaging exams of affected joints.

## GRANULOMATOUS AMEBIC ENCEPHALITIS

### Description

*Acanthamoeba* cause a fatal brain infection called granulomatous amebic encephalitis. Some of the infective species include *A. culbertsoni, A. polyphaga, A. castellanii, A. healyi, A. astronyxis, A. hatchetti,* and *A. rhysode. Acanthamoeba* can be found in soil, dust, lakes, rivers, hot springs, and hot tubs. Additionally, *Acanthamoeba* have been found in the nose and throat of both healthy individuals. *Acanthamoeba* can enter the skin through a cut, wound, or through the nostrils. Once inside the body, amebas can travel to the lungs and through the bloodstream to other parts of the body, especially the central nervous system (*Acanthamoeba infection,* 2004).

### Signs and Symptoms

Granulomatous amebic encephalitis is characterized by headaches, stiff neck, nausea, vomiting, fatigue, confusion, loss of balance, loss of motor control, seizures, and hallucinations.

### Treatment

Eye and skin infections caused by *Acanthamoeba* are treatable with propamidine isethionate and neomycin-polymyxin B-gramicidin. Although minor infections are treatable, granulomatous amebic encephalitis is almost always fatal.

### Testing

In *Acanthamoeba* infections, the diagnosis can be made from microscopic examination of stained smears of biopsy specimens (e.g., brain tissue, skin, cornea) or of corneal scrapings, which may detect trophozoites and cysts. Cultivation of the causal organism, and its identification by direct immunofluorescent antibody, may also occur.

## GRAVES' DISEASE

### Description

Graves' disease is an autoimmune disorder, in which antibodies are produced that stimulate growth of the thyroid gland. The thyroid growth results in the excess secretion of thyroid hormone (Sidhaye, 2004b). Similar antibodies may cause excessive growth of the tissues in the eye

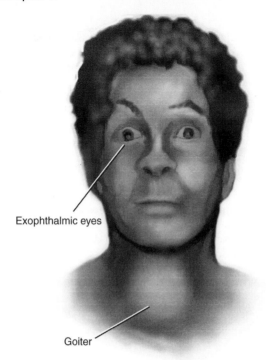

Exophthalmic eyes

Goiter

**Figure 2-35** Graves' disease

and the skin on the front of the lower leg. Graves' disease is the leading cause of an overactive thyroid gland, which is a disorder referred to as hyperthyroidism.

## Signs and Symptoms

Graves' disease is characterized by fatigue, weight loss, restlessness, rapid pulse, changes in sex drive, muscle weakness, heat intolerance, tremors, enlarged thyroid gland, and blurred vision. One of the most common signs of Graves' disease is bulging of the eyeballs, which is known as exoph-thalmia, as indicated in Figure 2-35. Graves' disease and goiters are more prevalent in developing countries that do not add iodine to their salt, as is done in the United States. Goiters are common in mountainous regions of the world like the Himalayas and the Andes.

## Treatment

Beta-blockers such as propranolol are often used to treat the symptoms of Grave's disease. The eye problems related to Graves' disease usually resolve when the hyperthyroidism is effectively treated with antithyroid medications, radiation, or surgery. Sometimes prednisone is used to reduce eye irritation and swelling. Taping the eyes closed at night to pre-vent drying may sometimes be required. Sunglasses and eyedrops may lessen irritation of the eyes, although surgery is needed in some cases of Graves' disease to return the eyes to their normal position.

## Testing

Tests used to diagnose Graves' disease indicate decreased serum TSH levels, elevated levels of serum T3 and free T4, and increased levels of radioactive iodine uptake.

## GUILLAIN-BARRE SYNDROME

## Description

Guillain-Barre syndrome is an acute nerve inflammation involving progressive muscle weakness or paralysis, often following an infection (Campellone, 2004f). A healthy neuron is illustrated in Figure 2-36.

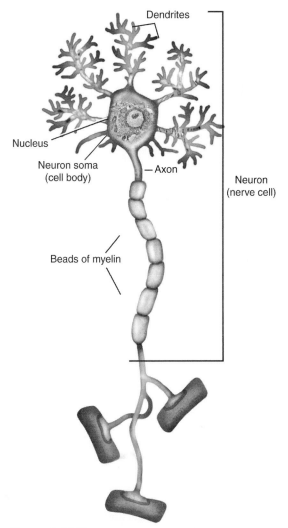

Dendrites

Nucleus

Neuron soma
(cell body)

Axon

Neuron
(nerve cell)

Beads of myelin

**Figure 2-36** Neuron

The damage usually includes loss of the myelin sheath of the nerve, which is known as demyelination, which slows the conduction of impulses through the nerve. The damage may include destruction of the axon of the nerve cell, which is known as denervation, which stops nerve function entirely.

The exact cause of Guillain-Barre syndrome is unknown, although it is known to follow minor infections, particularly respiratory infections or gastrointestinal infections. Guillain-Barre syndrome may occur in association with jejuni infection or viral infections like mononucleosis, AIDS, and herpes simplex. Sometimes Guillain-Barre occurs following surgery, vaccinations, trauma, or in association with systemic lupus erythematosus or Hodgkin's disease.

### Signs and Symptoms

Guillain-Barre syndrome progresses within days to a few weeks, causing weakness or paralysis equally on both sides of the body. Paralysis begins in the lower legs and spreads to the arms, while tingling, foot pain, hand pain, and clumsiness are experienced. The beginning phase of the illness is a rapid worsening that may take only a few hours to reach the most severe symptoms, which may last up to three weeks. This is followed by a period of no changes, then a phase of improvement. If the cranial nerves are involved, facial droop, double vision, slurred speech, and difficulty swallowing may be present (Cha-Kim, 2004).

### Treatment

Before treatment was available, many patients recovered completely with time. Plasmaphoresis may decrease the severity of the symptoms and facilitate a more rapid recovery. In this procedure, blood plasma is removed from the body and replaced with intravenous fluids or antibody-free donated plasma. Intravenous immune globulin may also reduce the severity and duration of the symptoms.

### Testing

Tests used in the diagnosis of Guillain-Barre syndrome include a nerve conduction velocity indicating demyelination, an EMG indicating lack of nervous stimulation, a cerebrospinal fluid exam indicating an increase in protein without an increase in white blood cell count, and an abnormal ECG.

## GUINEA WORM DISEASE

### Description

Dracunculiasis, more commonly known as guinea worm disease, is a preventable infection caused by the parasite *Dracunculus medinensis*. Infection affects poor communities in remote parts of Africa that do not have safe water to drink. Since 1986, when an estimated 3.5 million people were infected, guinea worm disease has been eradicated in much of the world by institutions like The Global 2000 program of The Carter Center of Emory University, UNICEF, the CDC, and the World Health

Organization (WHO). In 1998, 78,338 cases of guinea worm disease were reported. Most of those cases were from Sudan, where the ongoing civil war makes it impossible to eradicate the disease. Infection occurs by drinking water contaminated with *Dracunculus* larvae. In the water, the larvae are swallowed by small copepods "water fleas." *Dracunculiasis* occurs now in only 13 countries in Africa that lie in a band between the Sahara and the equator (*Dracunculiasis,* 2004).

## Signs and Symptoms

After ingesting contaminated water, stomach acid digests the water flea, but not the guinea worm. In approximately one year, during which the infected person shows no signs of illness, the guinea worm matures to a length of approximately three feet, after which it migrates to the surface of the body. An ulcer forms at the site where the worm will emerge, which is normally on the feet or legs, and the guinea worm releases millions of eggs through this ulcer when the infected person immerses the skin in water for relief of pain, which recontaminates the water supply.

## Treatment

Treatment for guinea worm disease requires that once the worm emerges from the wound, it be pulled out a few centimeters each day and wrapped around a small stick. Complete removal typically takes weeks or months.

## Testing

The clinical presentation of dracunculiasis is so typical and well known to the local population that it does not need laboratory confirmation. In addition, the disease occurs in areas where such confirmation is unlikely to be available. Examination of the fluid discharged by the worm can show rhabditiform larvae. No serologic test is available.

## GYNECOMASTIA

### Description

Gynecomastia is the development of breast tissue in males, which is common during puberty (Jain, 2004a; Segu, 2004). Gynecomastia during puberty is self-limiting over a period of months. Gynecomastia also may be associated with chronic liver disease, thyroid disease, kidney failure, and exposure to estrogens, androgens taken for body building, marijuana, and certain medications. Rare causes include tumors, Klinefelter syndrome, trauma to the testicles, viral infection in the testicles, or an overactive thyroid.

### Signs and Symptoms

Gynecomastia may occur in one or both breasts and begins as a small lump beneath the nipple, which may be tender. The breasts often enlarge unevenly.

### Treatment

Although spontaneous resolution is normal, persistent breast enlargement may be embarrassing for an adolescent boy. In these cases, gynecomastia may be treated with surgery for emotional reasons.

### Testing
Testing is not necessary, except to rule out other diseases.

## HAIRY CELL LEUKEMIA

### Description
Hairy cell leukemia is a rare cancer of immune cells (i.e., B lymphocytes) that leads to low blood counts (Besa, 2004). Hairy cell leukemia is caused by abnormal growth of B cells that have fine projections coming from their surface giving them a hairy appearance under the microscope. Hairy cell leukemia is more common in men, with an average age of onset of 55.

### Signs and Symptoms
Hairy cell leukemia is characterized by weakness, fatigue, weight loss, easy bruising, easy bleeding, recurrent infection, excessive sweating, and feeling full after eating only a small amount.

### Treatment
Early in the course of the disease, no treatment may be necessary, although an occasional blood transfusion may be required due to low blood counts. Removal of the spleen may improve blood counts as well. Chemotherapy drugs (e.g., cladribine and pentostatin) and interferon may be used to treat hairy cell leukemia, but they are unlikely to cure the disease. Most patients with hairy cell leukemia can expect to live 10 years or longer with the disease.

### Testing
Tests associated with the diagnosis of hairy cell leukemia may include a bone marrow biopsy, a peripheral blood smear, a tartrate-resistant acid phosphatase test, CBC, and an abdominal CT scan.

## HALLUX VALGUS

### Description
Hallux valgus is a type of bunion that displaces the big toe toward the other toes of the foot, which causes a bump on the edge of the foot at the joint of the big toe (Frank, 2004). Bunions are often caused by narrow-toed, high-heeled shoes. The condition may become painful as extra bone and a fluid-filled sac grow at the base of the big toe. Bunions occur more frequently in women and sometimes run in families.

### Signs and Symptoms
Hallux valgus is characterized by red, calloused skin along the foot at the base of the big toe, a bony bump on the side of the foot at the base of the big toe, pain over the joint, and a deformation of the big toe turned toward the other toes.

### Treatment
There are over 100 different surgical techniques that have been described to treat hallus valgus. Each is designed to realign the toe and remove the bunion.

## Testing

Hallux valgus is diagnosed by a physical exam coupled with imaging exams of the foot.

## HAND, FOOT, AND MOUTH DISEASE

### Description

Hand, foot, and mouth disease is a common illness of infants and children caused by viruses belonging to a group called enteroviruses (Goldenring, 2003a). Hand, foot, and mouth disease should not be confused with foot-and-mouth disease, which is a disease of cattle, sheep, and swine caused by a similar, but different, virus. The two diseases are not related. The most common cause of hand, foot, and mouth disease is coxsackievirus A16, and sometimes enterovirus 71, or other enteroviruses. The enterovirus group includes polioviruses, coxsackieviruses, echoviruses, and other enteroviruses. Hand, foot, and mouth disease is mildly contagious, and it is spread through contact with infected persons (*Hand, foot, and mouth disease*, 2001).

### Signs and Symptoms

Hand, foot, and mouth disease is characterized by fever, sores in the mouth, and a rash with blisters. The disease begins with a mild fever, loss of appetite, fatigue, and sore throat. Within two days after the fever begins, painful sores develop on the tongue, gums, and inside of the cheeks beginning as small red spots that blister and evolve into ulcers. A skin rash develops concomitantly exhibiting flat or raised red spots with some blistering. The rash does not itch and is usually located on the palms of the hands, soles of the feet, and on the buttocks.

### Treatment

Hand, foot, and mouth disease is usually mild and self-resolving, although it has been known to lead to severe meningitis. Treatment with antibiotics is not effective. Saltwater rinses may be soothing. Ensure an adequate fluid intake. The best fluids are cold milk products, especially ice cream, because they do not irritate the ulcers like juices and sodas may. Generally, complete recovery occurs within a week.

### Testing

There is no test needed to diagnose hand, foot, and mouth disease.

## HANSEN'S DISEASE

### Description

Hansen's disease, which is a type of leprosy, is a chronic infectious disease caused by the bacillus *Mycobacterium leprae*, affecting the skin and peripheral nerves, but with a wide range of possible clinical manifestations. *Mycobacterium leprae* multiplies slowly and affects the skin, nerves, and mucous membranes. In 2002, there were about 750,000 new cases of Hansen's disease worldwide with 96 cases occurring in the United States. In the same year, the World Health Organization listed Brazil, Madagascar,

Mozambique, Tanzania, and Nepal as having 90 percent of the world's cases of Hansen's disease. Worldwide, 1 million to 2 million persons are permanently disabled as a result of Hansen's disease (*Hansen's disease*, 2004; Smith, 2003d).

## Signs and Symptoms

Hansen's disease is characterized by one or more lesions that are lighter in their center than the surrounding tissue. These lesions have decreased sensation to touch, heat, or pain, and they do not heal after several weeks to months. Additionally, there is a numbness or absence of sensation in the hands and arms, or feet and legs. Muscle weakness may also result in the toe dragging when the foot is lifted to take a step.

## Treatment

Medications used in the treatment of Hansen's disease may include dapsone, rifampin, clofazimine, and ethionamide. Aspirin, prednisone, or thalidomide are used for the control of inflammation (e.g., erythema nodosum leprosum) that may occur with therapy.

## Testing

Lepromin skin test can be used to distinguish lepromatous from tuberculoid leprosy but is not used for diagnosis. Skin scraping examination for acid-fast bacteria may also be conducted to diagnose Hansen's disease.

## HANTAVIRUS PULMONARY SYNDROME

### Description

Hantavirus belongs to the bunyavirus family, which contains five genera of viruses that are each made up of single-stranded RNA viruses. Hantavirus is the only virus in the bunyavirus family that is rodent-borne; all the others are arthropod-borne. Hantavirus causes a respiratory disease known as Hantavirus Pulmonary Syndrome (HPS), or just Hantavirus disease. HPS is spread through contact with rodent droppings, especially mice. To date, HPS has been identified in 31 states (All about hantavirus, 2003; Kotton, 2003a).

### Signs and Symptoms

Hantavirus disease is characterized by difficulty breathing; fever; muscle pain; headache; chills; dizziness; nonproductive cough; nausea; vomiting; diarrhea; low blood pressure; irregular heartbeat; and pain in the joints, back, and abdomen.

### Treatment

There is no specific treatment or cure for hantavirus infection. The mortality rate of HPS is 38 percent.

### Testing

Blood tests, X-rays, and serological testing for hantavirus may all be used in diagnosis.

## HASHIMOTO THYROIDITIS

### Description

Chronic thyroiditis is an inflammation of the thyroid gland that results in hypothyroidism, which results in the insufficient production of thyroid hormones (Odeke, 2003; Rennert, 2004a). Chronic thyroiditis or Hashimoto's disease can occur at any age, but it is most often seen in middle-aged women. It is caused by a reaction of the immune system against the thyroid gland. The onset of the disease is slow, and it may take months or even years for the condition to be detected. When Hashimoto's disease occurs with adrenal insufficiency and type 1 diabetes mellitus, the condition is called type 2 polyglandular autoimmune syndrome (PGA II). Less commonly, Hashimoto's disease occurs with hypoparathyroidism, adrenal insufficiency, and fungal infections of the mouth and nails in a condition called type 1 polyglandular autoimmune syndrome (PGA I).

### Signs and Symptoms

Hashimoto's disease is characterized by an intolerance to cold, weight gain, fatigue, constipation, goiter, dry skin, hair loss, heavy and irregular menses, facial swelling, and difficulty concentrating. Late in the disease, the thyroid gland may atrophy. There may be no symptoms in some people.

### Treatment

Replacement therapy with thyroid hormone (e.g., levothyroxine) is given.

### Testing

Hashimoto's disease may be diagnosed by a free T4 test, a serum TSH test, a T3 test, and tests for the presence of antithyroid peroxidase antibody or antithyroglobulin antibody.

## HEAD LICE

### Description

Head lice are technically known as *Pediculus humanus capitis,* and having head lice is common. They spread through either direct or indirect contact with infected persons. Preschool and elementary-age children, between ages 3 and 10, are infested most often. In the United States, African Americans rarely get head lice.

There are three forms of lice. Nits are head lice eggs, and they are hard to see and are often confused for dandruff or hair spray droplets. Nits are found firmly attached to the hair shaft. They are oval and usually yellowish white. Nits take about one week to hatch into nymphs, which resemble adult head lice, but they are smaller. It takes another 7 days for nymphs to mature into adult head lice. The adult louse is about the size of a sesame seed, has six legs, and is tan to grayish-white. Adult lice can live up to 30 days on a person's head, and they die within two days if they fall off a person's head. Head lice are typically found on the scalp behind the ears and near the neckline at the back of the neck.

## Signs and Symptoms

Signs and symptoms of head lice may begin with a tickling feeling of something moving in the hair. Head lice also may cause itching, due to an allergic reaction to the bites. Children with head lice may become irritable, and they may develop sores on their head due to scratching. Head lice spread through direct contact with infected people, sharing infected clothing, and the sharing of combs, brushes, or towels. Head lice may also spread through contact with a bed, couch, pillow, carpet, or stuffed animal of an infected person.

## Treatment

Head lice can be effectively treated through physical removal and medicated shampoo. Over-the-counter lotions and shampoos containing permethrin are usually effective. Medications used for lice are insecticides; therefore, they should be used exactly as directed. Eggs may be removed with a nit comb. Washing all clothes and bed linens helps prevent reinfestation and head lice from spreading to others.

## Testing

There is no need for tests to diagnose head lice.

## HEMOLYTIC ANEMIA

## Description

Hemolytic anemia results from the hemolysis, or rupturing, of red blood cells prematurely (Cohen, 2003a). Hemolytic anemia may be a congenital disorder, or it may be due to the effects of poisons. The hemoglobin separates into heme and globin prematurely, reducing the available amount of hemoglobin in the blood to transport oxygen. Causes of hemolytic anemia include infection, certain medications, autoimmune disorders, and inherited disorders. Types of hemolytic anemia include sickle-cell anemia, paroxysmal nocturnal hemoglobinuria, hemoglobin SC disease, hemolytic anemia due to G6PD deficiency, hereditary elliptocytosis, hereditary spherocytosis, hereditary ovalocytosis, idiopathic autoimmune hemolytic anemia, nonimmune hemolytic anemia caused by chemical or physical agents, secondary immune hemolytic anemia, and thalassemia (Anemia, 2003).

## Signs and Symptoms

Hemolytic anemia is characterized by chills, fatigue, pallor, difficulty breathing, rapid heart rate, jaundice, dark urine, and enlarged spleen.

## Treatment

Folic acid, iron replacement, and corticosteroids may be used to treat hemolytic anemia. In emergencies, transfusion of blood may be necessary.

## Testing

There are specific tests that identify the specific types of hemolytic anemia, and they are performed after hemolysis has been established. Direct measurement of the red-cell life span by isotopic tagging techniques shows a decreased life span. Tests may include measures of bilirubin levels, serum haptoglobin levels, hemoglobin in the urine, hemosiderin in the urine, reticulocyte counts, red blood cell counts, urine and fecal urobilinogen levels, and serum lactate dehydrogenase (LDH) levels.

## HEMOLYTIC DISEASE OF THE NEWBORN

### Description
Hemolytic disease of the newborn—formerly known as erythroblastosis fetalis—occurs when a child is conceived of an Rh-positive father and an Rh-negative mother. The disorder only occurs if the child inherits the Rh-positive factor from the father. Although the blood of the fetus and the mother do not mix, occasionally leakage can occur. When the fetus's Rh-positive blood mixes with the Rh-negative blood of the mother, the mother produces antibodies against the Rh factor. During the pregnancy, enough time will usually not pass to allow the development of Rh factor antibodies, which might cause harm to the fetus. If a second Rh-positive fetus is conceived, however, the Rh factor antibodies can cross the placental barrier and endanger the fetus. The administration of a drug to the mother, after the birth of her first Rh-positive infant, prevents her from making the anti-Rh antibodies, protecting any future fetuses.

### Signs and Symptoms
Initial signs at birth may include an enlarged liver and spleen, generalized swelling, jaundice, and anemia.

### Treatment
Hemolytic disease of the newborn may be fatal, but it also may be treated in utero by medication or intrauterine transfusion. After birth, depending on the severity, a transfusion may be performed.

### Testing
Diagnosis of hemolytic disease of the newborn is determined by an Rh blood test.

## HEMOPHILIA

### Description
Hemophilia is an inherited disease characterized by a tendency toward excessive and sometimes spontaneous bleeding (Cohen, 2004a). There are two types of hemophilia: A and B. Hemophilia B is also known as Christmas disease. Both types are caused by low levels or complete absence of a blood protein essential for blood clotting to take place. Hemophilia A is due to a lack of the blood clotting protein factor VIII, and hemophilia B is due to a lack of factor IX. Although females transmit the disease, almost always only males develop hemophilia (*Hereditary bleeding disorders*, 2004).

## Signs and Symptoms

Hemophilia is characterized by bruising and spontaneous bleeding. There is also internal bleeding into joints, the gastrointestinal tract, and the urinary tract, which results in bloody urine and bloody stool. Prolonged bleeding from cuts, tooth extraction, and surgery may also occur.

## Treatment

Standard treatment of hemophilia is infusion of factor VIII concentrates to replace the defective clotting factor. Mild hemophilia may be treated with infusion of cryoprecipitate or desmopressin (DDAVP), which causes release of factor VIII stored within the lining of blood vessels. Although it is possible for hemophiliacs to die from internal bleeding, the administration of blood clotting factors has proven to be an effective method of resolving this disorder.

## Testing

Many blood clotting tests are performed if the person tested is the first one in the family to have a bleeding disorder, after which other family members will need less testing to diagnose the disorder. Tests related to hemophilia indicate prolonged prothrombin time (PTT), normal prothrombin time, normal bleeding time, normal fibrinogen levels, and low serum factor VIII activity.

## HEMORRHOIDS

### Description

About half of the American population will develop hemorrhoids by the age of 50 (Hart, 2003b). Figure 2-37 illustrates hemorrhoids, which are inflamed veins around the anus or lower rectum, which often result from straining to defecate. They may also be associated with pregnancy, aging, chronic constipation or diarrhea, and anal intercourse. Hemorrhoids are common during pregnancy because the pressure of the fetus and hormonal changes cause the hemorrhoidal vessels to enlarge; although hemorrhoids are temporary for most pregnant women.

### Signs and Symptoms

The most common characteristics of internal hemorrhoids are bright red rectal bleeding and painful swelling around the anus. Hemorrhoids may result from excessive straining, rubbing, or cleaning around the anus, which may all result in further inflammation and the development of more hemorrhoids. Other disease characteristics associated with hemorrhoids may include anal itching; anal pain; blood in the stool; painful bowel movements; and the presence of hard, tender lumps near the anus.

### Treatment

Hemorrhoids are usually not dangerous or life-threatening, with symptoms subsiding in a few days. Exercise and increased fiber in the diet helps reduce constipation and straining by producing feces that are softer and easier to pass. Good sources of fiber are fruits, vegetables, and whole

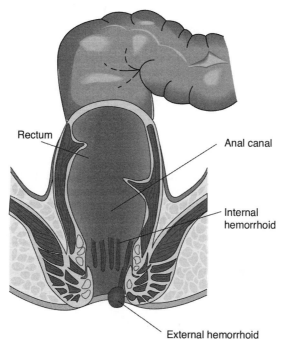

Rectum

Anal canal

Internal hemorrhoid

External hemorrhoid

**Figure 2-37** Hemorrhoids

grains. Drinking six to eight glasses of water daily also reduces constipation and strain during defecation. Corticosteroid creams and creams with lidocaine can reduce pain and swelling. Witch hazel can reduce itching, and a sitz bath can help reduce inflammation by sitting in warm water for 10 to 15 minutes. Stool softeners help reduce straining and constipation. In severe cases, surgical hemorrhoidectomy may be necessary.

## Testing

Hemorrhoids are diagnosed through physical exm. Diagnosis can be confirmed by stool guaiac, sigmoidoscopy, and anoscopy.

## HENDRA AND NIPAH VIRUS INFECTIONS

### Description

Hendra virus, which was formerly called equine morbillivirus, and Nipah virus are the causative agents of extremely rare respiratory and neurological diseases. Although they are both members of the *Paramyxoviridae* family of viruses, they are not identical. The natural reservoir for Hendra and Nipah viruses are bats of the genus *Pteropus*. Both of these viruses were spread in previous outbreaks of illness through contact with infected animals and their secretions. In the case of Hendra virus, the infected animals were horses; in the case of Nepah virus, the infected animals were pigs (*Hendra virus*, 2004).

## Signs and Symptoms

Hendra virus disease is characterized by a respiratory illness with severe flulike signs and symptoms. Infection with Nipah virus is characterized by an encephalitis accompanied by fever and drowsiness, coma, seizures, and inability to maintain breathing. Nipah virus disease begins with fever and headache followed by drowsiness, disorientation, and confusion. Within two to four days, these signs and symptoms can progress to coma and respiratory illness.

## Treatment

The drug ribavirin has been shown to be effective against the viruses in laboratory tests; however, controlled drug investigations have not been performed and the clinical usefulness of this drug is uncertain. In two of the three known cases of Hendra virus disease, the patients died, and during the Nipah virus disease outbreak in 1998, about 40 percent of the patients died from the illness.

## Testing

Procedures for the laboratory diagnosis of Nipah virus infections include serology, histopathology, immunohistochemistry, electron microscopy, polymerase chain reaction (PCR), and virus isolation.

## HENOCH-SCHONLEIN PURPURA

### Description

Henoch-Schonlein is an idiopathic inflammation of the blood vessels caused by an abnormal response of the immune system, resulting in purple spots on the skin, joint pain, gastrointestinal symptoms, and glomerulonephritis (Clowse, 2003a; Scheinfeld, 2004). Henoch-Schonlein syndrome is usually seen in children, but people of any age may be affected. It is more common in boys than in girls, and it is associated with the presence of a recent upper respiratory illness.

### Signs and Symptoms

Henoch-Schonlein is characterized by large bruises over the lower legs, buttocks, and elbows (see Color Plate 34). This is accompanied by hives, joint pain, abdominal pain, nausea, vomiting, diarrhea, bloody stools, and painful menstruation.

### Treatment

There is no specific treatment for Henoch-Schonlein, but most cases resolve spontaneously without treatment.

### Testing

In cases of Henoch-Schonlein, a physical examination reveals skin lesions and joint tenderness, urinalysis reveals bloody urine, and skin biopsy indicates vasculitis.

## HEPATITIS

### Description

Hepatitis is inflammation of the liver, and it can be caused by infections from parasites, bacteria, or viruses. Hepatitis may also be caused by illicit drugs or poisonous mushrooms (Hart, 2003c). An overdose of acetaminophen in combination with excessive alcohol can also cause a fatal form of hepatitis. The body's immune system can also attack the liver, causing autoimmune hepatitis. Table 2-5 identifies certain medications that can contribute to hepatitis. Additionally, hepatitis may be associated with inherited diseases like cystic fibrosis, or it may be due to excess levels of copper in the body (Viral Hepatitis A, 2003; Viral Hepatitis B, 2003; Viral Hepatitis C, 2003).

**Hepatitis A.** Hepatitis A, which is also known as infectious hepatitis, is spread via the fecal-oral route by the ingestion of contaminated water and food. The hepatitis A virus (HAV) infects the intestine and then spreads to the blood, kidneys, liver, and spleen. HAV is resistant to normal levels of chlorine in water. Mollusks, such as oysters, which live in contaminated water, may be a source of infection when eaten undercooked. The incubation period averages about four weeks, and there is no chronic form of HAV infection. By the time the symptoms of hepatitis A are observable, individuals are no longer infectious.

**Hepatitis B.** Hepatitis B (see Figure 2-38), or serum hepatitis, is spread through contaminated body fluids. Nearly 10,000 health-care workers are infected with HBV each year. HBV has been isolated in numerous bodily fluids (e.g., blood, saliva, breast milk, semen, vaginal secretion). Hepatitis B is a chronic, sometimes rapidly progressive disease. The sharing of needles during intravenous drug abuse, contaminated tattoo needles, and unprotected sex all lead to higher incidences of HBV infection.

**Hepatitis C.** Hepatitis C is caused by the hepatitis C virus (HCV), which is spread through direct contact with blood or other body fluids. Hepatitis

**Table 2-5** Medications Contributing to Hepatitis

| Medication | Use |
| --- | --- |
| Methyldopa | Used to treat hypertension |
| Isoniazid | Used to treat tuberculosis |
| Valproate or phenytoin | Used to treat seizures |
| Chlorpromazine or Amiodarone | Used to treat irregular heartbeat |
| Trimethoprim-sulfamethoxazole or erythromycin | Antibiotics used to treat infections |
| Methotrexate | Used to treat cancer and, in smaller doses, arthritis |

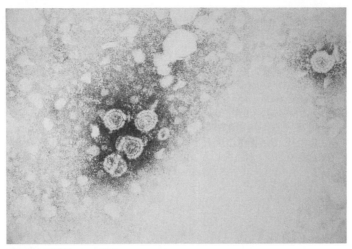

**Figure 2-38** Hepatitis B virus (Courtesy of the CDC)

C is subclinical in 80 percent of cases. Half of the cases progress to chronic hepatitis. The characteristics of hepatitis C infection are similar to hepatitis B infection. Most cases of hepatitis C are transmitted through the use of illegal injected drugs. There is no vaccine for hepatitis C.

## Signs and Symptoms

**Hepatitis A.** Although most cases of hepatitis A are subclinical, disease conditions may include loss of appetite, fatigue, nausea, diarrhea, fever, jaundice, and chills.

**Hepatitis B.** Hepatitis B may cause jaundice, fatigue, abdominal pain, loss of appetite, nausea, vomiting, and arthritis.

**Hepatitis C.** Hepatitis C causes jaundice, fatigue, dark urine, abdominal pain, loss of appetite, and nausea.

## Treatment

**Hepatitis A.** There is no specific treatment for hepatitis A. Over 85 percent of people with hepatitis A recover within three months, and over 99 percent of people recover by six months.

**Hepatiis B.** Hepatitis B is treated with interferon as well as lamivudine and adefovir dipivoxil. About 90 percent of acute hepatitis B infections end in complete recovery.

**Hepatitis C.** There is no cure for hepatitis C, although some patients with hepatitis C benefit from treatment with interferon alpha or a combination of interferon alpha and ribavirin. Liver transplantation is used to treat end-stage chronic hepatitis. There is a vaccine available for hepatitis A and hepatitis B.

## Testing

Laboratory tests for hepatitis may include hepatitis virus serologies, liver function tests, autoimmune blood markers, abdominal ultrasound, liver biopsy, and paracentesis in cases of fluid in the abdomen.

## HERNIAS

### Description

Hernias are protrusions of an organ through the wall of the cavity containing the organ, as illustrated in Figure 2-39. Two common sites of hernias are in the groin and in the diaphragm (Hart, 2003d). Abdominal hernias are associated with pregnancy, heavy lifting, obesity, tumors, weakness from debilitating illness, and coughing. Hernias are more common in men because the abdominopelvic cavity is weak at the level at which the testicles descend. Coughing during a physical examination increases the intra-abdominal pressure exerted against the lower abdominal wall, allowing health-care providers to feel a hernia. Hiatal hernias occur when digestive system organs protrude through the diaphragm (Figure 2-40).

### Signs and Symptoms

Inguinal hernias are characterized by groin discomfort or groin pain aggravated by bending or lifting, a tender groin lump or scrotum lump, and a nontender bulge or lump in children. Hiatal hernias are characterized by indigestion, abdominal pain, and shortness of breath.

### Treatment

Most hernias are repaired surgically.

### Testing

Hernias can be confirmed during a physical exam without lab tests (Hart, 2003e).

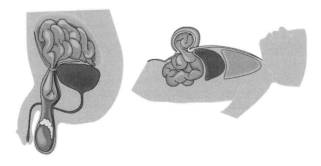

Inguinal                        Umbilical

**Figure 2-39** Hernias

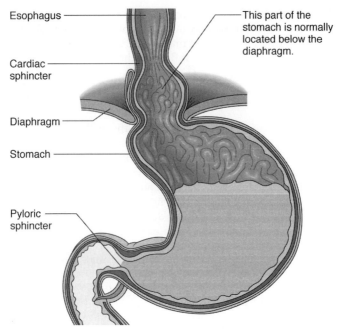

Esophagus

This part of the stomach is normally located below the diaphragm.

Cardiac sphincter

Diaphragm

Stomach

Pyloric sphincter

**Figure 2-40** Hiatal hernia

## HERPES

### Description

Herpes is both a sexually transmitted disease and an infectious disease of the integument. The herpes simplex 1 virus causes fever blisters and cold sores, and the herpes simplex 2 virus causes sexually transmitted herpes infections (Levy, 2004g). Figure 2-41 pictures the herpes simplex virus.

Genital herpes, a sexually transmitted disease, is caused by the herpes simplex 2 virus. According to Wener (2004g), nationwide, 45 million people ages 12 and older are infected with herpes simplex 2 virus. Genital herpes is more common among African Americans (45.9 percent) than Caucasians (17.6 percent). The largest increase in the rate of genital herpes is currently occurring among young, Caucasian teens. Condom use offers uncertain protection, however, because the blisters appear on the external genitalia of women and at the base of the penis on men, which condoms do not cover. Condom use, however, greatly reduces the spread of genital herpes (Genital herpes, 2001).

### Signs and Symptoms

Most individuals have no signs or symptoms from herpes infection. When signs do occur, they typically appear as one or more blisters on or around the genitals or rectum (Figure 2-42). The blisters break, leaving tender sores that may take two to four weeks to heal. Another outbreak can

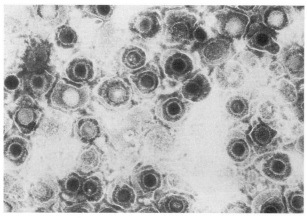

**Figure 2-41** Herpes simplex virus (Courtesy of the CDC)

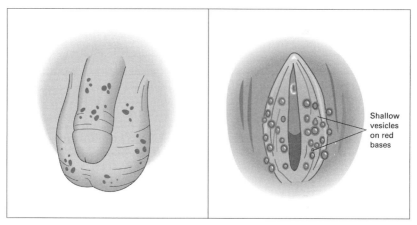

Shallow
vesicles
on red
bases

**Figure 2-42** Genital herpes

appear weeks or months after the first, but it almost always is less severe
and shorter than the first episode.

## Treatment

There is no cure for genital herpes, although there are medications that
may limit the number and severity of recurrences of the symptoms of the
disease—for example, acyclovir (Zovirax), famciclovir (Famvir), penciclovir (Denavir), and valacyclovir (Valtrex). Foscarnet (Foscavir), a power-
ful antiviral agent, is the first choice for treatment of herpes strains that
have become resistant to acyclovir and similar drugs.

## Testing

Tzanck test of skin lesions is consistent with herpes virus infection.
Detection of the herpes simplex virus DNA by PCR from the blister fluid
is positive.

## HETEROPHYIASIS

### Description

Heterophyiasis is an infection caused by one of the smallest trematodes infecting humans, *Heterophyes heterophyes*. Heterophyiasis is contracted through the ingestion of raw fish. Heterophyiasis is most commonly found in parts of Africa, the Middle East, southeast Asia, the Far East, and Hawaii (*Heterophyes heterophyes*, 2004; *Heterophyiasis*, 2004).

### Signs and Symptoms

The primary symptoms of heterophyiasis are diarrhea and abdominal pain. The infection is most serious when eggs of *Heterophyes heterophyes* migrate to the heart causing potentially fatal heart damage. Other organs that may become involved include the liver and brain.

### Treatment

Praziquantel is used to treat heterophyiasis.

### Testing

The diagnosis of heterophyiasis is based on the identification of eggs in the stool.

## HIRSCHSPRUNG'S DISEASE

### Description

Hirschsprung's disease is an obstruction of the large intestine caused by inadequate motility resulting from a congenital condition (Muir, 2003b; Neville, 2003). In cases of Hirschsprung's disease, the nerve ganglia necessary for peristalsis are missing, from the rectum or colon. The obstruction causes the bowel and abdomen to become distended. If the condition is severe, the newborn may fail to pass meconium, which is the first bowel movement. Unlike constipation, children with Hirschsprung's disease experience soiling and overflow incontinence.

### Signs and Symptoms

Hirschsprung's disease is characterized by failure to pass meconium shortly after birth, failure to pass a first stool within 24 to 48 hours after birth, constipation, abdominal distention, vomiting, watery diarrhea, poor weight gain in babies, slow growth prior to five years of age, and malabsorption. Hirschsprung's disease is fatal 25 to 30 percent of the time due to enterocolitis, which is characterized by abdominal pain, fever, foul-smelling/bloody diarrhea, and vomiting.

### Treatment

Most cases of Hirschsprung's disease require surgery to create a temporary colostomy (Figure 2-43). Antibiotics are given if perforation of the intestine or enterocolitis occurs.

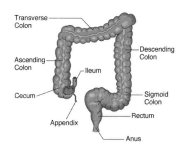

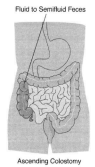 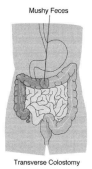 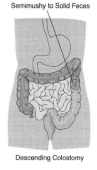 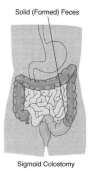

**Figure 2-43** Sites of a colostomy

## Testing

Tests used in the diagnosis of Hirschsprung's disease include abdominal X-ray, barium enema, anal manometry in which a balloon is dilated in the rectum to measure the anal sphincter pressure, and rectal biopsy showing absence of ganglion nerve cells.

## HISTOPLASMOSIS

### Description

Histoplasmosis is a fungal infection of the respiratory system (Levy, 2004k). Its other names include reticuloendothelial cytomycosis, cave disease, spelunker's disease, and Darling's disease. It is caused by the fungus *Histoplasma capsulatum*. In the United States, rates of histoplasmosis are highest in Ohio, Missouri, and the Mississippi Delta. *H. capsulatum* is found in bats and in the fecal material of birds. The high nitrogen content of bird droppings makes a good breeding ground for this fungus. The disease is acquired from airborne spores, which may enter the ventilation system of buildings where birds nest (*Histoplasmosis*, 2003).

### Signs and Symptoms

In most cases of the disease, there are no symptoms. This disease is not spread from contact with infected persons. In symptomatic cases, the fungus affects the lungs causing lesions, and any organ of the body may be affected as the disease progresses systemically. The clinical relevance of histoplasmosis is primarily of importance in immunocompromised cases. Once the disease reaches the systemic level, it causes fatal chronic obstructive pulmonary disease (COPD).

## Treatment

Histoplasmosis is treated with antifungal therapy. Medications used in the treatment of histoplasmosis may include itraconazole, ketoconazole, and amphotericin B.

## Testing

Tests may include analysis of the organism in sputum, lung tissue, blood, cerebrospinal fluid, or bone marrow tissue, as well as antigen tests performed on blood, urine, or cerebrospinal fluid.

## HODGKIN'S LYMPHOMA

### Description

Hodgkin's lymphoma, which is also known as Hodgkin's disease, is an idiopathic lymphatic cancer (Grund, 2004b). The primary difference between Hodgkin's disease and non-Hodgkin's lymphoma is the presence of Reed-Sternberg cells. B-cells should produce antibodies that guide the immune system in defense of invading bacteria, but Reed-Sternberg cells are a malignant, nonfunctional form of B lymphocyte.

### Signs and Symptoms

Complications due to Hodgkin's lymphoma include swollen glands, pain after drinking alcohol, night sweats, loss of appetite, weight loss, fever, and general itching over the entire body.

### Treatment

Chemotherapy and radiation therapy are the two main methods of treating Hodgkin's disease.

### Testing

Tests for Hodgkin's lymphoma include lymph node biopsy, bone marrow biopsy, and detection of Reed-Sternberg cells by biopsy. Blood tests and imaging tests are used to evaluate the staging of tumors.

## HOOKWORM INFECTION

### Description

Hookworm infections occur mostly in tropical and subtropical climates and are estimated to infect about 1 billion people globally (Levy, 2003b). Hookworm infection is a disease caused by several species of parasites that, in early stages of disease, travel through the body in the larvae form, which is referred to as larva migrans. Hookworm infections are spread from animals, like puppies and kittens, that are especially likely to have hookworm infections. The infected animals pass hookworm eggs in their feces, which contaminates the soil and surrounding environment. One of the most common species of hookworm, *Ancylostoma duodenale,* is found in southern Europe, northern Africa, northern Asia, and parts of South America. A second species, *Necator americanus,* was once widespread in the southeastern United States but has largely been controlled in recent years (*Hookworm infection,* 1999).

### Signs and Symptoms

Hookworm sometimes has no symptoms. In other cases, hookworm infection begins with mild diarrhea or cramps but may lead to serious health problems for newborns, children, pregnant women, and persons who are malnourished. As the larvae move through the skin, painful and itchy skin infections may develop. While in the intestine, the larvae cause bleeding, inflammation, swelling, and abdominal pain. Other symptoms include cough, fever, coughing up blood, loss of appetite, nausea, vomiting, pallor, fatigue, and eggs and blood in the stool.

### Treatment

Hookworm infection is treated with medications such as mebendazole or albendazole.

### Testing

Hookworm infection is detected by stool ova and parasite examination and alterations in the results of a D-xylose absorption test.

## HUNTINGTON'S CHOREA

### Description

Huntington's disease, which is also known as Huntington's chorea, is a progressive disorder involving degeneration of nerve cells in the brain, and it is inherited as a single faulty gene on chromosome 4 (Kiriakopoulos, 2003c; Revilla & Grutzendler, 2004). The disease may occur earlier and more severely in succeeding affected generations. Every child of a parent with the disorder has a 50 percent chance of inheriting Huntington's disease. Symptoms usually appear between the ages 35 and 50. The incidence of Huntington's disease is highest in Lake Maracaibo region of Venezuela, the island of Mauritius off the coast of South Africa, and in Tasmania. It occurs least frequently in Finland and Japan.

### Signs and Symptoms

In children, Huntington's disease may appear to be Parkinson's disease with rigidity, slow movements, and tremor. There is progressive loss of mental function, personality changes, loss of cognitive functions, and speech dysfunction. Abnormal facial and body movements develop, including quick jerking movements. The term *chorea* means dance and refers to the typical movements that develop.

## Treatment

There is no cure for or means of slowing the progress of Huntington's disease. Dopamine blockers such as haloperidol or phenothiazine medications may reduce abnormal behaviors and movements. Drugs like tetrabenazine and amantadine are used to try to control extra movements. There has been some evidence to suggest that coenzyme Q10 may minimally decrease progression of the disease. Antipsychotics may also be prescribed.

## Testing

A head CT scan may show atrophy, especially of deep brain (caudate) structures. Other tests may include a head MRI scan, a Positron Emission Tomography (PET) (isotope) scan of the brain, and DNA marker studies. Genetic testing may also be conducted.

## HYDROCELE

### Description

According to Gilbert (2003b), hydrocele is a collection of fluid in the scrotum. Specifically, the serous fluid accumulates in the scrotum as a result of either a defect or an irritation of the tunica vaginalis or the spermatic cord within the scrotum. Most hydroceles are congenital, and they are most common in children between the ages of 1 and 2. In adult males, most cases of hydrocele are observed in those over the age of 40. In adults, hydrocele is most commonly the result of cancer, infections, trauma to the testicles, hernias, or damage to the circulatory system within the male reproductive system.

### Signs and Symptoms

Only about 1 percent of all males experience hydroceles. Most hydroceles are asymptomatic; however, they may be accompanied by a sensation of heaviness or dragging. A painless enlargement of the scrotum is also a common sign of hydrocele. Hydroceles may also cause mild discomfort that radiates from the scrotum to the mid-lower back. Hydroceles occur on both sides of the scrotum in about 7 to 10 percent of the cases.

### Treatment

Hydroceles are usually not dangerous and are self-resolving. They are usually only treated when they cause discomfort or embarrassment or if they threaten the testicles' blood supply. One option is to remove the fluid in the scrotum via needle aspiration; however, aspiration can cause infection, and it is common for the fluid to reaccumulate. Medications used to treat hydrocele include tetracycline and sodium tetradecyl sulfate. Hydrocelectomy is a surgical procedure in which an incision is made in the scrotum or the lower abdomen and a scrotal drainage tube is inserted.

### Testing

During a physical exam, a light can be shined through the scrotum, outlining the testicle and indicating the presence of clear fluid. An ultrasound may be done to confirm the diagnosis.

## HYDROCEPHALUS

### Description

Hydrocephalus is a degenerative disorder of the nervous system. Hydrocephalus is a condition in which the cerebrospinal fluid fails to be properly drained or absorbed, causing the ventricles of the brain to fill with cerebrospinal fluid. The condition may be caused by developmental anomalies, infection, injury, or brain tumors. In infants, hydrocephalus may cause extreme distention and disfigurement of the head because the cranial sutures have not yet formed (Hydrocephalus, 2003).

### Signs and Symptoms

Hydrocephalus is characterized by enlargement of the head, bulging fontanelles, separation of cranial sutures, and vomiting. Later symptoms may include irritability; poor temper control; muscle spasm; decreased mental function; delayed development; difficulty moving; weakness; urinary incontinence; and brief, shrill, high-pitched crying. In older children, symptoms may include headache, vomiting, vision changes, crossed eyes, loss of coordination, poor gait, and mental aberrations.

### Treatment

Surgical interventions are the primary treatment of hydrocephalus. This includes direct removal of the obstruction, if possible. Surgical placement of a shunt within the brain may allow cerebrospinal fluid to bypass the obstructed area and be redirected to the right atrium of the heart or to the abdominal peritoneum (Figure 2-44). Surgical cautery or removal of the

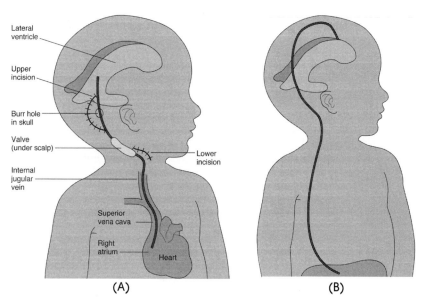

**Figure 2-44** (A) A ventriculoatrial shunt drains spinal fluid into the heart. (B) The ventriculoperitoneal shunt drains spinal fluid into the abdomen.

parts of the ventricles that produce cerebrospinal fluid may, theoretically, reduce cerebrospinal fluid production. Untreated hydrocephalus has a 50 to 60 percent fatality rate, with the survivors having varying degrees of intellectual, physical, and neurologic disabilities (Goldenring, 2004d).

## Testing

Tapping with the fingertips, which is known as percussion, on the skull may show abnormal sounds associated with thinning and separation of skull bones. A neurologic examination may show focal neurologic deficits, and reflexes may be abnormal for the age of the child. Other tests may include transillumination of the head to show abnormal fluid accumulation, a head CT scan, skull X-rays, brain scan using radioisotopes, arteriography of brain blood vessels, an EEG, and a radionuclide cisternogram scan.

## HYDRONEPHROSIS

### Description

Hydronephrosis is a condition that occurs as part of a disease; it is not a disease itself (Gilbert, 2004c). Hydronephrosis occurs when anatomic or functional processes interrupt the flow of urine, causing a kidney to become distended due to a backup of urine, as illustrated in Figure 2-45. When both kidneys are involved, the condition is called bilateral hydronephrosis; the involvement of a single kidney is referred to as unilateral hydronephrosis. Hydronephrosis may accompany pregnancy, or it may be

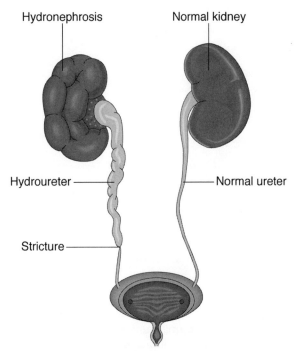

**Figure 2-45** Hydronephrosis

caused by obstruction of the renal system, backflow of urine from the bladder into the ureter and kidney, and kidney stones. Occasionally, unilateral hydronephrosis may not present any signs or symptoms.

## Signs and Symptoms

Hydronephrosis is characeterized by flank pain, an abdominal mass, nausea, vomiting, urinary tract infections, fever, disruptions of urinary output, frequency of urination, and urgency to urinate. The lower extremities may swell, and the bladder may distend (Manian & Resnick, 2004).

## Treatment

Hydronephrosis may be treated by inserting a stint that allows urination; however, this only allows the removal of excess urine. The original cause of the hydronephrosis must still be treated, as prolonged hydronephrosis eventually results in renal failure.

## Testing

Tests used in the diagnosis of hydronephrosis may include an intravenous pyelogram (IVP), isotope renography, ultrasound of the kidneys, CT scan of the abdomen, and an abdominal MRI.

## HYMENOLEPIASIS

### Description

Hymenolepiasis is caused by the dwarf tapeworm (*Hymenolepis nana*) and by rat tapeworm (*Hymenolepis dimnuta*). *Hymenolepis nana* is the most common global cause of all cestode infections, and in temperate areas its incidence is higher in children and institutionalized groups. *Hymenolepis diminuta,* though less frequent, has been reported from various areas of the world. Hymenolepiasis is spread to humans through ingestion of contaminated food or water and contact with contaminated surfaces through the fecal-oral route (*Hymenolepiasis,* 2004; Smith, 2003c).

### Signs and Symptoms

Hymenolepiasis is often an asymptomatic illness, but severe infection may result in weakness, headaches, loss of appetite, abdominal pain, and diarrhea.

### Treatment

Praziquantel is the current treatment of choice for hymenolepiasis.

### Testing

Examination of the stool for eggs and parasites confirms the diagnosis.

## HYPEREMESIS GRAVIDARUM

### Description

Hyperemesis gravidarum is extreme, persistent nausea and vomiting during pregnancy that may lead to dehydration (Michelini, 2004; Rein, 2003). Morning sickness is common to most pregnant women, especially during the first trimester due to drastic hormone level changes. Extreme nausea and vomiting during pregnancy may indicate multiple pregnancy or, rarely, hydatidiform mole, which is abnormal tissue growth that results from conception but does not give rise to a viable fetus.

## Signs and Symptoms

Hyperemesis gravidarum is characterized by pregnancy, nausea, and vomiting. Some mothers experience lightheadedness and fainting.

## Treatment

It is important for pregnant woman to maintain their fluid intake during times when they are least nauseated. Medication to prevent nausea is reserved for cases where vomiting is persistent and severe enough to present potential maternal and fetal risks. Nausea and vomiting usually peaks between 2 and 12 weeks' gestation and resolves by the second half of a pregnancy. With adequate identification of symptoms and careful follow-up, this sickness rarely presents serious complications for the infant or mother. Drinking seltzers or sparkling water may be soothing.

## Testing

Blood tests may be used to determine the level of dehydration.

## HYPERTENSION

## Description

Hypertension, which is commonly referred to as high blood pressure, can contribute to coronary artery disease, strokes, kidney failure, and sudden rupture of the aorta. In addition, chronic high blood pressure associated with hypertensive heart disease can cause acute cardiac failure and result in sudden death. Although there are no rigid rules for determining high blood pressure, a sustained systolic pressure of over 140 or a sustained diastolic pressure of over 90 is considered hypertension (Koren, 2003b). Normal blood pressure should be near 120 over 80.

There are several reasons why scientists believe that individuals develop high blood pressure, although 90 to 95 percent of the cases of hypertension have no known cause. These idiopathic cases of high blood pressure are believed to be related to social factors such as stress, obesity, smoking, physical inactivity, and diets high in salt. Beside its other detrimental effects, high blood pressure ultimately damages the lining of blood vessels. This damage to the blood vessels increases risk for both rupture of blood vessels in the brain, causing stroke, and rupturing the aorta, causing uncontrolled internal bleeding.

## Signs and Symptoms

Usually, no symptoms are present other than a mild headache. More severe symptoms may include tiredness, confusion, vision changes, chest pain, heart failure, bloody urine, ringing in the ears, and nosebleed.

## Treatment

Medications used to treat hypertension may include diuretics, beta-blockers, calcium-channel blockers, angiotensin-converting enzyme (ACE) inhibitors, angiotensin receptor blockers (ARBs), or alpha-blockers. Medications such as hydralazine, minoxidil, diazoxide, or nitroprusside may be required if the blood pressure is extremely high.

## Testing

Hypertension may be suspected when the blood pressure is high at any single measurement. It is confirmed through blood pressure consistently elevated over 140 systolic or 90 diastolic.

## HYPERTENSIVE HEART DISEASE

### Description

Uncontrolled blood pressure can result in several severe disorders, specifically in the brain, kidneys, and heart (Hart, 2003f). When the left ventricle of the heart enlarges in combination with a history of high blood pressure, the individual is diagnosed with hypertensive heart disease. As the wall of the left ventricle increases in size, its demand for nutrients also increases; however, the ability of the heart to deliver nutrient-rich blood diminishes as the heart enlarges. As the wall of the left ventricle hypertrophies, it becomes tighter and less efficient at pumping, reducing the overall cardiac output of blood. Chronic hypertension also predisposes individuals to atherosclerosis, which can cause coronary artery disease (Riaz & Forker, 2003).

### Signs and Symptoms

Hypertensive heart disease is characterized by difficulty breathing, rapid and irregular pulse, heart palpitations, cough, coughing up blood, fatigue, swelling of the feet, increased urination at night. Other symptoms may include nausea, chest pain, sweating, and dizziness.

### Treatment

Medications used to treat hypertensive heart disease include thiazide diuretics, potassium replacements, alpha and beta blockers, calcium-channel blockers, angiotensin-converting enzyme (ACE) inhibitors, angiotensin II receptor antagonists, and direct vasodilators such as hydralazine. Diazoxide and nitroprusside are intravenous medications that may be prescribed if hypertension is extremely severe and intensive care is necessary.

### Testing

Tests used in the diagnosis of hypertensive heart disease include blood pressure, use of a stethoscope to reveal sounds of fluid, an ECG, an echocardiogram, chest X-ray, and a coronary angiogram.

## HYPOSPADIAS

### Description

Hypospadias is an idiopathic, congenital defect in which the opening of the urethra is on the underside, rather than at the end, of the penis (Gatti, 2003;

Gilbert, 2004a). In most cases, the opening of the urethra is located near the tip of the penis on the glans, but in more severe cases, the opening is at the midshaft of the penis, base of the penis, or in the scrotum or perineum. Hypospadias is often associated with chordee, which is a downward curvature of the penis during erection. Erections are common with infant boys. Infants with hypospadias should not be circumcised because the foreskin will be used in surgery.

## Signs and Symptoms

Hypospadias is characterized by the opening of the urethra being displaced to the underside of the penis, which may exhibit a marked curvature downward. The penis appears hooded due to malformation of the foreskin.

## Treatment

Hypospadias is treated surgically before the child starts school—preferably before 18 months of age. During the surgery, the penis is straightened and the hypospadias is corrected using grafts from the foreskin. Surgical treatment is usually positive, although multiple surgeries may be necessary.

## Testing

Diagnosis is made on physical examination, but imaging tests may be necessary to look for other anomalies.

## ICHTHYOSIS

## Description

Ichthyosis vulgaris, which is also known as fish scale disease, is a common inherited skin disorder causing dry, scaly skin. It occurs in approximately 1 in 300 persons. Ichthyosis vulgaris may begin in early childhood, before a child is four. In most cases one parent and one-half of the children will be affected. Ichthyosis is most severe over the legs but may involve the arms, hands, and trunk, especially on the extension surfaces but absent from the flexor surfaces. Often there are many fine lines over the palm of the hand, and the condition is often more noticeable in the winter. Ichthyosis seldom affects medical health and usually improves during adulthood, but it may recur when a person becomes elderly. Secondary bacterial skin infection may develop if scratching causes openings in the skin (Drayer, 2003b).

## Signs and Symptoms

Ichthyosis is characterized by a skin rash with a scaly appearance, scales, and thick, dry skin. There is also a mild itching associated with the rash. The forehead and cheeks may be involved early on, but the scaling diminishes quickly in these areas. Ichthyosis is aggravated during the summer months (Okulicz & Schwartz, 2005).

## Treatment

Creams and ointments are more effective than lotions, and they are best applied to wet skin immediately after bathing. The use of mild, nondrying soaps is encouraged. Use of moisturizing creams that contain keratolytic agents, which are chemicals that help skin to shed normally (e.g., lactic acid, salicylic acid, urea), are often helpful.

## Testing

The diagnosis is made primarily on the basis of the skin appearance, and tests are therefore unnecessary.

## IMPETIGO

### Description

*S. pyogenes* not only causes Strep throat, but it is also the causative agent of impetigo (M. Lehrer, 2003a). In addition, *Staphylococcus aureus* may also cause impetigo, which is a localized skin infection that begins with small blisters that progress into weeping lesions (see Color Plate 35). After several days, a crust forms when the lesions dry. Children between two and five are most commonly infected. The disease spreads through insect bite, small abrasions in the skin, and contaminated hands on the face.

### Signs and Symptoms

Impetigo is characterized by skin lesions on the face, arms, or legs, that spread to other areas. Impetigo lesions begin as a cluster of tiny blisters that burst, followed by oozing and the formation of a thick honey- or brown-colored crust that is firmly stuck to the skin. Other symptoms include itching and lymphadenopathy.

### Treatment

Mild impetigo infections are treated with antibacterial creams such as bactroban and oral antibiotics like erythromycin or dicloxacillin. The skin should be gently washed several times a day with an antibacterial soap to remove crusts and drainage. Use of a clean washcloth and towel each time will help prevent the spread of infection. Impetigo has a high cure rate, but recurrence is common in young children. The sores of impetigo heal slowly and seldom scar.

### Testing

Diagnosis is based primarily on the appearance of the skin lesion. A culture of the skin or mucosal lesion usually grows streptococcus or staphylococcus.

## INCLUSION DISEASE

### Description

Inclusion disease is a viral infection caused by the cytomegalovirus (CMV). CMV is a herpesvirus that causes cellular swelling resembling an owl's eyes. CMV infection is chronic. The virus is shed in body fluids like saliva, urine, semen, vaginal secretions, and breast milk. It is estimated that 80 percent of the United States carries CMV, which is harbored in the parotid salivary glands and causes fever, sore throat, swollen lymph glands, and fatigue (Cytomegalovirus infection, 2002; Wener, 2004b).

## Signs and Symptoms

Inclusion disease is characterized by malaise, cough, difficulty breathing, fever, loss of appetite, night sweats, muscle aches, and joint pain.

## Treatment

Inclusion disease is treated with antiviral agents such as ganciclovir or foscarnet. Antiviral medications stop the replication of the virus but do not destroy it. Oxygen therapy and ventilatory support may initially be necessary to maintain oxygenation until the infection is brought under control.

## Testing

Tests used in the diagnosis of inclusion disease include urine culture, blood culture, CMV serology by indirect fluorescent antibody (IFA), bronchoscopy, tissue biopsy, tissue stains, tissue culture for CMV, and chest X-rays.

## INFLUENZA

### Description

The flu, or influenza, is an acute, viral, inflammatory disease of the respiratory system (Greene, 2003). The influenza virus consists of eight weakly linked RNA segments enclosed in a layer of protein and an outer bilayer of lipids. Because of the influenza virus's ability to recombine, it is able to spread through a variety of human and animal strains. Migratory birds are mixing vessels that carry the virus over large geographic areas. Some of the more common types of influenza viruses are swine flu, Hong Kong flu, Asiatic flu, avian flu, and equine flu. Although Americans refer to stomach flu, this disorder is most likely a bacterial infection of the digestive tract and is not viral influenza at all (Influenza, 2003).

### Signs and Symptoms

Influenza is characterized by fever, chills, loss of appetite, headache, muscle pain, nasal congestion, cough, sore throat, and extreme fatigue. Diarrhea is not usually found in cases of influenza.

### Treatment

If influenza is diagnosed within 48 hours of the onset of symptoms, antiviral medications are available that may shorten the duration of symptoms by approximately 1 day. These medications include amantadine or rimantadine (active against influenza A only) and oseltamivir and zanamivir (active against influenza A and B). Treatment is usually not necessary for children, but in certain cases, oseltamivir (Tamiflu) may be used to treat children. In otherwise healthy people, influenza fully resolves within 10 days.

### Testing

Laboratory tests used to diagnose influenza may include CBC, blood cultures, sputum cultures, and antigen detection tests.

## INFLUENZAL MENINGITIS

### Description

*Haemophilus influenzae* is the causative agent of influenzal meningitis. *H. influenzae* is a highly virulent gram-negative, nonmotile bacterium. Its high virulence is a function of its unique capsule and antigens on its outer membrane, which have been shown to paralyze the sweeping motion of the tiny hairs on the cells that line the respiratory tract (i.e., ciliated respiratory epithelium). Influenzal meningitis is found in approximately 45 percent of the reported cases of meningitis in the United States each year. *H. influenzae* received its name erroneously because it was thought to be the causative agent of the influenza pandemic of 1918. It is now understood that the presence of this bacterial rod in nasal and lung cultures taken from infected individuals was actually the result of a secondary infection. Influenza is actually caused by a virus and not the *H. influenzae* bacterium. Influenzal meningitis occurs primarily between the age of six months and six years old, and it is the primary cause of childhood arthritis (*Haemophilus influenzae*, 2003).

### Signs and Symptoms

Influenzal meningitis is characterized by arthritis, irritability, poor feeding in infants, fever, severe headache, stiff neck, nausea, vomiting, back pain when the chin is flexed toward the chest, unusual body posture, and sensitivity to light.

### Treatment

Treatment of meningitis is started as soon as the diagnosis is suspected. *H. influenzae* meningitis is treated with antibiotics. Steroid medication may also be used, mostly in children. Steroids are given to reduce hearing loss, which is a common complication of meningitis. The outcome is good with early treatment, but influenzal meningitis has a 5 percent fatality rate.

### Testing

Tests for influenzal meningitis may include cerebrospinal fluid culture, blood serology indicating recent exposure to *H. influenzae,* and blood culture indicating *H. influenzae.*

## INHALATION ANTHRAX

### Description

Inhalation anthrax, which is also called Woolsorter's disease or pulmonary anthrax, is acquired when *Bacillus anthracis* spores are inhaled into the lungs (Levy, 2003c). Anthrax commonly affects hoofed animals such as sheep and goats; humans contract inhalation anthrax by breathing spores from industrial processes such as tanning hides and processing wool. Anthrax is a potential agent for use as a biological weapon, but experts have concluded that inhalation anthrax would be difficult to use on a large scale as a weapon. At least 17 nations are believed to have a biological weapons program, but it is unknown how many nations or groups are working with anthrax.

## Signs and Symptoms

Upon inhalation, anthrax spores move to the lymph nodes, germinate, and release toxins. This results in hemorrhage, swelling, and tissue death. There are usually two stages of inhalation anthrax. The first stage can last from a few hours to days and is similar to a flulike illness with fever, headache, cough, shortness of breath, and chest pain. The second stage often develops suddenly and is notable for shortness of breath, fever, and shock. This second stage is fatal in 90 percent of cases. It may take only 24 hours before death occurs. It is important to note that exposure does not equate to infection. Simply inhaling spores does not mean a person will become ill. The spores must germinate, and antibiotic treatment of spores in nasal passages can prevent the illness.

## Treatment

Antibiotics used to treat inhalation anthrax include penicillin, clindamycin, doxycycline, and ciprofloxacin (Cipro). For outbreaks, the antibiotic of choice is ciprofloxacin, until it is known whether the anthrax strain is resistant to other antibiotics. The length of treatment is usually 60 days, because that is the required time for spore germination. In the event of a bioterrorist attack, the United States National Pharmaceutical Stockpile is available to provide antibiotics.

## Testing

Tests used in the diagnosis of inhalation anthrax include chest X-ray, blood cultures, and sputum cultures. Initial chest X-rays are likely to show abnormalities such as fluid surrounding the lungs or abnormally wide space between the lungs. Samples may need to be sent to a special lab for more definitive testing, including PCR, immunoflourescence, and immunohistochemistry. A spinal tap for cerebrospinal fluid culture and a Gram stain may also be performed.

## INTERSTITIAL CYSTITIS

### Description

Interstitial cystitis is a recurring condition characterized by discomfort and pain in the bladder and the surrounding pelvic region. Interstitial cystitis is idiopathic (Interstitial cystitis, 2002; Levy, 2004u).

### Signs and Symptoms

Symptoms of interstitial cystitis include an urgent need to urinate, a need to urinate as many as 60 times a day, and increasing pain as the bladder fills with urine or as it empties. Women's symptoms worsen during menstruation. Through time, the bladder wall may become irritated or scarred, and pinpoint bleeding caused by recurrent irritation may appear on the bladder wall.

## Treatment

Currently there is no cure for interstitial cystitis, and antibiotics are not effective in its treatment. The common treatment is to drink large amounts of fluids to increase urine output, which will aid in the removal of the infection mechanically.

## Testing

Tests used in the diagnosis of cystitis may include urine analysis, ultrasound of the kidneys, and a pyelogram.

## ISOSPORIASIS

### Description

Isosporiasis is an intestinal infection of humans caused by the protozoan *Isospora belli*. This parasite causes isosporiasis in tropical and subtropical areas of the world, and it has resulted in outbreaks of isosporiasis in institutionalized groups in the United States. Isosporiasis normally presents as a mild diarrheal disease in otherwise healthy individuals, but it can cause severe infection in AIDS patients. Humans are the only known natural host for *Isospora belli*, which is spread through the fecal-oral route by ingesting contaminated food or water or contact with contaminated surfaces (Minnaganti, 2002).

### Signs and Symptoms

Isosporiasis is characterized by abdominal pain; vomiting; malaise; loss of appetite; weight loss; low-grade fever; and profuse, watery, nonbloody diarrhea, which may contain mucus.

### Treatment

Trimethoprim-sulfamethoxazole is used to treat isosporiasis.

### Testing

Tests used in the diagnosis of isosporiasis include microscopic examination for oocysts in the stool. The oocysts may be passed in small amounts and intermittently, requiring repeated stool examinations and concentration procedures. If stool examinations are negative, examination of duodenal specimens by biopsy or string test (Enterotest®) may be needed. The oocysts can be visualized on wet mounts by microscopy with bright-field, differential interference contrast (DIC), and epifluorescence. They can also be stained by modified acid-fast stain.

## KAPOSI'S SARCOMA

### Description

Kaposi's sarcoma is a malignant tumor of the connective tissue, often associated with AIDS due to an interaction between HIV, immunosuppression, and human herpesvirus-8 (HHV-8). In AIDS patients, Kaposi's sarcoma can develop aggressively and involve the skin, lungs, gastrointestinal tract, and other organs (Grund, 2004c). The tumors consist of bluish-red or purple nodules made up of vascular tissue (Color Plate 36). Early lesions may start on the feet or ankles and spread to the arms and hands. The appearance of Kaposi's sarcoma is a poor prognostic sign for individuals with HIV infection (Fishman, 2002).

## Signs and Symptoms

Kaposi's sarcoma is characterized by bluish-red macules or bumps with an irregular shape, bleeding with gastrointestinal lesions, difficulty breathing due to pulmonary lesions, and coughing up blood.

## Treatment

Treatment of Kaposi's sarcoma depends on the extent and location of the lesions, as well as the person's symptoms and degree of immunosuppression. Antiretroviral therapy against the AIDS virus can shrink the lesions, and radiation therapy or cryotherapy can be used for lesions in certain areas.

## Testing

Tests used in the treatment and diagnosis of Kaposi's sarcoma include skin lesion biopsy, endoscopy, and an EGD (esophagogastroduodenoscopy).

## KASABACH-MERRITT SYNDROME

### Description

Kasabach-Merritt syndrome is a tumor of the blood vessels (i.e., capillary hemangioma) associated with bruising due to low platelet count (i.e., thrombocytopenic purpura) (Krafchik, 2003). In lay terms, Kasabach-Merritt syndrome is a disease in which tumors develop in the blood vessels under the skin and the blood fails to clot properly, resulting in bruising and bleeding. The disease gets its name from Kasabach and Merritt, who, in 1940, described a male infant with a discolored raised lesion on the left thigh that rapidly grew and invaded the entire left leg, scrotum, abdomen, and thorax, and who exhibited severe thrombocytopenia. Kasabach-Merritt syndrome, which is uncommon in the United States, is fatal 10 to 37 percent of the time.

### Signs and Symptoms

Kasabach-Merritt syndrome is characterized by reddish-brown lesions, hemorrhaging, profound thrombocytopenia, severe infections, and bruising.

### Treatment

Treatment of Kasabach-Merritt syndrome includes a mixture of medication and surgical therapy. Corticosteroids, interferon alpha, vincristine, epsilon-aminocaproic acid, aspirin, dipyridamole, pentoxifylline, and cryoprecipitate have been used to treat Kasabach-Merritt syndrome.

### Testing

Tests used in the diagnosis of Kasabach-Merritt syndrome include CBC, fibrinogen levels, fibrin split products, and D-dimers. MRI or CT scan may reveal a vascular mass that can be difficult to differentiate from a vascular malformation or solid tumor.

## KAWASAKI SYNDROME

### Description
Kawasaki syndrome is an idiopathic, acute, febrile disease that primarily affects boys and children younger than five years of age. It was first described in Japan by Tomisaku Kawasaki in 1967, and the first cases outside Japan were reported in Hawaii in 1976 (*Kawasaki syndrome*, 2003; Peng, 2003b).

### Signs and Symptoms
Kawasaki syndrome is characterized by fever; rash; swelling of the hands and feet; irritation and redness of the whites of the eyes; swollen lymph glands in the neck; and irritation and inflammation of the mouth, lips, and throat. Kawasaki syndrome may also result in coronary artery enlargement and aneurysms, and it is a leading cause of acquired heart disease in the United States.

### Treatment
Treatment for Kawasaki syndrome includes intravenous immunoglobulins and asprin, which help reduce the disease's effects on the heart.

### Testing
Tests used in the diagnosis of Kawasaki syndrome include CBC, ESR, chest X-rays, and urinalysis. EKG and echocardiography, which may reveal signs of myocarditis, pericarditis, arthritis, aseptic meningitis, and coronary vasculitis.

## KERATOACANTHOMA

### Description
Keratoacanthoma is a benign tumor of the skin that grows quickly from the hair follicle (Chuang, 2003a). It is more common in men and in smokers. Keratoacanthoma has a mound-shaped body with a central keratin-filled crater. The lesion resembles squamous cell carcinoma.

### Signs and Symptoms
Keratoacanthomas are solitary and begin as firm, round, skin-colored or reddish bumps that rapidly progress to dome-shaped nodules with a smooth shiny surface and a central keratin plug. Keratoacanthomas resemble a horn.

### Treatment
Keratoacanthomas may heal spontaneously, but they may require surgical excision.

### Testing
Keratoacanthoma is diagnosed through tumor biopsy.

## KIDNEY STONES

### Description

Nephrolithiasis is a condition in which one or more kidney stones are present in the urinary system (Agha, 2003d; Koren, 2001b). The technical name for kidney stones is renal calculi. Kidney stones may form when the urine becomes over concentrated with substances like calcium, oxalates, phosphates, and carbonate. Stones are often asymptomatic until they begin to move down the ureter, causing pain that starts in the abdominal flank and leads to the groin. Kidney stones are common, and recurrence is common, especially if a person has had more than two episodes of kidney stones. Premature infants are likely to develop kidney stones, and some types of stones tend to run in families.

### Signs and Symptoms

Kidney stones are characterized by nausea, vomiting, urinary frequency, bloody urine, severe pelvic and abdominal pain, fever, chills, and discoloration of the urine.

### Treatment

Most kidney stones are passed spontaneously through the urine; however, surgical removal of stones may be required. An alternative to surgery may be lithotripsy, which is illustrated in Figure 2-46. Ultrasonic waves are used to break up stones, so that they may be expelled in the urine or removed with an endoscope, which is inserted into the kidney through a small incision.

### Testing

Tests used in the diagnosis of kidney stones may include ultrasounds, IVP, abdominal X-rays, retrograde pyelograms, abdominal CT scans, and abdominal MRIs.

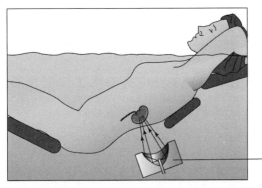

Shock wave generator

**Figure 2-46** Lithotripsy to treat kidney stones

## KLINEFELTER SYNDROME

### Description

Klinefelter syndrome is a chromosome abnormality that affects only men and causes hypogonadism (H. Chen, 2003a; Stewart, 2003g). Klinefelter syndrome affects about 1 in 500 men, and it causes a male to have two X chromosomes and one Y chromosome, rather than the normal singular X chromosome and Y chromosome. The defect usually becomes apparent in puberty, when secondary sexual characteristics fail to develop. Testicular changes result in infertility in most cases. Klinefelter syndrome is not inherited, and it is more common when mothers give birth at an older age. Klinefelter syndrome may be accompanied by autoimmune disorders such as lupus, Sjögren syndrome, and rheumatoid arthritis.

### Signs and Symptoms

Klinefelter syndrome is characterized by a simian crease in the palm, small penis, small firm testicles, enlarged prostate, diminished secondary hair, sexual dysfunciton, gynecomastia, tall stature, abnormal body proportions (i.e., long legs, short trunk), and learning disabilities.

### Treatment

There is no treatment for the infertility associated with Klinefelter syndrome, although testosterone therapy improves the development of secondary sexual characteristics. Gynecomastia can be treated with plastic surgery, if it is disfiguring.

### Testing

Tests for Klinefelter syndrome include karyotyping, semen exam indicating low sperm levels, decreased serum testosterone levels, increased serum luteinizing hormone, increased serum follicle stimulating hormone, and increased serum estradiol levels.

## KRABBE DISEASE

### Description

Krabbe disease, which is also known as Globoid cell leukodystrophy or galactosylcerebrosidase, is an inherited disorder characterized by a deficiency of the enzyme galactocerebroside beta-galactosidase, which is also known as galactosylcereamidase. It is most common among people of Scandinavian descent and among the Druze community in Israel. It generally affects about 1 in 100,000 infants. Absence of the enzyme galactocerebroside beta-galactosidase causes destruction of the myelin that surrounds nerve axons and ultimate destruction of the nervous system (Stewart, 2003h; Tegay & Fallet, 2004).

### Signs and Symptoms

Krabbe disease has an early onset form and a late onset form. In the early form, symptoms begin in the first months of life with feeding problems and failure to thrive, unexplained fevers, and vomiting. Changes in muscle tone are frequent. Seizures may begin early and are severe. Visual and hearing losses are progressive. Affected children eventually assume an unusual, rigid body position called decerebrate posturing. Death follows shortly thereafter, usually before the second year of life. The late onset form of the disease begins in late childhood or early adolescence. Visual problems progressing to blindness may be the first symptom. Walking disturbance and muscle rigidity lead to progressive disability.

## Treatment
There is no specific treatment for Krabbe disease. Bone marrow transplantation and enzyme replacement therapy are being developed and attempted. Prevention by prenatal genetic testing is available. The prognosis is poor, with infantile-onset cases often dying before two years of age and later-onset cases surviving into adulthood but with neurologic dysfunction.

## Testing
Galactocerebroside beta-galactosidase levels can be measured from the serum, white blood cells, chorionic villi, and fibroblasts. There is an increase in the total protein in the cerebrospinal fluid, and abnormal white matter in the brain can be observed by an MRI or CT of the head. Nerve conduction velocity tests show delayed nerve conduction and evidence of demyelination. There is also the presence of abnormal Globoid cells in biopsied tissue of the nervous system. Genetic testing may be available for the glycosylceramidase gene (GALC).

## KWASHIORKOR

### Description
Kwashiorkor is a form of malnutrition caused by inadequate protein intake in the presence of normal total calorie intake with swelling present. Kwashiorkor occurs most commonly in areas of famine, limited food supply, and areas with inadequate knowledge of proper diet. The incidence of kwashiorkor in children in the United States is extremely low. This is typically a disease of impoverished countries. Estimates suggest that as many as 50 percent of elderly persons in nursing homes in the United States suffer from kwashiorkor. Malnutrition is estimated to affect two-thirds of children in Asia and one-fourth of children in Africa (Grigsby, 2003).

### Signs and Symptoms
Early symptoms of any type of malnutrition include weakness and irritability. As protein deprivation continues, growth failure, loss of muscle mass, generalized swelling occur. The immune system is also affected. A large, protuberant belly is common. Skin conditions (e.g., dermatitis, changes in pigmentation, thinning of hair, vitiligo) are common. Severe kwashiorkor may leave a child with permanent mental and physical

disabilities. Malnutrition early in life permanently decreases IQ. Kwashiorkar can be fatal (Blackman, 2004d).

## Treatment

Calories are given first in the form of carbohydrates, simple sugars, and fats. Because the person will have been without food for a long period of time, starting oral feedings must be reintroduced slowly, and the diet must not be too high in calories at first. Proteins are added to the diet last. Many malnourished children will be intolerant to milk sugar and will need to be given supp'ements to aid them in digesting milk products. Vitamin and mineral supplements are essential.

## Testing

Total protein levels from a chemistry profile show insufficient amounts of albumin proteins. CBC demonstrates presence of anemia. Tests for decreased kidney function include urinalysis, serum creatinine, creatinine clearance, BUN, serum potassium, and arterial blood gases.

## LASSA FEVER

### Description

Lassa fever is an acute viral illness that was discovered in Nigeria, West Africa, in 1969. Lassa fever is a significant cause of illness and death in endemic regions of Africa. Symptoms are often mild or absent in about 80 percent of infected people. During occasional epidemics, the fatality rate of Lassa fever has reached as much as 50 percent. The reservoir of Lassa virus is a rodent known as the multimammate rat. This rat belongs to the genus *Mastomys,* and it is uncertain which species of *Mastomys* rodents are associated with Lassa virus transmission. Humans contract the virus from infected rodents through contact with urine and feces. The virus may also be inhaled, and *Mastomys* are also sometimes consumed by humans as a food source. Infected humans pass the Lassa virus to other humans through contaminated body fluids. Lassa fever is not spread, however, through casual contact. Lassa fever can be spread through nosocomial infection (*Lassa fever,* 2004).

### Signs and Symptoms

Lassa fever is characterized by fever, chest pain, sore throat, back pain, cough, abdominal pain, vomiting, diarrhea, conjunctivitis, facial swelling, proteinuria, and mucosal bleeding. Other disease conditions may include hearing loss, tremors, and encephalitis.

### Treatment

Ribavirin has been used with success in Lassa fever patients. It is most effective when given early in the course of the illness.

### Testing

Lassa fever is most often diagnosed by using enzyme-linked immunosorbent serologic assays (ELISA), which detect IgM and IgG antibodies as well as Lassa antigen.

## LEGG-CALVE-PERTHES

### Description

Legg-Calve-Perthes disease is an inflammatory disorder of the bone and connective tissue of the femur (A. Chen, 2003b; Harris, 2004). The blood flow to the femur is interrupted, and the bone dies within about three weeks. The head of the femur flattens, and may eventually collapse. Legg-Calve-Perthes disease occurs most frequently in boys 4 to 10 years old, and it may occur after an accident.

### Signs and Symptoms

Legg-Calve-Perthes disease is characterized by a lurching motion when walking, knee pain, persistent thigh or groin pain, a painless limp, atrophy of the muscles of the upper thigh, shortening of the leg, hip stiffness, difficulty walking, and limited range of motion of the hip and leg.

### Treatment

Legg-Calve-Perthes disease is treated by protecting the bone and joint from further stress and injury while the healing process takes place. Bedrest or crutches may be needed during the initial phase. A brace, cast, or splint to immobilize the hip's position may be used while bone regrowth takes place. Surgery may be performed to keep the hip in its socket.

### Testing

Diagnosis of Legg-Calve-Perthes disease includes X-rays of the hip and conducting a roll test. With the patient lying in the supine position, the examiner rolls the hip of the affected extremity into external and internal rotation, which should invoke guarding or spasm, especially with internal rotation.

## LEGIONNAIRES' DISEASE

### Description

Legionellosis is a disease of the respiratory tract caused by a bacterial infection of *Legionella pneumophilia*. Legionellosis, or Legionnaires' disease, received its name from a group of men from the American Legion who died after attending the same meeting in 1976. *L. pneumophilia* is found in the water of air-conditioning cooling towers, water faucets, shower heads, humidifiers, and contaminated respiratory therapy equipment, suggesting that it has an airborne transmission. The bacterium is resistant to chlorine for long periods (Legionellosis, 2001; Levy, 2003d).

### Signs and Symptoms

Legionnaires' disease is characterized by high fever, cough, and symptoms of pneumonia. Other symptoms include muscle pain, arthritis, difficulty breathing, chest pain, diarrhea, loss of energy, loss of muscle control, and headache. Legionnaires' disease may be fatal due to cardiovascular collapse.

## Treatment

Legionnaires' disease is treated with antibiotics. Treatment is started as soon as Legionnaire's disease is suspected, without waiting for confirmation by culture results. The antibiotic commonly used is a quinolone (ciprofloxacin, levofloxacin, moxifloxacin, or gatifloxacin) or a macrolide (azithromycin, clarithromycin, or erythromycin). The mortality for patients who develop Legionnaires' disease while hospitalized is close to 50 percent, especially when antibiotics are started late.

## Testing

Tests used in the diagnosis of Legionnaires' disease include listening to the chest with a stethoscope for fine crackles, sputum direct fluorescent antibody staining for Legionella, culture of the airway for Legionella, a positive urine antigen test, the presence of pneumonia on chest X-rays, CBC indicating increased WBC counts, low serum sodium, and moderate elevation of liver function tests.

## LEIOMYOMAS

## Description

Leiomyomas are benign tumors that arise from smooth muscle and may develop wherever smooth muscle is present. For example, leiomyomas may originate from the tunica media within the walls of arteries and veins, muscle of the male scrotum or the labia majora of the vagina, or the erectile muscles of the nipple. Uterine leiomyomas are the most common neoplasms of the female genital tract. They are frequent in women over 30, rare in woman younger than 18, and they are less likely after menopause. They are one of the most frequent reasons for major surgery during women's reproductive years (Miethke & Raugi, 2003; Vanni, 2002).

## Signs and Symptoms

Leiomyomas are characterized by a sensation of fullness or pressure in the lower abdomen, pelvic cramping or pain with periods, abdominal fullness, increased urinary frequency, heavy menstrual bleeding accompanied by the passage of blood clots, and sudden, severe pain. Often, however, there are no disease characteristics associated with leiomyomas.

## Treatment

Treatment of leiomyomas may consist of simply monitoring the rate of growth of the fibroids with periodic pelvic exams or ultrasound. Nonsteroidal anti-inflammatory medications (e.g., ibuprofen or naprosyn) may be recommended for lower abdominal cramping or pain with menses. Iron supplementation will help to prevent anemia in women with heavy periods. Hormonal treatment, involving drugs such as injectable Depo-Leuprolide, causes fibroids to shrink, but can also cause significant side effects. Hysteroscopic resection of fibroids may be appropriate for women with fibroids growing within the uterine cavity. Uterine artery embolization is a procedure in which small catheters are placed through veins in the pelvis and advanced to the arteries that supply the uterus with blood. Materials are then injected to block these arteries permanently, which decreases the blood supply to the uterus and fibroids. The removal of just the fibroids by myomectomy is frequently the chosen treatment for premenopausal women who want to bear more children. Hysterectomy is a curative option for women beyond childbearing age.

## Testing

A pelvic examination reveals an irregularly shaped, lumpy, or enlarged uterus. Tests used to diagnose leiomyomas may include a transvaginal ultrasound, pelvic ultrasound, a D & C, or a pelvic laparoscopy to rule out other conditions.

## LEIOMYOSARCOMAS

### Description

A leiomyosarcoma is a malignant neoplasm of smooth muscle that commonly metastasizes to the lungs, although leiomyosarcomas in the digestive system are more likely to spread to the liver. Although leiomyosarcomas can develop at any site in the body, the most common sites are the uterus and the stomach (What Is Leiomyosarcoma?, 2001).

### Signs and Symptoms

Leiomyosarcomas usually start as rapidly growing, painless swellings in the wall of an organ or a blood vessel.

### Treatment

The treatment for leiomyosarcoma is surgery, radiation therapy, and chemotherapy.

### Testing

Diagnosis is based primarily on imaging tests.

## LEISHMANIASIS

### Description

Leishmaniasis is a parasitic disease spread by the bite of infected sand flies, and the two most common forms of the disease are cutaneous leishmaniasis and visceral leishmaniasis. It is estimated that there are approximately 1.5 million new cases of cutaneous leishmaniasis and approximately 500,000 new cases of visceral leishmaniasis annually. More than 90 percent of the world's cases of visceral leishmaniasis are in India, Bangladesh, Nepal, Sudan, and Brazil. Leishmaniasis is not found in Australia or islands in the Pacific. Rarely, cases of cutaneous leishmaniasis have been present in rural southern Texas, but no cases of visceral leishmaniasis are known to have been acquired in the United States (*Leishmania infection*, 2004; Wener, 2004h).

## Signs and Symptoms

Cutaneous leishmaniasis is characterized by the presence of skin sores that change in size and appearance over time. The sores often resemble volcanos with raised edges and a central crater, and they may be covered with a scab. It is not uncommon for swelling of the lymph glands to occur near the site of sores. In contrast, visceral leishmaniasis is characterized by fever, weight loss, enlarged spleen, and enlarged liver, with the spleen being larger than the liver. In addition, visceral leishmaniasis may result in anemia, thrombocytopenia, and leukocytopenia.

## Treatment

Antimony compounds are the principal medications used to treat leishmaniasis. These include meglumine antimonate and sodium stibogluconate. Other drugs may include pentamidine and amphotericin B. Surgery may be required to correct disfigurement by destructive facial lesions. A splenectomy may be required in drug-resistant cases. Cure rates for leishmaniasis are high with antimony compounds.

## Testing

Tests used in the diagnosis of leishmaniasis may include Montenegro skin tests, skin biopsy, bone marrow biopsy, lymph node biopsy, tissue cultures, indirect immunofluorescent antibody tests, and a direct agglutination assay.

## LENTIGO

## Description

Lentigo is a flat brown-black spot that usually occurs in sun-exposed areas of the body (Lehrer, 2003c; Okulicz & Jozwiak, 2002). They are also known liver spots, although they are unrelated to liver function. Lentigines are brought on by aging and exposure to sun or other forms of ultraviolet light. Liver spots are common after 40 years of age.

## Signs and Symptoms

Lentigines are skin lesions that are painless, flat patches with a light brown or black color. They are most often on the back of the hands, forearms, shoulder, face, and forehead. Lentigos are harmless and painless.

## Treatment

For cosmetic reasons, bleaching creams, or laser treatment may be used to remove liver spots. Malanocytes, the cells that give skin its color, are susceptible to freezing with liquid nitrogen, so cryosurgery is effective.

## Testing

Diagnosis is based on the appearance of the skin, and no tests are required.

## LEPTOSPIROSIS

### Description

Leptospirosis is primarily a disease of animals, although it can cause liver and kidney disease in humans (Levy, 2004j). *Leptospira interrogans* is the spirochete that causes leptospirosis. *L. interrogans* has a hooked end when viewed under a microscope. Humans become infected with the bacterium when they come in contact with the contaminated waste of infected animals or infected water or soil. Dogs, rats, and other rodents are the most common reservoirs for *L. interrogans* in the United States. The leptospires live in the lumen of renal tubules and are excreted in the urine. Leptospires can survive in neutral waters for months. There are about 50 cases of leptospirosis reported each year in the United States. Leptospires are most likely to enter humans through nonintact skin or mucous membranes (Leptospirosis, 2001).

### Signs and Symptoms

The symptoms of leptospirosis, which typically subside within a few days, are headache, muscle ache, chills, and fever. A more severe, systemic infection known as Weil's disease, may also result from this spirochete. Weil's disease, which may be fatal, may include renal infection, hepatic infection, or central nervous system infection.

### Treatment

Penicillins, tetracyclines, chloramphenicol, and erythromycin can be given to treat leptospirosis. Treatment generally has a positive outcome, although deaths do occur in complicated cases if not treated promptly.

### Testing

Tests used to diagnose leptospirosis include CBC, creatine kinase tests, liver enzymes tests, serologic tests, dark field microscopy, silver stain, fluorescent microscopy, blood culture, urine culture, and cerebrospinal fluid culture.

## LESCH-NYHAN SYNDROME

### Description

Lesch-Nyhan syndrome is an inherited disorder that affects how the body builds and breaks down purines, which are units in RNA and DNA. Lesch-Nyhan syndrome is inherited as an X-linked trait, so it is seen mainly in males. It was first detailed clinically by Michael Lesch and William Nyhan in 1964 (Blackman, 2004e; Jinnah, 2002).

### Signs and Symptoms

Lesch-Nyhan syndrome is characterized by the overproduction of uric acid, neurological disability, and behavior problems. There is an absence of the enzyme hypoxanthine guanine phosphoribosyltransferase (HGP). Males with Lesch-Nyhan have delayed motor development followed by bizarre movements and increased deep tendon reflexes. Lesch-Nyhan

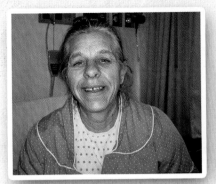

**PLATE 1:**
Acromegaly (Courtesy of Matthew C. Leinung, M.D., Acting Head, Division of Endocrinology, Albany Medical College, Albany, NY)

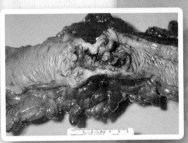

**PLATE 2:**
Adenocarcinoma of the colon (Courtesy of the CDC, Dr. Edwin P. Ewing, Jr.)

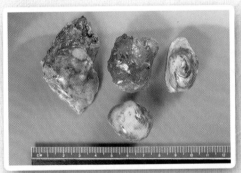

**PLATE 3:**
Alveolar hydatid disease in lung tissue (Courtesy of the CDC, Dr. Kagan)

**PLATE 4:**
Extraintestinal amebiasis involving the right flank (Courtesy of the CDC)

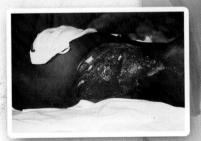

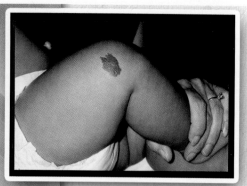

**PLATE 5:**
Angioma

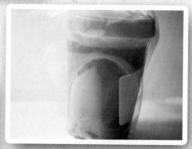

**PLATE 6:**
Rice-water stool due to cholera

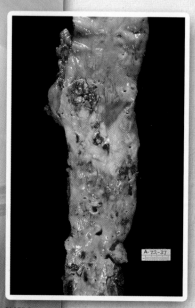

**PLATE 7:**
Atherosclerosis of the aorta (Courtesy of
the CDC, Dr. Edwin P. Ewing, Jr.)

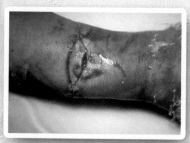

**PLATE 8:**
Wound botulism involvement of a compound
fracture of the right ulna (Courtesy of the CDC)

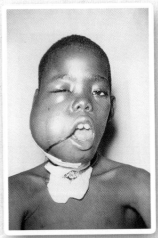

**PLATE 9:**
Facial tumor due to malignant
Burkitt's lymphoma (Courtesy of
the CDC, Robert S. Craig)

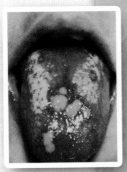

**PLATE 10:**
Thrush on the tongue

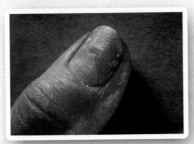

**PLATE 11:**
Fungal Candidiasis infection of the
fingernail (Courtesy of the CDC)

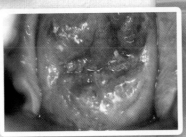

**PLATE 12:**
Cervical carcinoma (Courtesy of the CDC)

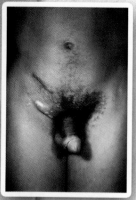

**PLATE 13:**
Chancroid infection (Courtesy of the CDC, Renelle Woodball)

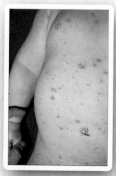

**PLATE 14:**
Chickenpox (Courtesy of Robert A. Silverman, M.D., Pediatric Dermatology, Georgetown University)

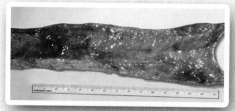

**PLATE 15:**
Typhoid fever cholecystitis with an ulceration and perforation of the gallbladder into the intestine (Courtesy of the CDC and the Armed Forces Institute of Pathology, Charles N. Farmer)

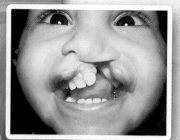

**PLATE 16:**
Cleft lip (Courtesy of Dr. Joseph Konzelman, School of Dentistry, Medical College of Georgia)

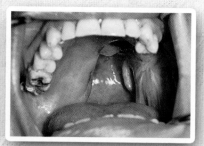

**PLATE 17:**
Cleft palate (Courtesy of Dr. Joseph Konzelman, School of Dentistry, Medical College of Georgia)

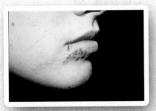

**PLATE 18:**
Cold sores (Courtesy of Robert A.
Silverman, M.D., Pediatric Dermatology,
Georgetown University)

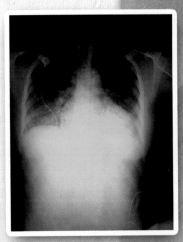

**PLATE 19:**
Congestive heart failure in a 28-year-old female
due to chronic high blood pressure
(Courtesy of the CDC, Dr. Thomas Hooten)

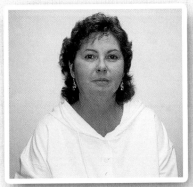

**PLATE 20:**
Cushing's syndrome (Courtesy of Matthew
C. Leinung, M.D., Acting Head, Division of
Endocrinology, Albany Medical College,
Albany, NY)

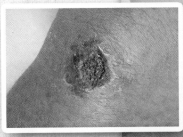

**PLATE 21:**
Skin lesion on the forearm due to
cutaneous anthrax (Courtesy of the CDC)

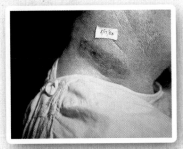

**PLATE 22:**
Skin lesion on the neck due to cutaneous
anthrax (Courtesy of the CDC)

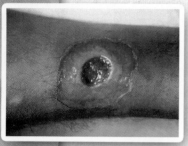

**PLATE 23:**
Diphtheria skin lesion on the leg
(Courtesy of the CDC)

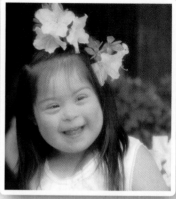

**PLATE 24:**
Down syndrome (Courtesy of Marijane
Scott, Marijane's Designer Portraits,
*Down Right Beautiful 1996 Calendar*)

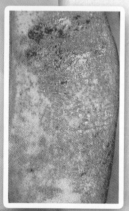

**PLATE 25:**
Eczema (Courtesy of the CDC)

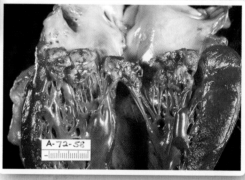

**PLATE 26:**
Bacterial infection of the lining of the heart
(Courtesy of the CDC, Dr. Edwin P. Ewing, Jr.)

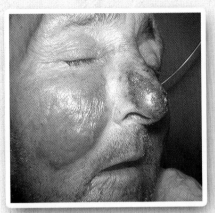

**PLATE 27:**
Facial erysipelas (Courtesy of the CDC)

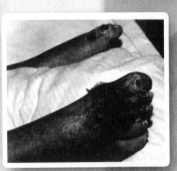

**PLATE 28:**
Gas gangrene

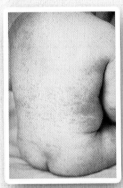

**PLATE 29:**
German measles (Courtesy of
the CDC)

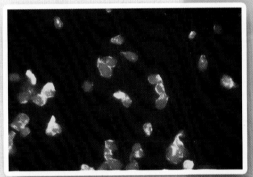

**PLATE 30:**
*Giardia lamblia* parasites using indirect immunofluorescence
test (Courtesy of the CDC, Dr. Visvesvara)

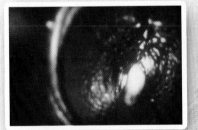

**PLATE 31:**
Discharge from penis due to gonorrhea
(Courtesy of the CDC, Susan Lindsley)

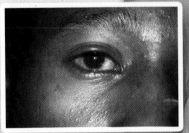

**PLATE 32:**
Gonorrheal infection of the eye
(Courtesy of the CDC, Joe Miller)

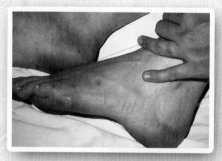

**PLATE 33:**
Foot lesions due to gonorrhea infection (Courtesy of the CDC, J. Pledger, Dr. S.E. Thompson, VDCD)

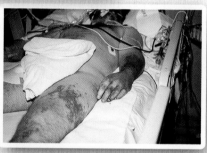

**PLATE 34:**
Purpura (Courtesy of Dr. Mark Dougherty, Lexington, Ky.)

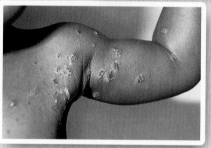

**PLATE 35:**
Impetigo (Courtesy of Robert A. Silverman, M.D., Pediatric Dermatology, Georgetown University)

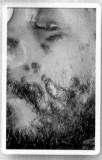

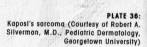

**PLATE 36:**
Kaposi's sarcoma (Courtesy of Robert A. Silverman, M.D., Pediatric Dermatology, Georgetown University)

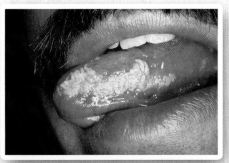

**PLATE 37:**
Hairy leukoplakia (Courtesy of the CDC, J.S. Greenspan, B.D.S., University of California, San Francisco; Sol Silverman, Jr., D.D.S.)

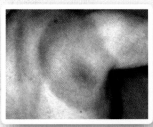

**PLATE 38:**
Bull's eye rash due to Lyme disease (Courtesy of the CDC)

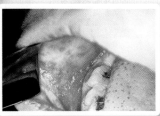

**PLATE 39:**
Koplik's spots in the mouth due to measles (Courtesy of the CDC)

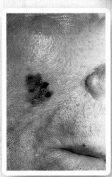

**PLATE 40:**
Malignant melanoma (Courtesy of Robert A. Silverman, M.D., Pediatric Dermatology, Georgetown University)

**PLATE 41:**
Four-month-old child with gangrene due to meningococcemia (Courtesy of the CDC, Mr. Gust)

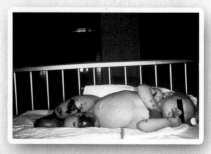

**PLATE 42:**
Mucormycosis, fungal infection of the eye (Courtesy of the CDC, Dr. Thomas F. Sellers, Emory University)

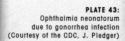

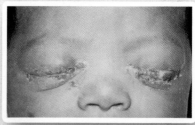

**PLATE 43:**
Ophthalmia neonatorum due to gonorrhea infection (Courtesy of the CDC, J. Pledger)

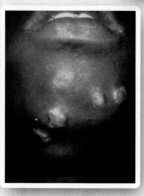

**PLATE 44:**
Papilloma on the chin (Courtesy of the CDC, Dr. Peter Perine)

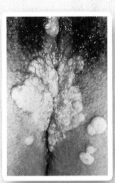

**PLATE 45:**
Genital warts
(Courtesy of the CDC)

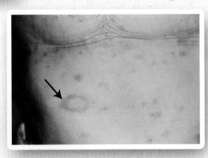

**PLATE 46:**
Pityriasis rosea patch
on the abdomen
(Courtesy of the CDC)

**PLATE 47:**
An axillary bubo in a person with plague
(Courtesy of the CDC, Margaret Parsons,
Dr. Karl F. Meyer)

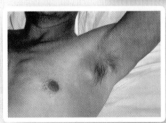

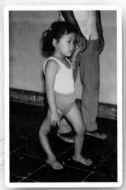

**PLATE 48:**
Deformity of the right leg due to poliovirus infection
(Courtesy of the CDC)

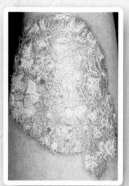

**PLATE 49:**
Psoriasis (Courtesy of Robert A. Silverman, M.D., Pediatric Dermatology, Georgetown University)

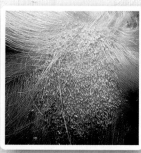

**PLATE 50:**
Cradle cap (Courtesy of Robert A. Silverman, M.D., Pediatric Dermatology, Georgetown University)

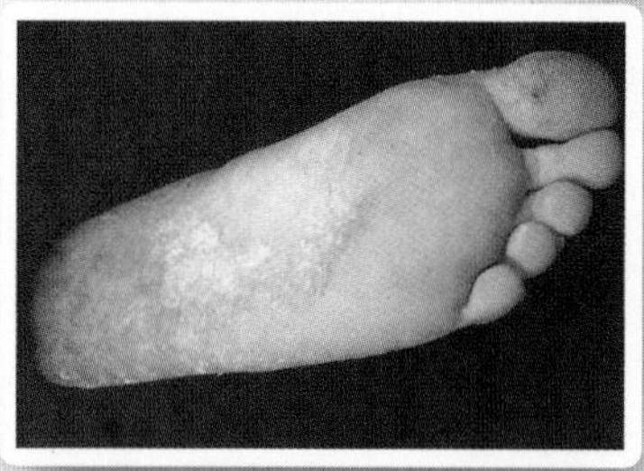

**PLATE 51:**
Athlete's foot (Courtesy of the CDC)

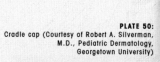

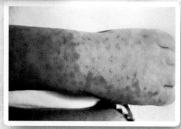

**PLATE 52:**
Rocky Mountain spotted fever rash (Courtesy of the CDC)

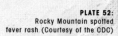

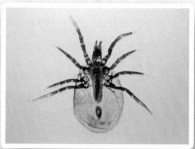

**PLATE 53:**
Mite (Courtesy of the CDC)

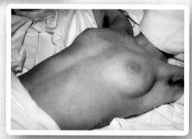

**PLATE 54:**
Scarlet fever rash
(Courtesy of the CDC)

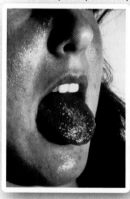

**PLATE 55:**
Strawberry tongue due to scarlet fever
(Courtesy of the CDC)

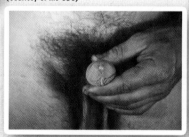

**PLATE 56:**
Epidermoid cyst occluding the urethra
(Courtesy of the CDC, William R.Smart,
San Rafael, California/Susan Lindsley)

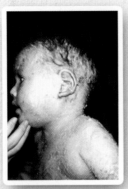

**PLATE 57:**
Seborrheic dermatitis
(Courtesy of the CDC, Susan Lindsley)

**PLATE 58:**
Shingles (Courtesy of Robert A.
Silverman, M.D., Pediatric Dermatology,
Georgetown University)

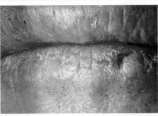
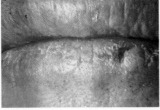

**PLATE 59:**
Squamous cell carcinoma on the lower
lip (Courtesy of Dr. Joseph Konzelman,
School of Dentistry, Medical College
of Georgia)

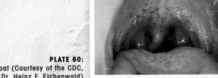

**PLATE 60:**
Strep throat (Courtesy of the CDC,
Dr. Heinz F. Eichenwald)

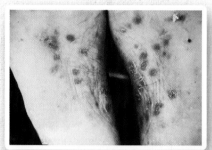

**PLATE 61:**
Rash on the feet during secondary stage of syphilis (Courtesy of the CDC, Dr. Gavin Hart)

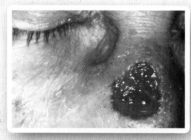

**PLATE 62:**
Gumma on the nose of a person in tertiary stage of syphilis (Courtesy of the CDC, J. Pledger)

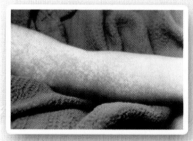

**PLATE 63:**
Rash on the arm 3 to 5 days after onset of Toxic Shock Syndrome (Courtesy of the CDC)

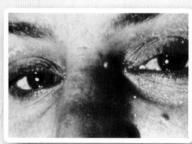

**PLATE 64:**
Infection in the eyes due to Toxic Shock Syndrome (Courtesy of the CDC)

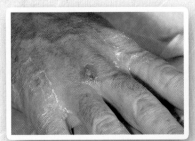

**PLATE 65:**
Tularemia lesion on the hand
(Courtesy of the CDC, Dr. Brachman)

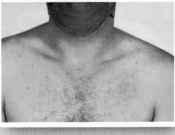

**PLATE 66:**
Rose spots on the chest due to
typhoid fever (Courtesy of the CDC,
Armed Forces Institute of Pathology,
Charles N. Farmer)

**PLATE 67:**
Swelling due to nephrosis
(Courtesy of the CDC,
Dr. Myron Schultz)

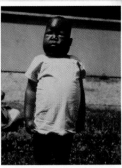

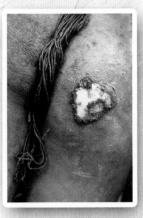

**PLATE 68:**
Yaws lesion on the buttocks of a 13-year-old girl
(Courtesy of the CDC, Clement Benjamin)

syndrome is also characterized by chewing off fingertips and lips. The excess uric acid levels cause goutlike swelling in the joints and renal dysfunction.

## Treatment

No specific treatment exists for Lesch-Nyhan syndrome. Allopurinol decreases the uric acid concentrations, but it has no effect on the neurological outcome.

Some symptoms may be relieved with the drugs carbidopa/levodopa, diazepam, phenobarbital, or haloperidol. Baclofen and tizanidine may also be helpful. The gene responsible for the production of HGP can now be cloned. The outcome is poor, even with attempts to treat the condition.

## Testing

The carrier state of the mother may be determined by culture of skin fibroblasts. Half the fibroblasts will have normal levels of the HGP enzyme and the remaining half will have deficient or absent HGP. Genetic tests of the HPRT gene may indicate the mutation.

## LEUKEMIA

### Description

Leukemia is a cancer of the white blood cells or the tissues that synthesize white blood cells. The types of white blood cells are described in Figure 2-47. The primary sign of leukemia is a white blood cell count elevated 10 to 100 times that of the normal range. Leukemia is more frequent in combination with Down syndrome, exposure to radiation, or among persons being treated aggressively with chemotherapy. Leukemia is categorized by its acute or chronic nature, and by the type of white blood cell affected. The four major forms of leukemia are acute myelocytic leukemia (AML); acute lymphocytic leukemia (ALL); chronic myeloid leukemia (CML); and, chronic lymphocytic leukemia (CLL).

### Signs and Symptoms

Each form of leukemia has its own disease characteristics, but, in general, immature blood cells multiply at the cost of normal blood cells. As the normal blood cells are depleted, anemia, infection, hemorrhage, and death occur.

### Treatment

Although each form of leukemia is treated differently at different stages of disease, the typical treatments for leukemia are chemotherapy and radiation. Treatment may also include bone marrow transplant, blood transfusions, or platelet transfusions. Without treatment, leukemia is fatal.

### Testing

Tests included in the diagnosis of leukemia include a CBC, bone marrow aspiration, tests for the presence of the Philadelphia chromosome, and tests for leukocyte alkaline phosphatase levels.

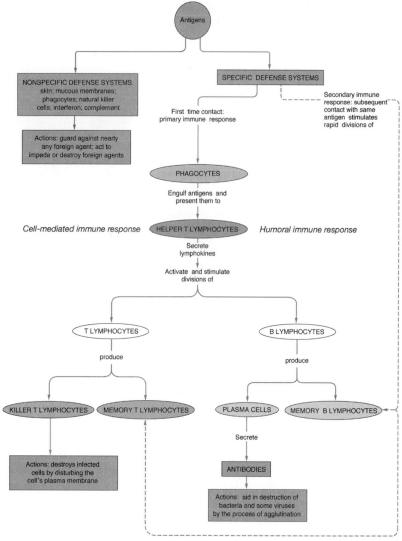

**Figure 2-47** Immune system defenses

## LEUKOPLAKIA

### Description

Leukoplakia is a precancerous lesion of the tongue, the female external genitalia, or inside the cheek. Leukoplakia is caused by chronic irritation, which may result from rough teeth or rough places on dentures, fillings, or crowns, especially among the elderly (Grund, 2004d). Pipe smoking increases the risk of leukoplakia. Chewing tobacco or snuff use also increases risk. Approximately 3 percent of leukoplakia lesions develop cancerous changes. Hairy leukoplakia of the mouth is an unusual form of leukoplakia among HIV-positive individuals, consisting of fuzzy white patches on the tongue resembling thrush. Hairy leukoplakia may be one of the first signs of infection with HIV (see Color Plate 37).

## Signs and Symptoms

The primary symptom of leukoplakia is a skin lesion on the tongue or inside of the cheek. The lesion is usually white or gray, although, in cases of erythroplakia, it may be red. The lesions are thick, slightly raised, and have a hard surface. In contrast, the lesions associated with hairy leukoplakia are painless, fuzzy, white patches on the tongue.

## Treatment

The treatment of leukoplakia begins with removal of the source of irritation. Surgical removal of the lesion may be necessary.

## Testing

An oral brush biopsy of the lesion confirms diagnosis in cases of leukoplakia. Using this computer-assisted tool, a pathologist can detect 1 or 2 abnormal cells in several hundred thousand in the epithelium (Scully, 2005).

## LICHEN PLANUS

### Description

Lichen planus is a disorder of the skin and mucous membranes resulting in inflammation, itching, and distinctive skin lesions (Chuang & Stittle, 2003; Lehrer, 2003b). The exact cause is unknown, and lichen planus is an immune reaction after exposure to allergens such as medications, dyes, and chemicals. Symptoms are increased with changes in the immune system during stress. Lichen planus may last for weeks to months, resolve, then recur for years. Lichen planus may be associated with several other disorders, most notably hepatitis C. Chemicals or medications associated with development of lichen planus include gold (used to treat rheumatoid arthritis), antibiotics, arsenic, iodides, chloroquine, quinacrine, quinidine, antimony, phenothiazines, and diuretics such as chlorothiazide. The rash usually appears on the mucous membranes, upper extremities, or on the genitals.

### Signs and Symptoms

Lichen planus is characterized by symmetric lesions on the wrist, legs, torso, or genitals. The lesions itch, may be singular or clustered, are approximately two to four centimeters in size, and have sharp borders. The bumps become clustered into a plaque or large, flat-topped groups. They may be covered with fine, white streaks or linear scratch marks called Wickham's striae. The lesions are shiny, scaly, dark colored, and may blister or ulcerate. Lesions on the skin are purple; mouth lesions are gray. Other symptoms include nail abnormalities, dry mouth, metallic taste in the mouth, and hair loss.

## Treatment

If symptoms of lichen planus are mild, no treatment may be needed. Other treatment may include antihistamines, lidocaine mouth washes, corticosteroids (e.g., triamcinolone acetonide cream or prednisone), retinoic acid cream (a form of vitamin A), and ultraviolet light therapy.

## Testing

Lichen planus is diagnosed by the physical appearance of the lesions. A tissue biopsy may help confirm diagnosis. Immunofluorescence studies indicate globular deposits of immunoglobulin M.

## LISTERIOSIS

## Description

*Listeria monocytogenes* is a gram-positive, non–spore-forming bacillus, which is a foodborne pathogen (Smith, 2003e). Listeriosis is usually a mild, symptomless disease in healthy adults. Among those with compromised immune system function, however, it can be fatal. *L. monocytogenes* is capable of surviving within the white blood cells even after it has been engulfed by them. The bacillus can move from one macrophage to a neighboring macrophage, and infection frequently leads to fatal meningitis (Listeriosis, 2003).

   *L. monocytogenes* thrives at refrigerator temperatures and has been isolated from a variety of foods, including raw milk, cheese made from unpasteurized milk, hot dogs, and prepackaged meat products. Because *L. monocytogenes* is shed in the feces of infected animals, it is widely found in soil and water. Among infected pregnant women, there is a fetal mortality rate of 60 percent. Uterine infection may also result in a high rate of spontaneous abortion and stillbirths.

## Signs and Symptoms

Listeriosis is characterized by fever and chills, nausea, and, if the infection spreads to the nervous system, headache, stiff neck, confusion, loss of balance, and convulsions. Pregnant women may experience only mild, flulike illness, but the infection can lead to miscarriage, stillbirth, or serious health problems for her newborn child. The incubation period for listeriosis is approximately three weeks.

## Treatment

Antibiotics used in the treatment of listeriosis include ampicillin, gentamicin, and trimethoprim-sulfamethoxazole. Infection of the fetus with *L. monocytogenes* results in a poor outcome with approximately a 50 percent death rate, and the late infant onset form also has a high death rate. Healthy older children and adults have a lower death rate.

## Testing

Tests used in the diagnosis of listeriosis include cultures of amniotic fluid, blood cultures, clean catch urine cultures, and cerebrospinal fluid cultures.

# LIVER CANCER

## Description

Hepatocellular carcinoma sometimes begins as a single tumor that grows by expanding, and only metastasizes to the rest of the liver late in the disease (Grund, 2004a). Another form of hepatocellular carcinoma begins as many tumors that spread tentacle-like growths throughout the liver, almost from the beginning of their formation. This form of liver cancer is most common among individuals with liver cirrhosis. Another form of liver cancer is cholangiocarcinoma, which starts in the bile ducts within the liver. The risk of developing cholangiocarcinoma is higher in the presence of gallstones, gallbladder inflammation, or chronic ulcerative colitis.

Most liver cancers do not originate in the liver; they spread from cancers in other places in the body. These tumors are named after their primary site. The liver is a common site of secondary metastasis of cancer because the blood is filtered by the liver. When the liver filters out the spreading malignant cells, the cells grow within the liver causing the formation of secondary malignant tumors.

## Signs and Symptoms

Liver cancer is characterized by abdominal pain or tenderness in the right-upper quadrant, enlarged abdomen, easy bruising, easy bleeding, and jaundice.

## Treatment

Chemotherapy and radiation are not usually effective in the treatment of liver cancer, although they may be used to shrink large tumors prior to surgery. Liver transplant may also be a treatment option. Under 20 percent of hepatocellular carcinomas can be removed completely using surgery, and liver cancer is fatal within three to six months, if the cancer cannot be completely removed.

## Testing

Tests used in the diagnosis of liver cancer may include liver biopsy, serum alpha fetoprotein levels, abdominal CT scan, tests of liver enzyme levels, urine porphyrins, PBG, serum and urine leucine aminopeptidase level tests, gallbladder radionuclide scan, delta-ALA tests, urine tests for bilirubin levels, AST, ALT, Alpha-1 antitrypsin, and 5'-N'Tase tests.

# LOBAR PNEUMONIA

## Description

The most common cause of bacterial pneumonia is *Streptococcus pneumonia*. Lobar pneumonia is isolated to the individual lobe of the lung where the infection occurs, although it can become systemic. If two lobes are involved, the resultant infection is known as double pneumonia. Lobar pneumonia is not usually a primary infection, rather it results from disturbance of the normal defense barriers of the body. Predisposing conditions include

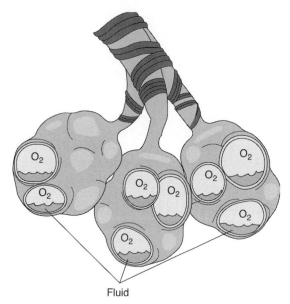

Fluid

**Figure 2-48** Lung alveoli fill with fluids.

alcoholism, anesthesia, malnutrition, and viral infection of the respiratory system. Lobar pneumonia involves the bronchi and the alveoli where fluids are produced (Figure 2-48). The local production of fluid in the alveoli contributes to the infection's localization within the lobe of the lung.

## Signs and Symptoms
Lobar pneumonia is characterized by acute onset fever, chills, difficulty breathing, chest pain, and coughing up blood. In addition, rapid respiration, abnormal breathing sounds via percussions on the chest wall, and crackles heard through a stethoscope are characteristic signs of pneumonia.

## Treatment
There is a vaccine available for pneumococcal pneumonia, used primary for the elderly. Treatment may also include steroid medications, antibiotics, or respiratory treatments.

## Testing
Tests used in the diagnosis of pneumonia include chest X-rays, sputum cultures, CBC, thoracic CT scan, pulmonary ventilation/perfusion scan, and pleural fluid culture.

## LUNG ABSCESS

### Description
A lung abscess is an area of inflamed, pus-filled tissue in the lung caused by infection. A lung abscess is usually caused by bacteria that have been inhaled from the nose and mouth, resulting in an infection. Periodontal

gum diseases are frequently the cause of a lung abscess. A lung abscess may also be associated with a tumor in the lung, or it may be associated with pneumonia. Although most people develop only one lung abscess, multiple lung abscesses have been noted in IV drug users who use contaminated needles. In these cases, the infection begins at the site of injection and spreads to the lungs through the blood.

## Signs and Symptoms

A lung abscess will eventually rupture, causing the formation of a cavity filled with fluid and air in the lung. The rupture of an abscess produces a large quantity of pus, fluid, and blood that is coughed up and expectorated. If the lung abscess ruptures into the pleural space, pus may fill the space causing empyema. Symptoms of a lung abscess may include cough, fever, loss of appetite, and weight loss. Foul-smelling sputum is also present in about half of the cases of lung abscess, but it is not always present because anaerobic infections do not produce a foul smell.

## Treatment

Traditionally penicillin alone was used, but there is now an increasing incidence of penicillin resistance in oropharyngeal anaerobes. Metronidazole alone has also failed due to lack of activity against micro-aerophilic streptococci. Clindamycin is the most popular antimicrobial for treatment of lung abscesses; beta-lactams and imipenem are also used against anaerobes.

## Testing

Tests for the presence of a lung abscess may include needle aspiration biopsy, open lung biopsy, tissue culture, fluid culture, and imaging exams of the chest.

## LUNG CANCER

## Description

Lung cancers are divided into two categories, labeled small-cell lung cancer and nonsmall-cell lung cancer. Small-cell carcinomas, which are also known as oat cell carcinomas, grow rapidly and spread quickly. The other type of lung cancer is nonsmall-cell cancers, which are categorized into squamous cell carcinoma, adenocarcinoma, and large-cell carcinoma (Green, 2003).

Lung cancer is rarely found in its early development because early-stage disease generally produces few, if any, symptoms. The lungs are especially well-supplied by the blood and lymph system, which promotes the spread of cancer. Although smoking accounts for the vast majority of lung cancer cases, exposure to certain compounds increases risk. These include asbestos, bischloromethyl ether and chloromethyl ether, chromium, beryllium, and arsenic (Fretz & Hughes, 2003).

## Signs and Symptoms

The characteristics of lung cancer may include difficulty breathing, hoarseness, coughing, coughing up blood, pneumonia, bronchitis, wheezing, swelling of the face or neck, headache, fever, and pain in the chest, shoulder, or arm.

## Treatment

Most patients with stage I and II nonsmall-cell tumors, and some patients with stage III tumors, can undergo surgery with the goal of being cured. Stage IV means the cancer has spread to other sites in the body (e.g., bone, brain, liver) and is usually not curable. Treatment consists of chemotherapy, radiation, or surgery.

## Testing

Tests used to diagnose lung cancer include imaging exams of the chest, bronchoscopy with washing and biopsy, pleural biopsy, open lung biopsy, CAT scan directed needle biopsy, and mediastinoscopy with biopsy.

## LUPUS ERYTHEMATOSUS

### Description

Lupus erythematosus is a chronic, inflammatory, autoimmune disorder that may affect many organ systems including the skin, joints, and internal organs (Lamont, 2001; Peng, 2004c). In cases of lupus, the body's defenses are turned against itself and immune cells attack healthy tissues. Although the cause of autoimmune diseases is unknown, researchers suspect it occurs following infection with an organism that looks similar to particular proteins in the body. Lupus affects nine times as many women as men, and African Americans and Asians are affected most often.

### Signs and Symptoms

Symptoms may include fever, fatigue, weight loss, a butterfly rash covering the face, aggravation of the rash by sunlight, sensitivity to sunlight, arthritis, swollen glands, muscle pain, nausea, vomiting, pleuritic chest pain, seizures, and psychosis. Other symptoms may include bloody urine, coughing up blood, nosebleed, difficulty swallowing, skin rash, Raynaud's phenomenon, mouth sores, hair loss, abdominal pain, and vision disturbances.

### Treatment

There is no cure for lupus. Treatment may include NSAID and corticosteroids. Antimalarial drugs (hydroxychloroquine) are used to treat arthritis. Cytotoxic drugs (drugs that block cell growth) may be used in resistant cases of lupus. The 10-year survival rate for lupus patients exceeds 85 percent. People with severe involvement of the brain, lungs, heart, and kidney have the worst prognosis.

### Testing

The diagnosis of lupus is based upon the presence of at least 4 out of 11 characteristics of the disease. Tests may include antinuclear antibody panel, chest X-rays, urinalysis, CBC, kidney biopsy, and neurological exams. Other tests for lupus may include serum globulin electrophoresis, rheumatoid factor, protein electrophoresis, mononucleosis spot tests, ESR, cryoglubulins, Coomb's test, complement component 3, antithyroid micro-somal antibody, antithyroglobulin antibody, antimitochondrial antibody, and anti-smooth muscle antibody.

## LYME DISEASE

### Description

Lyme disease, or Lyme borreliosis, is caused by the gram-negative, highly flexible bacterial spirochete *Borrelia burgdorferi* (Kotton, 2003b). Lyme disease is named after Lyme, Connecticut, which is the geographic location in which it was first reported in the United States. All *Borrelia* are arthropod-borne, and *B. burgdorferi* is transmitted by ticks. Other insects may also harbor the spirochete. Nymphs, which are young ticks, transmit the disease directly into human tissue by regurgitating during feeding. Lyme disease occurs most frequently in the summer, when more people are outdoors (Lyme disease, 2001).

### Signs and Symptoms

Infection with *B. burgdorferi* causes a characteristic bull's-eye rash at the site of the bite (see Color Plate 38). About 60 percent of those infected exhibit this bull's eye rash, which is technically known as erythema migrans (EM). As the rash fades, flulike symptoms appear. If the disease enters a late stage, a pacemaker may be required to control damage caused to the heart. The nervous system may also become involved leading to paralysis of the face, meningitis, and encephalitis. Arthritis often accompanies cases of Lyme disease. Long-term Lyme disease cases resemble the later stages of syphilis, which is caused by a spirochete of the same family as *B. burgdorferi*.

### Treatment

Attached ticks should be removed immediately because pathogen transmission is related to the length of attachment. Antibiotics are prescribed based on disease stages and manifestations. Doxycycline, tetracycline, cefuroxime, ceftriaxone, and penicillin are some of the choices.

### Testing

Tests used in the diagnosis of Lyme disease include a test for antibodies to *B. burgdorferi* by immunofluorescence (IFA) or ELISA. ELISA tests are confirmed with a Western blot test.

## LYMPHADENITIS

### Description

Lymphadenitis is an infection of the lymph nodes (Levy, 2003e; Shaikh, 2003). A healthy lymph node is illustrated in Figure 2-49. Lymphadenitis may occur if the glands are overwhelmed by microorganisms, or it may occur as a result of circulating cancer cells. It commonly is a result of a cellulitis or other bacteria infection, usually infection by streptococci or staphylococci.

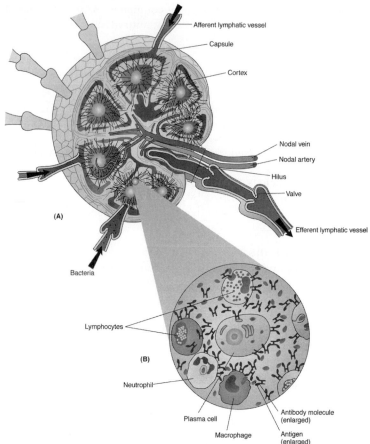

**Figure 2-49** (A) Section through a lymph node, showing the flow of lymph. (B) Microscopic detail of bacteria being destroyed within the lymph node.

## Signs and Symptoms

Lymphadenitis is characterized by swelling, tenderness, and hardening of the lymph nodes. They may feel smooth or irregular to touch, or soft and rubbery. Signs of inflammation (e.g., heat, redness, loss of function, pain, swelling) are also present.

## Treatment

Lymphadenitis may spread within hours. Treatment should begin promptly with antibiotics, when bacterial infection is diagnosed.

## Testing

Tests used to diagnose lymphadenitis may include blood cultures and a biopsy and tissue culture of the affected area.

## LYMPHADENOPATHY

### Description

The enlargement of lymph nodes is known as lymphadenopathy. The increased size is caused by proliferation of lymphocytes and leukocytes within the node or by the presence of a tumor in the node. Most frequently, lymphadenopathy occurs as a result of infections. Lymphadenopathy may also be due to cancer, inflammation of the thyroid, autoimmune diseases, or drug reactions. Lymphadenopathy is more common in young children because their immune systems are responding more frequently to newly encountered infections. In the United States, some possible causes of lymphadenopathy include infectious mononucleosis, cytomegalovirus infections, upper respiratory infections, and HIV infection. Internationally, however, lymphadenopathy is more commonly due to tuberculosis, typhoid fever, trypanosomiasis, schistosomiasis, and fungal infections.

### Signs and Symptoms

The most prominent sign of severe lymphadenopathy is extreme swelling in the lymph nodes.

### Treatment

Treatment is dependent upon the cause of the underlying disease.

### Testing

Diagnosis of lymphadenopathy is based on the physical exam, lab studies, and imaging exams to identify the underlying cause of the lymphadenopathy.

## LYMPHANGITIS

### Description

Lymphangitis is an inflammatory disorder of the lymph vessels, characterized by local and systemic pain. Lymphangitis results from a bacterial infection of the skin known as cellulites or from a skin abscess. The presence of lymphangitis suggests that an infection is progressing, and that bacteria may have migrated to the bloodstream. This fatal condition may be confused with blood clots in the veins of the legs.

### Signs and Symptoms

Lymphangitis is characterized by red streaks extending from the infected area to the axilla or groin, throbbing pain along the affected area, fever and chills, loss of appetite, headache, and muscle aches.

### Treatment

Lymphangitis may spread within hours, and antibiotic treatment should begin immediately. An abscess may require surgical drainage.

### Testing

Tests used to diagnose lymphangitis may include blood cultures and a biopsy and tissue culture of the affected area.

## LYMPHOCYTIC CHORIOMENINGITIS

### Description

Lymphocytic choriomeningitis is a rodent-borne, viral disease caused by the lymphocytic choriomeningitis virus, and the disease is characterized by meningitis, encephalitis, or meningoencephalitis. Although it is commonly recognizable as a neurological disease, it may also be present without symptoms or only as a mild febrile illness. Lymphocytic choriomeningitis is spread by the common house mouse, and, once infected, mice can become chonic carriers of the virus. The virus spreads to humans through inhalation of particles of infected rodent urine, feces, or saliva. Infection may also occur through ingestion of contaminated food or through contact with contaminated human body fluids (*Lymphocytic choriomeningitis*, 2004).

### Signs and Symptoms

The initial phase of illness begins with fever, malaise, loss of appetite, muscle pain, headache, nausea, and vomiting. Other less frequent symptoms may include sore throat, cough, joint pain, chest pain, testicular pain, and parotid pain. After a few days' remission, the second phase occurs, consisting of disease conditions of meningitis (e.g., fever, headache, stiff neck) or characteristics of encephalitis (e.g., drowsiness, confusion, sensory disturbances, and motor abnormalities, such as paralysis).

### Treatment

Lymphocytic choriomeningitis is rarely fatal. Aseptic meningitis, encephalitis, or meningoencephalitis requires hospitalization and supportive treatment. There is no specific drug therapy for lymphocytic choriomeningitis. Anti-inflammatory drugs, such as corticosteroids, may be considered.

### Testing

During the first phase of the disease, the most common laboratory abnormalities are a low white blood cell count (leukopenia) and a low platelet count (thrombocytopenia). Liver enzymes in the serum may also be mildly elevated. After the onset of neurological disease during the second phase, an increase in protein levels, an increase in the number of white blood cells, or a decrease in the glucose levels in the cerebrospinal fluid is usually found.

## LYMPHOGRANULOMA VENEREUM

### Description

*Chlamydia trachomatis* causes a sexually transmitted disease known as lymphogranuloma venereum (Levy, 2004k). There are between 4 million and 10 million new cases each year. Teenage girls have the highest rates of lymphogranuloma venereum infection; 15- to 19-year-old girls represent 46 percent of infections, and 20- to 24-year-old women represent another 33 percent. Approximately 75 percent of women and 50 percent of men with lymphogranuloma venereum are asymptomatic and fail to seek treatment. Untreated, chlamydia causes pelvic inflammatory disease, which may result in infertility and birth defects. Chlamydial infections also increase the chance of becoming infected with HIV if exposed. Untreated chlamydia in men typically causes urethral infection, but may also result in complications such as swollen and tender testicles (Chlamydia in the United States, 2001).

## Signs and Symptoms

Lymphogranuloma venereum appears 7 to 12 days after exposure when a blister appears on the genitals. This vesicle ruptures and heals painlessly. In one to eight weeks, the regional lymph nodes enlarge and may become infected with pus. Other symptoms may include inflammation of the skin over the inguinal lymph nodes, bleeding from the rectum, and pain during bowel movements.

## Treatment

Medications used in the treatment of lymphogranuloma venereum may include tetracycline, doxycycline, and erythromycin.

## Testing

Tests used to diagnose lymphogranuloma venereum include biopsy of the node, culture of a node aspirate for chlamydia, indirect immunofluorescence for chlamydia, and serology tests for lymphogranuloma venereum.

## MACULAR DEGENERATION

## Description

Macular degeneration is a disorder that affects the central part of the retina of the eye, which is known as the macula, causing decreased visual acuity and possible loss of central vision (Pons, 2001). The macula allows the eye to see fine details at the center of the field of vision. Degeneration results from a partial breakdown of the retinal pigment epithelium, which is the insulating layer between the retina and the choroid, which is the layer of blood vessels behind the retina. There are two types of macular degeneration: dry and wet. The dry form is characterized by small yellow spots. The wet form is caused by the abnormal growth of blood vessels that leak fluids into the eye. By age 75, almost 15 percent of people will develop macular degeneration, which may be associated with family history, cigarette smoking, and being Caucasian (Feinberg, 2004c).

## Signs and Symptoms

Macular degeneration is characterized by blurred vision, distored vision, dimmed vision, and absent central vision. Although macular degeneration causes central vision loss, it does not lead to complete blindness because it does not affect peripheral vision.

## Treatment

Macular degeneration may be treated with laser photocoagulation, which reduces leakage from choroidal blood vessels. Photodynamic therapy is another form of treatment, in which a light-sensitive medication called

Visudyne (verteporfin) is injected into a vein in the patient's arm. The drug circulates through the body to the eyes. When a nonthermal laser is shone into the eyes, Visudyne produces a chemical reaction that destroys abnormal blood vessels.

## Testing

Tests used in the diagnosis of macular degeneration may include tests of visual acuity, refraction tests, papillary reflex response, slit lamp examination, retinal exams, retinal photography, fluorescein angiography, indocyanine green angiography, and Amsler grid tests.

## MALABSORPTION SYNDROME

### Description

Malabsorption is a dysfunction in the digestion or absorption of nutrients from food substances, resulting from a variety of diseases (Frye & Tamer, 2002; Jonnalagadda, 2004a). Typically, malabsorption involves the failure to absorb specific sugars, fats, proteins, or vitamins. It can be caused by a disorder of the pancreas, enzyme deficiencies, an injury to the mucous lining of the intestine, and numerous infections.

### Signs and Symptoms

Malabsorption is characterized by the avoidance of specific foods, chronic diarrhea, bloating, flatulence, and growth failure in infants and children.

### Treatment

The treatments for malabsorption are dependent upon the underlying disease.

### Testing

Tests used in the diagnsosis and treatment of malabsorption are dependent upon the underlying disease.

## MALARIA

### Description

Malaria is a disease spread by the *Anopheles* mosquito, which is a biological vector. Malaria is caused by a protozoan of the genus *Plasmodium* (Levy, 2003f). The most common forms of malaria are caused by *P. falciparum, P. vivax, P. ovale,* and *P. malariae.* The mosquito carries the pathogen in its saliva and transmits it to the human host through its bite. Mosquito control in the United States has decreased the number of cases of malaria. Worldwide there are 300 million to 500 million people infected annually with malaria, resulting in about 3 million deaths each year (Malaria, 2002).

### Signs and Symptoms

Within 30 minutes of infection, the protozoon moves to the liver cells where it multiplies. Afterwards it reaches the red blood cells, where it multiplies again. When the infected red blood cells burst, the symptoms of chills and fever appear. These symptoms alternate every two to three days with asymptomatic periods. Malaria is characterized by chills and fever, headache, nausea, vomiting, muscle pain, anemia, blood stools, jaundice, convulsions, and coma.

## Treatment

Antimalarial drugs can be prescribed to people traveling to areas where malaria is prevalent. The types of antimalarial medications prescribed will depend on the drug-resistance patterns in the areas to be visited. According to the CDC, travelers going to South America, Africa, the Indian subcontinent, Asia, and the South Pacific should take mefloquine, doxycycline, chloroquine, hydroxychloroquine, or Malarone, which is a combination of atovaquone and proguanil. To treat active infections, chloroquine is the most common antimalarial medication, but quinidine or quinine, or the combination of pyrimethamine and sulfadoxine, are given for chloroquine-resistant infections. The outcome is positive in most cases of malaria with treatment, but poor in Falciparum infection with complications. Falciparum malaria, can be fatal within a few hours after the initial symptoms appear.

## Testing

Malaria is diagnosed based on physical examination revealing enlarged liver and enlarged spleen. Malaria blood smears taken at 6- to 12-hour intervals confirm the diagnosis.

## MARBURG HEMORRHAGIC FEVER

## Description

Marburg hemorrhagic fever is a rare disease affecting both humans and nonhuman primates caused by a genetically unique zoonotic RNA virus. Marburg virus belongs to the same family as the Ebola virus, and it was first recognized in 1967 during outbreaks of hemorrhagic fever in laboratories in Marburg and Frankfurt, Germany, and Belgrade, Serbia. The virus was transmitted from African green monkeys being used for polio vaccine research. Marburg virus is indigenous to Africa, and the actual animal host for Marburg virus remains unknown. Marburg hemorrhagic fever can spread through contact with infected persons (*Marburg hemorrhagic fever,* 2004).

## Signs and Symptoms

The symptoms of Marburg hemorrhagic fever begin with an acute onset of fever, chills, headache, and muscle pain. About the fifth day after the onset of symptoms, a maculopapular rash may appear prominently on the trunk of the body, along with nausea, vomiting, chest pain, sore throat, abdominal pain, and diarrhea. Symptoms may progress to jaundice, pancreatitis, severe weight loss, delirium, shock, liver failure, massive hemorrhaging, and multiorgan dysfunction.

## Treatment

There is no specific treatment available for Marburg hemorrhagic fever. Sometimes treatment may include transfusion of fresh-frozen plasma and other preparations to replace the blood proteins important in clotting. A controversial treatment is the use of heparin, which blocks clotting, to prevent the consumption of clotting factors. The fatality rate for Marburg hemorrhagic fever is about 25 percent, and recovery is prolonged and may be accompanied by orchitis, recurrent hepatitis, transverse myelitis, or uveitis.

## Testing

Antigen-capture enzyme-linked immunosorbent assay (ELISA) testing, IgM-capture ELISA, polymerase chain reaction (PCR), and virus isolation can be used to confirm a case of Marburg hemorrhagic fever within a few days of the onset of symptoms. The IgG-capture ELISA is appropriate for testing persons later in the course of disease or after recovery. The disease is readily diagnosed by immunohistochemistry, virus isolation, or PCR of blood or tissue specimens from deceased patients.

## MARFAN'S SYNDROME

### Description

Marfan's syndrome is a disorder of connective tissue affecting the skeletal system, cardiovascular system, eyes, and skin (H. Chen, 2003b; Stewart, 2003i). Marfan's syndrome is inherited via a mutation in the gene fibrillin-1 (FBN1) located on *chromosome* 15q21.1, which functions in the elastic tissue in the body. Marfan's syndrome results in changes in elastic tissues, particularly in the aorta, eye, and skin. Mutations in fibrillin-1 also result in tall stature and long limbs. Estimates suggest that 200,000 people in the United States have Marfan's syndrome.

### Signs and Symptoms

Marfan's patients exhibit a tall, lanky stature with long limbs and spider-like fingers, chest abnormalities, curvature of the spine, and a particular set of facial features, including a highly arched palate and crowded teeth. They may also experience nearsightedness and dislocation of the lens of the eye. Marfan's syndrome causes cardiovascular abnormalities, such as dilatation of the root of the aorta, aortic regurgitation, prolapse of the mitral valve, and a dissecting aortic aneurysm.

### Treatment

There is not a single, curative treatment for Marfan's syndrome. Lifespan is shortened in most cases of Marfan's syndrome due to cardiovascular complications. The survival rate is into the 60s, but may be extended with good care and heart surgery.

### Testing

Various tests may be used in the diagnosis and treatment of Marfan's syndrome, including echocardiogram, eye exams, and fibrillin-1 mutation testing. Imaging of the chest and pelvis is also performed. An aortograph may also be conducted.

## MASTOIDITIS

### Description

According to Newman (2003c) and Donaldson (2003), mastoiditis is an infection of the mastoid bone of the skull that is usually a consequence of a middle ear infection. If the infection spreads from the ear to the mastoid bone of the skull, the mastoid bone fills with infected materials and its honeycomb-like structure may deteriorate. Mastoiditis most commonly affects children, and, before antibiotics, was one of the leading causes of death in children. Now it is a relatively uncommon and much less dangerous disorder.

### Signs and Symptoms

Mastoiditis is characterized by earache, pain behind the ear, inflammation of the ear, fever, headache, and drainage from the ear.

### Treatment

Mastoiditis may be difficult to treat because the infection is deep within the mastoid bone. It is treated with antibiotics, and may require repeated treatments. Surgeries to remove part of the bone, drain the mastoid, or drain the middle ear through the eardrum (i.e., myringotomy) may be needed to treat the underlying middle ear infection.

### Testing

Tests used in the diagnosis and treatment of mastoiditis may include imaging tests of the head and cultures of ear drainage.

## McCUNE-ALBRIGHT SYNDROME

### Description

McCune-Albright syndrome was first described by Fuller Albright in 1937. This genetic disease is caused by a mutation in the *GNAS1* gene. The mutation causes the body to produce excess proteins from its endocrine glands, causing premature puberty in females. McCune-Albright syndrome causes bone disorders, hormone imbalance, and premature sexual development. The disease is not inherited, so it is not passed along to children. McCune-Albright syndrome is rare, with an estimate of less than 3 percent of the world's population exhibiting the disease (Stewart, 2004c; Uwaifo & Sarlis, 2004).

### Signs and Symptoms

McCune-Albright syndrome is characterized by fibrous tissue in the bones, which causes bone fractures, bone pain, and deformities. Abnormal growth of the skull can cause blindness and deafness due to nerve compression. Deformed facial bones and the presence of café-au-lait spots on the back are common signs of McCune-Albright syndrome.

## Treatment

There is no specific treatment for McCune-Albright syndrome. Drugs that inhibit estrogen production (e.g., testolactone) and surgery to remove the adrenal gland in cases of Cushing's syndrome associated with McCune-Albright syndrome may be required. Gigantism and pituitary adenoma may be treated with hormone inhibitors or surgery.

## Testing

Tests used in the diagnosis and treatment of McCune-Albright syndrome may indicate the presence of hyperthyroidism, hyperparathyroidism, excess adrenal hormones, or excess blood prolactin or growth hormone. X-rays show fibrous dysplasia of multiple bones, and an MRI of the head may show an adenoma in the pituitary gland. Genetic testing may be available for the *GNAS1* gene.

## MEASLES

### Description

Rubeola virus is the cause of a dermatropic disease known as measles, and Figure 2-50 pictures its effect on normal cells. Measles is extremely contagious and is spread via the respiratory route. Rubeola is similar to chickenpox and smallpox in its development. The infection spreads from the respiratory system after approximately 10 to 12 days, causing the same symptoms as the common cold. A rash appears on the face and spreads to the trunk and then the extremities. Approximately one week after the rash appears, encephalitis may develop in some cases of measles (Measles, n/d).

Before widespread immunization, measles was so common that most people had been infected by age 20. Measles cases dropped over the last

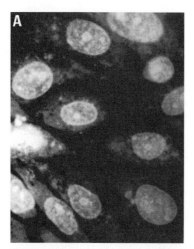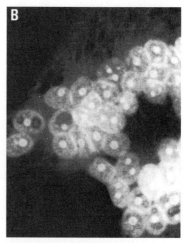

**Figure 2-50** (A) Normal cells. (B) Measles virus in cells. (Courtesy of Pfizer, Inc.)

several decades to virtually none in the United States and Canada because of widespread immunization. Rates are slowly rising because some parents refuse to vaccinate their children due to fears that the MMR vaccine causes autism (Banerjee, 2004b). The MMR vaccine protects against measles, mumps, and rubella, and large studies have found no connection between this vaccine and the development of autism. The danger to the public is that lower vaccination rates can cause serious outbreaks of measles, mumps, and rubella.

## Signs and Symptoms

Measles is a highly contagious viral illness characterized by a fever, cough, runny nose, muscle pain, bloodshot eyes, Koplik's spots inside the mouth (see Color Plate 39), photophobia, conjunctivitis, and a spreading rash. The rash appears around the fifth day of the disease and lasts about a week. It itches and usually begins on the head and spreads downward. Both flat, discolored areas and solid, red, elevated areas appear and later merge together.

## Treatment

There is no specific treatment of measles, though some children may require supplementation with vitamin A. Most cases of measles have an excellent outcome when treated, but pneumonia or encephalitis are possible complications.

## Testing

Tests for measles may include a measles serology or viral culture, although viral cultures are rarely done.

## MECKEL'S DIVERTICULUM

### Description

Meckel's diverticulum is a congenital disorder in which a small pouch called a diverticulum occurs in the wall of the small bowel (Molmenti, 2002; Shukla, 2002). The diverticulum may contain stomach or pancreatic tissue. Meckel's diverticulum is the result of remnants of structures within the fetal digestive tract not fully reabsorbing before birth.

### Signs and Symptoms

Meckel's diverticulum is characterized by diverticulitis and bleeding in the intestine. Symptoms include bloody stool, abdominal discomfort, and iron deficiency anemia. Symptoms often occur during the first few years of life but can occur in adults as well. Although 2 percent of the population has a Meckel's diverticulum, the majority are asymptomatic.

### Treatment

Surgery to remove Meckel's diverticulum is recommended if bleeding develops. Iron replacement may be needed to correct anemia, and blood transfusion may be necessary. Full recovery can be expected with surgery.

## Testing

Tests used in the diagnosis of Meckel's diverticulum include stool smears, hematocrit, hemoglobin, and technetium scans.

## MELANOMA

### Description

Melanoma is a serious form of skin cancer that begins in the melanocytes, which are the cells that make skin pigment called melanin (see Color Plate 40). Although melanoma accounts for about only 4 percent of all skin cancer cases, it causes most skin cancer–related deaths (Howard, 2003). The occurrence of melanoma is exacerbated by exposure to sunlight. Melanoma may occur in the skin, in the eye, and, rarely, in other areas where melanocytes are found, such as the digestive tract, meninges, or lymph nodes. Melanoma may metastasize, spreading cancer cells to the lymph nodes, liver, lungs, or brain.

### Signs and Symptoms

The signs of melanoma are as follows (Swetter, 2004):

- A notched border on a growth
- An asymmetric growth
- A growth that increases in size and appears brown, black, red, pink, or multicolored
- A mole that changes color, texture, shape, or grows larger than a pencil eraser
- A spot or growth that itches, hurts, crusts, scabs, erodes, or bleeds
- A sore that lasts for more than four weeks, or heals and then reopens
- A scaly bump that grows a projection similar to a small horn
- A diameter greater than 6 millimeters

There are four types of melanoma (Howard, 2003). Superficial spreading melanoma is flat and irregular in shape and color, with varying shades of black and brown. Nodular melanoma starts as a raised area that is dark blackish-blue or bluish-red, although some lack color. Lentigo maligna melanoma is characterized by abnormal skin areas that are large, flat, and tan with intermixed areas of brown occurring on the face, neck, and arms. Acral lentiginous melanoma occurs on the palms, soles, or under the nails and is more common in African Americans.

### Treatment

Melanoma is often curable if detected and treated in its early stages. A surgical lymph node biopsy may be necessary to see if the cancer has spread to nearby lymph nodes, which may need to be removed along with the tumors. Only the smallest and most shallow melanomas can be cured by surgery alone. Radiation therapy, chemotherapy, or immunotherapy may also be used to treat skin cancer. For patients with melanoma that has spread beyond the skin and lymph nodes to other organs, treatment is more difficult. For melanoma that has spread to other tissues and organs, the fatality rate is highest.

## Testing

A biopsy may be used to confirm diagnosis of skin cancer based on physical exam. The biopsy is used to determine tumor depth, ulcerations, level of invasion, presence of mitoses, regression, and lymphatic vessel invasion.

## MELASMA

### Description

Melasma is a dark skin discoloration found on sun-exposed areas of the face (e.g., cheeks, upper lips, chin, forehead). Young women with brownish skin tones (especially Hispanics and Asians) are at greatest risk (Kantor, 2004b). Melasma is often associated with the female hormones estrogen and progesterone, as it presents in pregnant women, women using oral contraceptives, and women taking hormone replacement therapy. It is particularly common in tropical climates where sun exposure is increased. Melasma is temporary and fades after stopping oral contraceptive use, hormone replacement therapy, or after delivering a child.

### Signs and Symptoms

Melasma is characterized by a uniform, symmetrical brown color over the cheeks, forehead, nose, or upper lip. Melasma does not cause systemic disease.

### Treatment

Melasma is treated with chemical peel, steroid creams, or with a combination of tretinoin cream and a bleaching cream containing hydroquinone. Severe cases may require laser treatments to remove the dark pigment. Frequently used medications include hydroquinone, azelex, and tretinoin (Montemarano, 2003).

### Testing

Diagnosis of melasma is based on the appearance of the skin, although a Wood's lamp may aid in diagnosis.

## MENIERE'S DISEASE

### Description

Meniere's disease is a disorder of the inner ear affecting balance and hearing, characterized by dizziness, loss of hearing, headache, difficulty walking, and ringing in the ears. In cases of Meniere's disease, the sac becomes inflamed causing balance and hearing problems due to an increase in the volume and pressure of the fluid in the inner ear. The exact cause of Meniere's disease is unknown; however, it may be related to middle ear infection, syphilis, head injury, viral illness, respiratory infection, or the use of certain drugs, including aspirin. About 100,000 people per year develop Meniere's disease (Campellone, 2004g; Lorenzo, 2004).

## Signs and Symptoms

Meniere's disease is characterized by dizziness that may be episodic, lasting from minutes to hours, and that worsens with movement. The dizziness also causes nausea and vomiting. Hearing loss and ringing in the ears is also a common sign of Meniere's disease. Profuse sweating and uncontrollable eye movements are also signs of Meniere's disease. Bright lights, TV, and reading may exacerbate symptoms during episodes.

## Treatment

There is no known cure for Meniere's disease. Medications such as antihistamines, anticholinergics, and diuretics may lower endolymphatic pressure by reducing the amount of endolymphatic fluid. Dizziness may be treated with sedatives/hypnotics and benzodiazepines like diazepam and antiemetics. Surgery on the labyrinth, endolymphatic sac, or the vestibular nerve may be required.

## Testing

A neurologic examination may show an abnormality of cranial nerve VIII. Tests used to distinguish Meniere's disease from other disorders may include imaging tests of the head, brain auditory evoked response (BAER), electronystagmography, and audiology tests. A caloric stimulation test of the reflexes of the eyes may also be used in the diagnosis of Meniere's disease. Both a Nylen-Bárány maneuver and a Hallpike maneuver, in which the patient is quickly moved about, indicate increased symptoms.

## MENINGITIS

### Description

According to Levy (2004l, 2004m, 2004n), meningitis is an infection of the cerebrospinal fluid, which is the fluid surrounding the spinal cord and brain. The meninges are illustrated in Figure 2-51. It is sometimes referred to as spinal meningitis, and it is usually caused by a virus or bacterium. Viral meningitis is usually less severe than bacterial meningitis. Before the 1990s, *Haemophilus influenzae* was the leading cause of bacterial meningitis, but today *Streptococcus pneumoniae* and *Neisseria meningitidis* are the leading causes of bacterial meningitis. A less common, but severe form of meningitis is fungal meningitis, which is also known as cryptococcal meningitis. Depending on the cause, meningitis can be contagious.

### Signs and Symptoms

Meningitis is characterized by stiff neck, headache, and high fever. In addition, symptoms of nausea, vomiting, discomfort under bright lights, confusion, and sleepiness may also signal meningitis. As meningitis progresses, seizures are common.

### Treatment

Meningitis is treated based on its underlying causes. Antibiotics will be prescribed for bacterial meningitis; but they are are ineffective in cases of viral meningitis. Early diagnosis and treatment of bacterial meningitis is

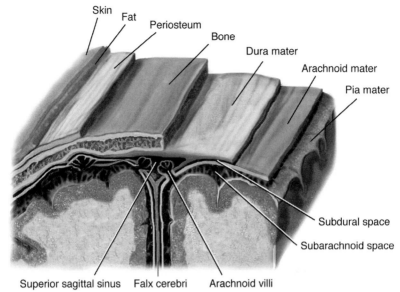

Skin  Fat  Periosteum  Bone  Dura mater  Arachnoid mater  Pia mater

Subdural space

Subarachnoid space

Superior sagittal sinus  Falx cerebri  Arachnoid villi

**Figure 2-51** Meninges: Membranes that sound the brain and spinal cord

essential to prevent permanent neurological damage, but viral meningitis is usually not serious, and symptoms should disappear within two weeks with no residual complications.

## Testing

Tests used in the diagnosis of meningitis may include a lumbar puncture with cerebrospinal fluid measurement and cell count, Gram stain and culture of cerebrospinal fluid, chest X-rays, and head CT scan looking for hydrocephalus, abscess, or swelling.

## MENINGOCOCCEMIA

### Description

Meningococcemia is an acute infection of the bloodstream and subsequent vasculitis caused by *Neisseria meningitidis*, which can infest the upper respiratory tract with no evidence of illness. Menigococcemia is often accompanied by meningococcal meningitis. Family members and those closely exposed to an infected individual are at increased risk. The infection occurs more frequently in winter and early spring, and it is transmitted via respiratory droplets (Meningococcal diseases, 2003).

### Signs and Symptoms

Meningococcemia may have few disease characteristics early in its progress, but early symptoms may include fever, petechial rash, irritability, and anxiety. As the disease progresses, it is characterized by acute illness, changing levels of consciousness, shock, large areas of hemorrhage under the skin, and large areas of thrombosis under the skin. The disease culminates in gangrene (see Color Plate 41).

## Treatment

Meningococcemia requires immediate admission to an intensive care unit for intensive monitoring and treatment. Patients are treated for shock, and antibiotics are administered. If corticosteroids are to be effective in the treatment of shock, they must be administered early. Clotting factors or platelet replacement may be needed if bleeding disorders develop. Respiratory isolation for the first 24 hours is also required to avoid spread to other patients. Patients who are treated early, and those who present with meningitis, have better outcomes (Levy, 2004g). Meningococcemia can be fatal.

## Testing

Tests used in the diagnosis and treatment of meningococcemia include CBC with differential, blood cluture, Gram stain of positive culture, skin biopsy and Gram stain, urinalysis, and clotting studies (PT and PTT).

## MESOTHELIOMA

### Description

Mesothelioma is a cancer of the membranes that surround the lungs (i.e., pleura) or the lining of the abdomen (i.e., peritoneum) (Tan, 2004). The cause of mesothelioma is usually a history of sustained exposure to asbestos. The extremely fine strands of asbestos are capable of reaching far down the respiratory tract, where they interact with immune cells to cause fibrous lesions. The latent period between asbestos exposure and onset of symptoms can be 20 to 50 years. Malignant mesothelioma tumors can spread rapidly to the pericardium, mediastinum, and opposite pleura.

### Signs and Symptoms

Malignant mesothelioma is characterized by progressive pain, difficulty breathing, cough, and weight loss. Pleural effusion, which is the production of fluids in the pleura by the tumors, is also a common symptom of malignant mesothelioma.

### Treatment

Results of treatment for malignant mesothelioma are disappointing. By the time patients become symptomatic, the cancer has often metastasized. When found in the early stages, however, surgery may result in cure. Chemotherapy and radiation may increase the chance of cure after surgery, but in advanced cases of mesothelioma they are not curative. A 2002 study showed that a chemotherapy regimen of cisplatin and pemetrexed appears promising in improving survival and decreasing symptoms. The median survival time varies from 4 to 18 months (Hart, 2004g).

## Testing

Tests used in the diagnosis and treatment of malignant mesothelioma include chest X-rays, thoracic CT scan, cytology from pleural fluid, and open lung biopsy.

## MOLLUSCUM CONTAGIOSUM

### Description

Molluscum contagiosum is a viral skin infection that causes a raised, pearl-like lesion on the skin, primarily among children. It is caused by *Molluscipoxvirus Molluscum contagiosum,* which is a member of the Poxvirus family. The rash may appear on the face, neck, axilla, arms, and hands, but may also occur anywhere on the body except the palms and soles. In adults, molluscum is seen on the genitals as a sexually transmitted disease. Molluscum produces no serious illness; therefore, it has not been treated as aggressively as other sexually transmitted diseases. This is not true among the growing population of immunocompromised people with AIDS, who may develop severe cases of molluscum contagiosum (Crowe, 2004; Lehrer, 2003d).

### Signs and Symptoms

The lesions of molluscum begin as a small bump that often has a dimple in its center and a waxy core. Scratching causes the bumps to spread, resulting in lines or in groups known as crops. The bumps are between 2 and 5 millimeters in diameter. Molluscum lesions are usually not inflamed, unless the patient has been scratching. Early lesions on the genitalia may be mistaken for herpes or warts, but unlike herpes, these lesions are painless.

### Treatment

Molluscum contagiosum lesions may persist from a few months to a few years, and they ultimately disappear without scarring. Individual lesions may be removed surgically, by scraping, de-coring, freezing, or through needle electrosurgery. Medications, such as those used to remove warts, may be helpful in removal of lesions (Crowe, 2004; Lehrer, 2003e).

### Testing

Diagnosis of molluscum contagiosum is based on the appearance of the skin lesion and can be confirmed by a skin biopsy.

## MONKEYPOX

### Description

Monkeypox is a viral disease with a clinical presentation in humans similar to smallpox. Unlike smallpox, monkeypox causes swollen lymph nodes. Vaccination against smallpox also gave protection against monkeypox. Children born after 1980 have not been vaccinated against smallpox. The number of cases of monkeypox in the United States has recently increased with 33 cases in the Midwestern states of Indiana, Illinois, and Wisconsin.

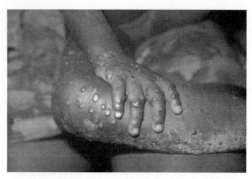

**Figure 2-52** Monkeypox lesions on the arm and leg (Courtesy of the CDC)

These cases are believed to have stemmed from contact with pet prairie dogs. The animals contracted the virus from an infected Gambian giant pouched rat, which came from Central or West Africa (Davey & Altman, 2003; *Monkey B Virus*, 1998; Monkeypox Fact Sheet, 1998).

## Signs and Symptoms
Monkeypox begins with fever, headache, muscle aches, backache, swollen lymph nodes, and exhaustion. Within three days after onset of fever, the patient develops a rash, often first appearing on the face. The lesions usually develop through several stages before crusting and falling off. The incubation period for monkeypox is about 12 days, and lasts for about four weeks. Figure 2-52 is a close-up of the monkeypox lesions on the arms and leg of an infected four-year-old.

## Treatment
There is no proven treatment for monkeypox. CDC is recommending that persons investigating monkeypox and involved in caring for infected individuals or animals receive a smallpox vaccination. The death rate from monkeypox is about 10 percent.

## Testing
Monkeypox is diagnosed by a skin culture.

## MONONUCLEOSIS

### Description
Mononucleosis, which is also known as both kissing disease and college disease, is an infectious inflammatory disease caused by the Epstein-Barr virus (EBV). Mononucleosis affects young adults between the ages of 15 and 25. Outside the United States, the disease is asymptomatic for most children because they are exposed to EBV at an early age. The disease is generally self-limiting and few fatalities occur. When the disease is fatal, the cause of death is usually a ruptured spleen during vigorous activity.

EBV is spread by transfer of saliva by contacts such as kissing, sharing drinking glasses, or drinking from public fountains. The incubation period for infectious mononucleosis is between four and seven weeks. EBV attacks the B memory cells within the immune system (Epstein-Barr, 2002; Hart, 2004h).

## Signs and Symptoms
EBV replicates in the parotid salivary glands until fever, sore throat, swollen lymph glands, enlarged spleen, muscle pain, and fatigue occur.

## Treatment
Most patients recover from mononucleosis within four weeks without medication. There is no specific treatment available for mononucleois. Antiviral medications do not help.

## Testing
Common tests for mononucleosis include a monospot test, EBV antigen by immunofluorescence, and EBV antigody titers.

## MORNING SICKNESS

### Description
Morning sickness is common (Hart, 2004i). Most pregnant women have at least some nausea, and about one-third have vomiting. Morning sickness usually begins during the first month of pregnancy and continues until the 16th week, although some women have nausea and vomiting through their entire pregnancy. Morning sickness does not hurt the baby in any way, and the degree of morning sickness during one pregnancy does not predict its occurrence in future pregnancies. The exact cause of morning sickness is unknown, but it may be caused by hormonal changes or lower blood sugar during early pregnancy (Yancey, 2001).

### Signs and Symptoms
Morning sickness is characterized by nausea and vomiting that often occurs in the morning during pregnancy.

### Treatment
It is important for pregnant woman to maintain their fluid intake during times when they are least nauseated. Medication to prevent nausea is reserved for cases where vomiting is persistent and severe enough to present potential maternal and fetal risks. Nausea and vomiting usually peak between 2 and 12 weeks of gestation and resolves by the second half of a pregnancy.

### Testing
Diagnostic tests that may be performed include blood tests, including CBC and blood chemistry (chem-20), urinalysis for ketones and severity of dehydration, and pregnancy tests.

## MORQUIO SYNDROME

### Description

Morquio syndrome is an inherited disease belonging to the group of mucopolysaccharide storage diseases (Baloghova, 2003; Stewart, 2003j). There is an absence of the enzyme galactosamine-6-sulfatase in Type A disease. There is also an excretion of keratan sulfate in the urine associated with Type A disease. Type B disease results from deficiency of the enzyme beta-galactosidase. In both types there is accumulation of large amounts of mucopolysaccharide.

### Signs and Symptoms

Morquio syndrome has several symptoms in common with other mucopolysaccharide storage diseases such as coarse facial features, short stature, and skeletal and joint abnormalities. Other symptoms include large head, bell-shaped chest, compression of the spinal cord, cloudy cornea, liver enlargement, curvature of the spine, and inguinal hernias. Like Sanfilippo syndrome, onset of symptoms is delayed until after the first year, and life expectancy may exceed 20 years. Unlike Sanfilippo syndrome, mental development is normal.

### Treatment

There is no specific treatment for Morquio syndrome. A spinal fusion may prevent irreversible spinal cord injury. Bone marrow transplantation or enzyme replacement therapy may be available in the future. Bone abnormalities represent a significant problem, and correction through surgery should be made where possible. For example, small vertebrae at the top of the neck can cause slippage that damages the spinal cord so that paralysis may result. Death may occur as a result of heart complications.

### Testing

Tests used in the diagnosis of Morquio syndrome include X-rays for skeletal defects, urine chemistry for increased keratosulfate or chondroitin sulfate, and culture of skin fibroblasts or white blood cells for deficient galactosamine-6-sulfatase or beta-galactosidase enzyme activity. Genetic testing may be available, and an echocardiogram may show thickened heart valves.

## MOUNTAIN SICKNESS

### Description

Mountain sickness is an illness that can affect travelers who ascend too rapidly to high altitudes, typically above 8,000 feet. It can be as mild as a headache or as severe as fluid in the lungs and brain. Reduced atmospheric pressure and a lower concentration of oxygen at high altitude are the causes of this illness. Approximately 20 percent of people will develop mild symptoms at altitudes between 6,300 to 9,700 feet, but pulmonary and cerebral swelling are extremely rare at these heights. Above 14,000 feet, however, a majority of people will experience at least mild symptoms;

approximately 10 percent will develop pulmonary swelling, and 2 percent will develop cerebral swelling (Johnson, 2004).

## Signs and Symptoms

Symptoms can range from mild to fatal. In severe cases fluid collects in the lungs causing pulmonary swelling, which results in shortness of breath and further decreasing oxygenation. This is referred to as HAPE, it is used for high altitude pulmonary edema. Swelling may also occur in the brain in the form of cerebral swelling, resulting in confusion, coma, and, if untreated, death. This is referred to as HACE, it is used for high altitude cerebral edema (Nazziola & Lafleur, 2004).

## Treatment

Treatment for all forms of altitude illness is to descend to lower altitude as rapidly and safely as possible. Supplemental oxygen should also be administered. Acetazolamide may be used to stimulate breathing and to speed acclimatization. Pulmonary swelling is treated with oxygen, mechanical ventilation, and nifedipine, which is a high blood pressure medication. For cerebral edema, the steroid drug dexamethasone may be used. A portable hyperbaric chamber (Gamor bag) may be used to simulate a lower altitude. Prochlorperazine may be prescribed for nausea.

## Testing

Diagnosis is based on case history, and imaging exams and blood gases may be used to confirm the severity of disease.

## MUCORMYCOSIS

## Description

Mucormycosis is a fungal infection of the sinuses, brain, or lungs that occurs primarily among the immunocompromised (Levy, 2004o; Yen & Yen, 2001). Common fungi found in soil and decaying vegetation cause mucormycosis especially those in the genera of *Mucor* or *Rhizopus*. Conditions associated with mucormycosis include diabetes mellitus, chronic steroid use, metabolic acidosis, organ transplantation, leukemia, lymphoma, treatment with deferoxamine, and AIDS.

## Signs and Symptoms

Mucormycosis is usually a medical emergency requiring surgery characterized by acute sinusitis, fever, eye swelling, visual changes, protrusion of the eye, and dark nasal scabbing (see Color Plate 42). Pulmonary mucormycosis may cause fever, cough, and difficulty breathing. Gastrointestinal mucormycosis causes abdominal pain and bloody vomit. Renal mucormycosis causes flank pain and fever. Cutaneous mucormycosis causes a single, painful, hardened area of skin exhibiting a black central area.

## Treatment

Treatment for mucormycosis is early surgical intervention to remove all dead and infected tissue, along with intravenous antifungal therapy.

Surgery may involve removal of the palate, nasal structures, or eye structures, but chances of survival are greatly decreased without this aggressive intervention. Mucormycosis has an extremely high mortality even with aggressive surgical intervention. Death rates range from 25 to 80 percent depending on the site involved.

## Testing

Tests used in the diagnosis of mucormycosis are dependent on the site of involvement, but CT scans or MRIs may be performed. To definitively diagnose mucormycosis, a tissue specimen must be obtained and analyzed.

## MULTIPLE MYELOMA

### Description

Multiple myeloma is a form of cancer in which excessive growth and malfunction of plasma cells in the bone marrow occur. This interferes with the production of red blood cells, white blood cells, and platelets. These blood cell changes result in anemia, susceptibility to infection, and increased bruising and bleeding. Patients typically exhibit bone pain, fractures, weakness, anemia, infections, excess calcium, spinal cord compression, or renal failure. Infections are often caused by pneumococcus. Multiple myeloma mainly affects older adults and is rare, with only three new cases per 100,000 people annually (Brose, 2004a; Grethlein, 2004).

### Signs and Symptoms

Multiple myeloma is characterized by bone pain, fractures, back pain, bleeding problems, increased infections, and symptoms of anemia, which include fatigue and difficulty breathing.

### Treatment

Complete remission in cases of multiple myeloma is unusual, so the goal of treatment is to relieve symptoms, because chemotherapy, radiation therapy, and bone marrow transplant rarely lead to permanent cure. The median for multiple myeloma is about three years, but this depends on the patient's age and the stage of disease.

### Testing

Tests that may be used in the diagnosis and treatment of multiple myeloma may include a CBC, bone marrow biopsy, serum protein electrophoresis, tests of serum calcium, total protein, and kidney function. A skeletal series of imaging tests is also used to diagnose multiple myeloma.

## MULTIPLE SCLEROSIS

### Description

Multiple sclerosis (MS) is an inflammatory disease of the central nervous system in which infiltrating lymphocytes, predominantly T cells and macrophages, degrade the myelin sheath of nerves. It is believed that MS is caused by viral infection. Persons with MS typically experience periods of exacerbation and remission of the disease. The location of the inflamed areas varies between episodes, but each time there is destruction of the myelin sheath in the affected area, leaving scar tissue (sclerosis). The average person with MS lives over 30 years with the disease; however, others die within a few months of its onset. There is usually a stepwise progression of the disorder, with episodes that last days, weeks, or months alternating with periods of remission. MS affects approximately 1 out of 1,000 people and usually begins between the ages of 20 and 40.

## Signs and Symptoms

The symptoms of MS vary greatly and differ with each episode. MS is characterized by weakness in the extremities, paralysis, tremors, muscle spasms, a slowly progressive movement dysfunction that begins in the legs, numbness, facial pain, vision disturbances in one eye at a time, loss of balance, dizziness, and urinary hesitancy and urgency. Mental function may also be altered, including memory loss, decreased spontaneity, impaired judgment, loss of abstract thought, decreased attention span, and inability to generalize. Other common symptoms include depression, slurred speech, and hearing loss. Symptoms may be exacerbated by fever, hot baths, and sun exposure. A history of at least two attacks separated by a period of reduced or no symptoms may indicate a pattern of attacks and remissions known as relapsing-remitting MS.

## Treatment

There is no known cure for multiple sclerosis. Patients with a relapsing-remitting course are placed on immune modulating therapy in the form of interferon (such as Avonex or Betaseron) or glatiramer acetate (Copaxone). Other medicines such as Lioresal (baclofen), tizanidine (Zanaflex), or one of the benzodiazepines may be used to reduce muscle spasticity. Cholinergic medications may be helpful to reduce urinary problems. Antidepressant medications can also help with mood or behavior symptoms, and amantadine may be given for fatigue. Although the disorder is chronic and incurable, life expectancy can be normal or nearly so (Campellone, 2004h).

## Testing

Tests used in the diagnosis and treatment of MS may include a head MRI scan, a spine MRI, a lumbar puncture, a cerebrospinal fluid oligoclonal banding test, and a cerebrospinal fluid immunoglobulin G index.

## MUMPS

### Description

Mumps, which is also known as epidemic parotitis, is an infectious disease of the parotid salivary glands caused by the mumps virus (Figure 2-53). The incubation period for epidemic parotitis is approximately 17 days. The mumps virus is spread via respiratory secretions and saliva. Children should be vaccinated with the MMR vaccine to reduce the occurrence of

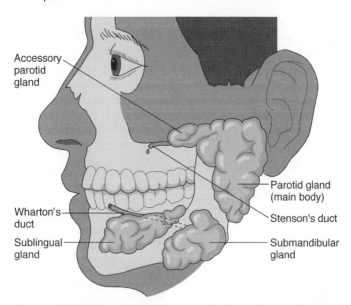

**Figure 2-53** Salivary glands

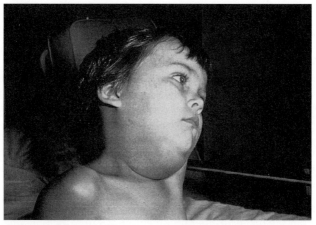

**Figure 2-54** Mumps (Courtesy of the CDC)

mumps. The MMR vaccine provides children with immunity for measles, mumps, and rubella (Mumps, n/d).

## Signs and Symptoms

The symptoms of mumps are swelling and pain in the parotid glands, headache, fever, and sore throat (Figure 2-54). In males, four to seven days after the onset of symptoms, inflammation of the testicles may occur. Inflammation of the testicles is known as orchitis, and it may lead to sterility. Mumps may also lead to meningitis, inflammation of the ovaries, and pancreatitis.

## Treatment

There is no specific treatment for mumps. Warm saltwater gargles, soft foods, and extra fluids may also help relieve symptoms. The probable outcome for mumps is good, even if other organs are involved (Banerjee, 2004c). After the illness, lifelong immunity to mumps occurs.

## Testing

Diagnosis of mumps is based on a physical exam, and no testing is usually required.

## MUSCULAR DYSTROPHY

### Description

Muscular dystrophy refers to a group of disorders characterized by progressive muscle weakness and loss of muscle tissue especially muscle fiber degeneration. Many muscular dystrophies are inherited disorders, such as Becker's MD, Duchenne MD, facioscapulohumeral MD, limb-girdle MD, Emery-Dreifuss MD, myotonic MD, and myotonia congenita. These disorders are distinguishable by the type of inheritance (e.g., sex-linked, dominant gene, recessive gene), age when symptoms appear, and disease characteristics (A. Chen, 2004a; Do, 2002).

### Signs and Symptoms

Symptoms vary by types of MD. Some are fatal (e.g., Duchenne MD); others have associated muscle weakness but cause little disability. The muscles primarily affected are around the pelvis, shoulder, and face. MD is characterized by progressive muscle weakness, frequent falls, delayed development of motor skills, difficulty walking, eyelid drooping, drooling, joint contractures, and scloiosis. Some types of MD also result in mental retardation.

### Treatment

There are no known cures for the various muscular dystrophies. In some cases, surgery on the spine or lower extremities may help improve function and slow deterioration. All types of MD progressively worsen, but the speed of decline and extent of disability they cause vary widely. Some types are fatal.

### Testing

Tests used in the diagnosis and treatment of MD may include a muscle biopsy, a blood DNA test, a serum CPK, an electromyogram, an electrocardiogram, a test of urine myoglobin, a test of serum myoglobin, an LDH, a creatinine level test, an AST, and an aldolase.

## MYASTHENIA GRAVIS

### Description

Myasthenia gravis is a neuromuscular disorder characterized by variable weakness of voluntary muscles, which often improves with rest and worsens with activity (Campellone, 2004i; Shah, 2004). Weakness occurs when an unexplainable, abnormal immune response produces antibodies that prevent muscle cells from receiving chemical neurotransmitters from nerve cells. In some cases, myasthenia gravis may be associated with tumors of the thymus. Myasthenia gavis increases the risk of having other autoimmune disorders (e.g., thyrotoxicosis, rheumatoid arthritis, systemic lupus erythematosus). Myasthenia gravis affects about 3 of every 10,000 people.

## Signs and Symptoms

Myasthenia gravis is characterized by double vision, eyelid drooping, difficulty swallowing, gagging, choking, weakness, paralysis, drooping head, difficulty climbing stairs or lifing objects, problems with speech, and difficulty chewing.

## Treatment

There is no known cure for myasthenia gravis. Some medications (e.g., neostigmine or pyridostigmine) improve communication between the nerve and the muscle. In severe cases, prednisone and other immunosuppressants (e.g., azathioprine or cyclosporine) may be prescribed. Plasmapheresis, a technique in which blood plasma containing antibodies against the body is removed from the body and replaced with fluids, may be used prior to surgery. A thymectomy may also be performed.

## Testing

Tests used in the diagnosis and treatment of myasthenia gravis may include an EMG and tests for acetylcholine receptor antibodies in the blood. A Tensilon test may be positive in some cases but must be interpreted carefully by an experienced doctor. Muscle function may improve after Tensilon (edrophonium), a medication that blocks the breakdown of acetylcholine, is administered.

## MYCETOMA

### Description

Mycetoma is a slow-growing bacterial or fungal infection focused in one area of the body, usually the foot (Ania, 2002; Turiansky, 2002). The first medical reports were from doctors in Madura, India, giving the disease its alternate name, Madura foot. Bacteria or fungi gain entry into the skin through a wound, and approximately one month after the injury, a painless nodule forms. Eventually, the nodule forms a tumor, containing sinuses that discharge blood and pus, along with colonies of microorganisms that look like tiny grains. As the infection continues, surrounding tissue becomes involved, with an accumulation of scarring and loss of function. Mycetoma may be complicated by secondary infections, in which new bacteria become established in the area and cause an additional set of problems.

### Signs and Symptoms

Mycetoma is characterized by an abnormal tissue mass beneath the skin, formation of sinuses within the mass, and a fluid discharge. As the infection progresses, it affects the muscles and bones; at this advanced stage, disability may result.

## Treatment

Treatment for mycetoma includes sulfones, trimethoprim, and sulfamethoxazole, or sulfonamides may benefit lesions caused by actinomycetes. If lesions are due to fungi, there is no specific treatment. Surgical removal of the growth may be required.

## Testing

In the early stages of mycetoma, prior to sinus formation, diagnosis may be more difficult and a biopsy, or microscopic examination of the tissue, may be necessary. If bone involvement is suspected, the area is X-rayed to determine the extent of the damage.

## *MYCOBACTERIUM AVIUM* COMPLEX

### Description

*Mycobacterium avium* complex (MAC) is a serious bacterial infection affecting persons with HIV. MAC is related to tuberculosis, and is sometimes called *Mycobacterium avium* intracellulare. MAC infection is usually found only in people with under 50 T4 cells, meaning that healthy individuals would not usually contract this disease. Atypical mycobacterial infection is an infection caused by a species of mycobacterium other than tuberculosis. Organisms causing MAC are commonly found in soil, water, and house dust. Coastal marshes have higher concentrations of the organisms than other areas. *M. avium* is a cause of disease in poultry and swine, but animal-to-human transmission has not been shown to be an important factor in human disease. The incidence of MAC has increased, however, owing to the prevalence of AIDS.

### Signs and Symptoms

MAC affects the intestines and inner organs first and is noted by weight loss, fever, chills, night sweats, swollen glands, abdominal pains, diarrhea, and fatigue. MAC can result in a wide variety of infections (e.g., abscesses, septic arthritis, osteomyelitis). MAC can also infect the lungs, lymph nodes, gastrointestinal tract, skin, and soft tissues.

### Treatment

Treatment of MAC depends upon the sensitivity of the infecting organism to specific antibiotics. As many as six drugs may be used to treat some infections, and treatment may require six months to two years. Certain lymph node infections and skin lesions can be surgically removed. The outcome of treatment depends upon the severity of the infection, the resistance of the organism, and the individual's immune status (*Mycobacterium avium* complex, 2003).

### Testing

Tests used in the diagnosis and treatment of MAC may include blood culture, sputum culture, lymph node culture, bone marrow culture, stool culture, and chest X-rays.

## MYELITIS

### Description

Myelitis is an inflammation of the spinal cord, resulting from an infection in the spinal cord, noninfectious necrosing of the spinal cord, or demyelination of the spinal cord. Transverse myelitis is an inflammatory disorder of the spinal cord, which occurs as a result of a process known as demyelination, which is the loss of the fatty tissue that surrounds the nerves. Transverse myelitis may be caused by viral infections, spinal cord injuries, immune reactions, or insufficient blood flow to the spinal cord. It may also occur as a complication of disorders like multiple sclerosis, smallpox, measles, or chickenpox.

### Signs and Symptoms

Myelitis is characterized by flaccid limb paralysis, incontinence, and weakness or numbness of the limbs. Transverse myelitis may have an acute onset, characterized by low back pain, spinal cord dysfunction, muscle spasms, headache, loss of appetite, and numbness or tingling in the legs.

### Treatment

Myelitis treatment varies based on cause. There is no treatment for transverse myelitis, except to treat the symptoms of the disorder. The prognosis for complete recovery from transverse myelitis is poor, with most individuals encountering considerable disability.

### Testing

The primary tests used in the diagnosis of myelitis are imaging exams (e.g., X-rays, MRI scans, CT scans, myelograms).

## MYOCARDIAL INFARCTION

### Description

A myocardial infarction (MI) is commonly referred to as a heart attack. An infarction is the formation of an area of dead tissue (i.e., necrosis) caused by obstruction in the artery supplying the area, although an infarct may also occur if the vein that drains the area of tissue becomes occluded. Most heart attacks are the result of a blood clot within the coronary artery that blocks the flow of blood to the heart muscle. Men are much more likely than women to experience an MI, and about half of all cases of MI are fatal due to acute cardiac failure. When a portion of the coronary artery is blocked, but blood is still allowed to flow to the myocardium, chronic cardiac failure ensues.

### Signs and Symptoms

The chest pain associated with heart attacks is referred to as angina pectoris. The pain is not usually described as stabbing or sharp, and it is not usually exacerbated by taking deep breaths, coughing, or swallowing. Angina pectoris may occur for days or weeks before an acute myocardial infarction; at which point, the pain is more severe and is exacerbated during physical activity, after eating a large meal, or during exposure to cold weather. MI is typified by a sensation of crushing pressure behind the breastbone and chest pain radiating to the neck, jaw, abdomen, shoulder, or left arm. Other symptoms include nausea, vomiting, difficulty breathing, and anxiety or fear.

## Treatment

A heart attack is a medical emergency. According to Hart (2004f and 2003b), a urinary catheter may be inserted to closely monitor fluid status. Oxygen is usually given, even if blood oxygen levels are normal. Nitroglycerin or other medicines (e.g., morphine) are given for pain and to reduce the oxygen requirements of the heart. Blood thining medications (e.g., streptokinase, tissue plasminogen activator, heparin, warfarin) may be administered. Antiplatelet medications (e.g., aspirin, ticlopidine [Ticlid], clopidogrel [Plavix]) may also be prescribed. Beta-blockers (e.g., metoprolol, atenolol, propranolol) are used to reduce the workload of the heart. ACE inhibitors (e.g., ramipril, lisinopril, enalapril, captopril) help prevent heart failure. Surgical procedures (e.g., angioplasty, coronary artery bypass surgery, implantation of an arterial stent) may also be necessary. The expected outcome of an MI varies with the amount and location of damaged tissue. The outcome is worse if there is damage to the electrical conduction system of the heart.

## Testing

Continuous electrocardiogram monitoring is started immediately, because life-threatening arrhythmias are the leading cause of death in the first few hours of an MI. Diagnostic tests may include an echocardiography, coronary angiography, and nuclear ventriculography.

## MYOCARDITIS

### Description

Myocarditis is an uncommon inflammation of the heart muscle caused by viral infections (e.g., coxsackievirus, adenovirus, echovirus). It may be associated with various infections (e.g., polio, influenza, rubella). Myocarditis may be caused by exposure to chemicals, allergic reactions, certain medications, or autoimmune diseases. Drugs may also cause myocarditis (e.g., cocaine, blood pressure drugs, and antiseizure drugs). The heart muscle becomes inflamed and weakened, causing symptoms of heart failure (Keller, 2004; Tang & Young, 2002).

### Signs and Symptoms

Myocarditis is characterized by a history of preceding viral illness, fever, chest pain, joint pain and swelling, abnormal heartbeat, fatigue, difficulty breathing, leg swelling, inability to lie flat, fainting, and decreased urine output. A total absence of symptoms is also common.

### Treatment

Treatment for myocarditis includes treatment of its underlying cause. Medications used in the treatment of myocarditis may include antibiotics, steroids, diuretics, and anti-inflammatories. Medications to treat heart failure, abnormal heart rhythm, and blood clotting dysfunction may also be administered. A pacemaker or defibrillator may also be needed. Some patients may recover completely; others may succumb to heart failure.

### Testing

Tests used in the diagnosis of myocarditis include electrocardiogram, chest X-rays, echocardiogram, blood cell counts, blood cultures, blood tests for antibodies, and a heart muscle biopsy.

## MYXEDEMA

### Description

Myxedema is the most severe form of hypothyroidism, and it is a medical emergency (Rennert, 2004b). Hypothyroidism is a condition in which the thyroid gland fails to produce enough thyroid hormone. Under the control of the pituitary, the thyroid gland secretes thyroxine (T4) and triiodothyronine (T3) hormones that control metabolism. Thyroid disorders may result from defects in the thyroid gland, the pituitary, or the hypothalamus.

### Signs and Symptoms

Myxedema occurs when the body's level of thyroid hormones becomes extremely low. In cases of myxedema, the body's normal rate of functioning slows, causing mental and physical sluggishness. Myxedema results in coma.

### Treatment

Myxedema is treated with intravenous thyroid replacement and steroid therapy. Supportive therapy of oxygen, assisted ventilation, fluid replacement, and intensive-care nursing may be indicated. With treatment, return to the normal state is usual. Myxedema coma can result in death.

### Testing

Tests used in the diagnosis of myxedema include T4 tests and serum TSH levels.

## NABOTHIAN CYST

### Description

A nabothian cyst is a mucus-filled cyst on the surface of the uterine cervix. The cervical canal is lined by glandular cells that normally secrete mucus. In cases of nabothian cyst, these glands are covered by the abnormal growth of squamous epithelium. As the glands fill with fluid, cysts form. They can occur singly or in groups, and they are not a threat to health. The cysts are more common among women who have children (Debemardo, 2004a).

### Signs and Symptoms

Nabothian cysts are rounded lumps just under the surface of the cervix that appear as small, white, pimplelike elevations. There are no systemic symptoms of nabothian cysts.

## Treatment

No systemic treatment is needed for nabothian cysts, but they do not spontaneously clear. They are usually treated by electrocautery or cryotherapy. There is no prevention known for nabothian cysts.

## Testing

Nabothian cysts are usually discovered upon routine pelvic examinations. Rarely, a colposcopic examination is necessary to distinguish nabothian cysts from other types of cervical lesions.

# NEPHRITIS

## Description

Nephritis is a kidney disorder caused by inflammation of the tubules and spaces between the tubules and glomeruli. Nephritis is classified as primary (e.g., primarily effecting the kidney itself) and secondary (e.g., systemic disorders that eventually involve the kidneys). Nephritis may be caused by the effects of various medications on the kidney. It may be chronic and progressive, resulting form infections. Nephritis is associated with analgesic nephropathy, and it can occur with reactions to a drug (e.g., penicillin, ampicillin, methicillin, sulfonamide, furosemide, NSAIDS, diuretics). Nephritis normally occurs two or more weeks after exposure to the medication (Agha, 2003c; Parmar, 2002). Nephritis is most severe in the elderly.

Metabolic acidosis may occur because of the inability to excrete acid. Patients may exhibit a pale appearance. High blood pressure and swelling occur.

## Signs and Symptoms

Nephritis is characterized by changes in urine output, fever, drowsiness, confusion, coma, nausea, vomiting, rash, uremia, swelling, and bloody urine.

## Treatment

Nephritis is treated by treating underlying causes and relieving symptoms by avoiding the suspect medications, dietary restriction of sodium intake, dietary restriction of proteins to control uremia and acute renal failure. Short-term dialysis may be required. Corticosteroids and NSAIDS may be administered. Treatment also includes diuretics (furosemide) and medications to control blood pressure (nefedipine, losartan, hydralazine, and captopril) (Neiberger, 2004).

## Testing

Tests used in the diagnosis of nephritis may include urinalysis, electrolytes, blood cell counts, BUN and creatinine levels, and kidney biopsies. Renal ultrasound rules out other diseases.

## NEURALGIA

### Description

Neuralgia is a condition in which pain follows the paths of affected nerves. Neuralgia may be due to a variety of causes (e.g., chemicals, trauma, surgery, tumors), but in many cases neuralgia is idiopathic. Trigeminal neuralgia is characterized by sudden attacks of severe pain on one side of the face. Neuralgia may also affect the glosso-pharyngeal nerve, causing shocklike pain in the throat. Neuralgia may occur after infections like shingles, syphillis, and Lyme disease. Diabetes causes neuraliga due to restricted blood flow to nerves. Neuralgia is also associated with kidney disorders (Campellone, 2004j).

### Signs and Symptoms

Neuralgia is characterized by pain located in the same location for subsequent episodes. The pain may be anywhere, but usually appears on the surface of the body. The pain may be a sharp, stabbing pain or a constant, burning pain. Neuralgia pain follows the path of a specific nerve causing impaired function, increased sensitivity of the skin, or numbness similar to the effects of a local anesthetic such as Novacaine.

### Treatment

Surgical removal of tumors or surgical separation of the nerve from blood vessels or other structures that compress it may be required. Analgesics may be prescribed; however, the effects of analgesics may be short-lived. Antiseizure medications (e.g., carbamazepine, gabapentin, lamotrigine, phenytoin) may be used to treat trigeminal neuralgia. Antidepressant medications (e.g., amitryptiline) may be prescribed. Other treatments may include nerve blocks, using local injections of anesthetic agents, or surgical procedures to decrease sensitivity of the nerve. Motor cortex stimulation consists of placing an electrode in the sensory cortex of the brain that is attached to a pulse generator under the skin. Neuralgia may be self-resolving.

### Testing

No tests are specific for neuralgia. Sometimes a nerve conduction study with electromyography (NCS/EMG) may confirm diagnosis. Blood tests to check blood sugar and kidney function are routinely used. A lumbar puncture is often used to diagnosis multiple sclerosis and other nerve disorders.

## NEURITIS

### Description

Neuritis is inflammation of a nerve or nerves. Some causes of neuritis include trauma, infection, and poisons. Trauma to the nerve causes it to become inflamed. Neuritis caused by infections may be either directly caused by an infection of the nerve, or it may be the result of complications due to infections (e.g., tuberculosis, tetanus, measles) (Campellone, 2004m).

## Signs and Symptoms

Neuritis symptoms depend on which type of nerve is affected. Sensory changes may include abnormal sensations, burning pain, numbness, or inability to determine joint position. Sensation changes often begin in the feet and progress toward the center of the body. Movement dysfunction may cause weakness, loss of muscle bulk, loss of desterity, cramps, and paralysis. Symptoms of autonomic nerve involvement include blurred vission, decreased ability to sweat, inability to control blood pressure, dizziness, fainting, heat intolerance, nausea, diarrhea, urinary incontinence, and impotence in males.

## Treatment

Nueritis treatment usually involves physical therapy and use of appliances such as wheelchairs, braces, and splints. Safety is an important consideration for people with neuritis due to dysfunction of muscle control and sensation. Patients may not notice injuries and should check their feet for bruises, open skin areas, or other lesions. Medications used to treat neuritis may include analgesics, anticonvulsants (e.g., phenytoin, carbamazepine, gabapentin), and tricyclic antidepressants. In cases where a medical condition can be identified and treated, the prognosis may be excellent; however, in other cases nerve damage can be permanent.

## Testing

Tests used in the diagnosis of neuritis may include EMG, nerve conduction tests, and nerve biopsy.

## NEUROBLASTOMA

### Description

Neuroblastoma is an idiopathic, malignant tumor of infants and children that develops from nerve tissue. It develops from tissues that form the sympathetic nervous system, which controls body functions such as heart rate, blood pressure, digestion, and hormone levels. Neuroblastoma usually begins in the adrenal gland and then metastasizes to the lymph nodes, liver, bones, and bone marrow. Neuroblastoma is typically diagnosed in children under five, and it occurs in about 1 in 100,000 children (Blackman, 2004).

### Signs and Symptoms

Symptoms of neuroblastoma may include pallor, dark circles around the eyes, chronic fatigue, diarrhea, enlarged abdomen, abdominal mass, fluid in the abdomen, bone pain, difficulty breathing, red skin, profuse sweating, rapid pulse, uncontrollable eye movement, paralysis, and irritability.

### Treatment

In some cases, surgery alone is enough, but often chemotherapy and radiation therapy are required. Neuroblastoma may go away on its own, or it may mature and develop into a benign ganglioneuroma that can be surgically removed. In other cases, the tumor spreads rapidly resulting in death.

## Testing

Tests used in the diagnosis and treatment of neuroblastoma include CT scans, MRI scans, chest X-rays, bone scans, bone marrow biopsy, hormone tests, blood cell counts, catecholamine levels in the urine and blood, and iodine-131-meta-iodobenzylguanidine (MIBG) scans.

## NEUROMAS

### Description

A neuroma is a benign tumor of nervous tissue. Acoustic neuromas usually grow slowly on the eighth cranial nerve leading from the brain to the inner ear over a period of years. The brain is not invaded by the growing tumor, but the tumor pushes the brain as it enlarges. Neuromas may also occur on the peripheral nerves of the feet.

### Signs and Symptoms

Acoustic neuromas may affect balance, hearing, and facial muscles. Neuromas can also press on the trigeminal nerve, affecting facial sensation. Even though a neuroma can occur at any site in the foot, the most common place is between the third and fourth toes. Almost 90 percent of the cases occur in women, and the most common complaint is a sharp pain in the ball of the foot with tingling and numbness traveling to the toes.

### Treatment

Treatment for neuromas typically includes surgical removal of the tumor. Chemotherapy and radiation therapy may also be used to control the growth of the tumor. Although it is rare, when neuromas cause severe pressure on the brain stem and cerebellum, they may be fatal.

### Testing

Imaging tests and tissue biopsy are used to diagnose neuromas. During the physical exam, when the foot is squeezed, a clicking sound may be heard called Mulder's sign.

## NEUROSARCOIDOSIS

### Description

Neurosarcoidosis is a complication of sarcoidosis involving the body's nervous system. Sarcoidosis is caused by the formation of abnormal immune system cells known as a granuloma. In the case of neurosarcoidosis, the granuloma results from the body's attempt to attack its own central nervous system tissues. Neurosarcoidosis is rare, but it can be life threatening. Neither the cause of sarcoidosis nor the cause of neurosarcoidosis is known (Bucurescu & Suleman, 2005; Campellone, 2004k; Kaufman, 2003).

## Signs and Symptoms

The disease characteristics of neurosarcoidosis are dependent upon the area of the body in which the affected nerve is located. Cranial nerve involvement may result in facial paralysis, impaired vision, impaired taste and smell, speech impairment, ringing in the ears, dizziness, and weakness of the trapezius and sternocleidomastoid muscles of the neck. Involvement of the area of the brain surrounding the pituitary gland can result in excessive thirst, increased urination, diabetes insipidus, obesity, shortness of breath, dementia, headaches, seizures, meningitis, and impotence.

## Treatment

There is no cure for neurosarcoidosis. Treatment may include corticosteroid therapy to suppress the immune system, radiation therapy, hormone replacement therapy, and antipsychotic drugs.

## Testing

Tests used in the diagnosis and treatment of neurosarcoidosis may include lab studies of cerebrospinal fluid (CSF) collected through a lumbar puncture and angiotensin-converting enzyme (ACE) levels in the blood. Antineutrophil cytoplasmic antibody (C-ANCA) titers may be determined to rule out other diseases like Wegener granulomatosis. Both imaging exams of the brain and nerve conduction tests may be performed. Muscle and nerve biopsy also are used to confirm diagnosis.

## NIEMANN-PICK DISEASE

### Description

Niemann-Pick disease, which is also known as sphingomyelinase deficiency, is caused by specific genetic mutations (McGovern, 2002; Stewart, 2004d). Types A and B Niemann-Pick are caused by deficiency of the enzyme acid sphingomyelinase. In the absence of acid sphingomyelinase, sphingomyelin accumulates within the cells, causing organ malfunction. Patients with type C Niemann-Pick disease are not able to metabolize cholesterol and other fats, resulting in accumulation of fats in the liver, brain, and spleen. Type C Niemann-Pick disease is most prevalent among Puerto Ricans of Spanish descent. Type D Niemann-Pick has only been found in the French Canadian population of Yarmouth County, Nova Scotia, and is believed to be a variant of type C. Geneological research indicates that Joseph Muise (c. 1679–1729) and Marie Amirault (1684–c. 1735) are common ancestors to all people with type D.

### Signs and Symptoms

Type A Niemann-Pick begins in the first few months of life and is characterized by feeding difficulties, enlarged abdomen, progressive loss of motor skills, and a cherry red spot in the eye. Type B is biochemically similar to type A, but the symptoms are more variable. Abdominal enlargement may be detected in early childhood, but there is almost no neurological involvement. Some patients may develop repeated respiratory infections. Type C Niemann-Pick usually affects children of school age, and is characterized by jaundice at birth, enlarged spleen, enlarged liver, vertical supranuclear gaze palsy, unsteady gait, dystonia, slurred speech, dementia, seizures, falls due to sudden loss of muscle tone, and tremors.

## Treatment

For types A and B Niemann-Pick, DNA testing and prenatal diagnosis is available. Research into treatments for types A and B has progressed rapidly since the early 1990s. Mount Sinai School of Medicine is conducting research on bone marrow transplantation, enzyme replacement therapy, and gene therapy. All these therapies have had some success against type B Niemann-Pick, but none has been effective against type A. No sp cific treatment is available for type C Niemann-Pick.

Type A Niemann-Pick is a severe neurologic disease, which leads to death by the age of three, whereas type B generally causes little or no neurologic involvement. A child showing signs of type C before one year of age may not live to school age. Children showing symptoms after entering school may live into their mid- to late teens, with few surviving into their 20s.

## Testing

Types A and B Niemann-Pick are diagnosed by measuring the acid sphingomyelinase activity in white blood cells. It is possible to diagnose types A and B carriers by DNA testing. Type C Niemann-Pick is initially diagnosed by skin biopsy. Additional tests might include slit-lamp eye exam, liver biopsy, bone marrow aspiration, and sphingomyelinase assays.

## NOCARDIOSIS

### Description

*Nocardia* is a genus of filamentous bacteria that cause pulmonary infections, brain abscesses, cellulitis, and systemic disease (Levy, 2004p). About 80 percent of the time, *Nocardia* cause pulmonary infections, and it is part of a complex of disorders related to HIV infection. In the United States, an estimated 500 to 1,000 new cases of *Nocardia* infection occur annually. Pulmonary and disseminated infections are spread through inhalation, whereas cutaneous infection is spread through contact with soil-contaminated wounds (*Nocardiosis*, 2004).

### Signs and Symptoms

Pulmonary nocardiosis is characterized by fever, coughing up blood, cough, and chest pain. Central nervous system nocardiosis results in headaches, fever, lethargy, confusion, seizures, and acute nerological deficit. Skin infections result in ulcers and mycetoma with draining tracts that can progress down to muscle and bone.

### Treatment

Long-term antibiotic therapy, usually with sulfonamides, is needed to treat nocardia. Surgery may be required in cases of mycetoma. Nocardia infection has a significant mortality rate if more than one site is involved (Kotton, 2002b).

## Testing

Nocardiosis is diagnosed by identification of the bacteria in culture. Depending on the site involved, this may involve obtaining a tissue sample for staining and culture by sputum culture, bronchoscopy, lung biopsy, skin biopsy, or brain biopsy.

## NON-HODGKIN'S LYMPHOMA

### Description

Non-Hodgkin's lymphomas are cancers of lymphoid tissue. Most arise within a lymph node, but some arise in areas other than nodes, such as the jaw or brain. Advances in molecular genetics have shown that non-Hodgkin's lymphoma is actually many diseases. Some of the non-Hodgkin's lymphomas more closely resemble leukemia than they do the Hodgkin's lymphomas. As more becomes known, some lymphomas that were categorized as non-Hodgkin's lymphomas may be reclassified with other cancers. Non-Hodgkin's lymphomas can be slow-growing (low-grade) or rapidly growing (high-grade). The incidence is 3 in 10,000 people (Brose, 2004d).

### Signs and Symptoms

Non-Hodgkin's lymphomas are characterized by enlarged lymph nodes, fever, night sweats, weight loss, and flank pain.

### Treatment

Treatment may include chemotherapy, radiation therapy, and bone marrow transplantation. The average survival is seven years for patients with low-grade lymphoma, and 30 percent of adults with high-grade lymphoma are cured.

### Testing

Tests used in the diagnosis of non-Hodgkin's lymphoma include a peripheral blood smear showing abnormal white blood cells, a CBC with differential, a lymph node biopsy, a bone marrow biopsy, a lymphangiogram, and a laparotomy or liver biopsy. Imaging tests of the torso may include X-rays, MRI scans, CT scans, or PET scans.

## NOONAN SYNDROME

### Description

Noonan syndrome is a genetic disorder causing abnormal development (Stewart, 2003k). It affects at least 1 in 2,500 children. *PTPN11* is the gene that causes Noonan syndrome, and it was discovered in 2001. Noonan syndrome used to be called male Turner syndrome and Turner-like syndrome because its symptoms are similar to Turner syndrome, which affects only females.

## Signs and Symptoms

Facial abnormalities may include low-set or abnormally shaped ears, sagging eyelids, wide-set eyes, folds above the eyes, and a small jaw. Mild mental retardation is present in about 25 percent of cases. Hearing loss may occur, puberty is delayed, and adult height is decreased. Males may have undescended testicles and a small penis. There is also a webbing of the neck, sunken chest, and congenital heart disease.

## Treatment

There is no single treatment for Noonan syndrome, except to treat its symptoms. Prognosis depends on the extent and severity of symptoms that are present, but most patients lead normal lives.

## Testing

There may be a bleeding tendency revealed by low platelet count or coagulation tests and measuring the levels of specific coagulation factors in the blood (factors XI-XIII). If there are signs of heart disease, an ECG, chest X-ray, or echocardiogram may be required.

## NOROVIRUS INFECTIONS

### Description

Noroviruses are a group of viruses causing gastroenteritis, and this group of viruses has several alternative names (e.g., Norwalk-like viruses, caliciviruses, and small round structured viruses). The incubation period for norovirus illness is between 12 and 48 hours, and the symptoms usually subside within 48 hours. Infection is spread through ingestion of contaminated food or water, contact with contaminated surfaces, or direct contact with infected persons, who may remain infectious between 3 and 14 days after recovery (*Norovirus*, 2003).

### Signs and Symptoms

Norovirus illnesses are characterized by acute onset and may include nausea, vomiting, diarrhea, abdominal cramping, low-grade fever, chills, headache, muscle pain, and lethargy.

### Treatment

Currently, there is neither an antiviral medication that works against norovirus nor is there a vaccine to prevent infection.

### Testing

Tests used in the diagnosis of norovirus illnesses include stool assays, which can identify the specific agent, and a stool culture, which is used to rule out other types of infection.

## NYSTAGMUS

### Description

Nystagmus is a rapid, involuntary movement of the eyes that may be from side to side (horizontal nystagmus), up and down (vertical nystagmus), or rotary. Nystagmus can occur in both eyes or in just one eye, and it is caused by abnormal function in the areas of the brain that control eye movements. The term "dancing eyes" has been used to describe nystagmus. The exact nature of nystagmus is poorly understood, and it may be either congenital or acquired. Congenital nystagmus is usually mild, does not change in severity, and is not associated with any other disorder. Affected people are not aware of the eye movements, although they may be noticed by a careful observer. A less common cause of nystagmus is disease or injury of the central nervous system. Among young people, head injuries during motor vehicle accidents are a common cause of nystagmus. In older people the most common cause is stroke (Bardorf, 2001; Kiriakopoulos, 2003a).

## Signs and Symptoms

Nystagmus may be observed through the following procedure. If the affected person spins around for about 30 seconds, stops, and tries to stare at an object, the eyes will first move slowly in one direction, then move rapidly in the opposite direction. The orientation of these alternating movements (side to side, up and down, or in a circular pattern) depends on the type of nystagmus.

## Treatment

Surgery for nystagmus may improve visual acuity. There is no therapy for most cases of congenital nystagmus. Availability of treatment for acquired nystagmus depends on the underlying cause, and in most cases nystagmus is irreversible.

## Testing

Tests used in the diagnosis of nystagmus may include CT scans of the head, MRI of the head, and electro-oculography.

## OPHTHALMIA NEONATORUM

## Description

Ophthalmia neonatorum is caused by *Neisseria gonorrhea*. During vaginal delivery, the infant's eyes may become infected from the presence of the bacteria in an infected mother's birth canal. The resultant infection can cause lesions on the eye and eventual blindness (see Color Plate 43). This can also cause joint infection or a life-threatening blood infection in the baby. Treatment of gonorrhea as soon as it is detected in pregnant women can lessen the risk of these complications. Ophthalmia neonatorum is rare in the United States because antimicrobial eyedrops or silver nitrate is placed in newborns' eyes upon delivery. Gonorrhea may cause perforation of the cornea and significant destruction of the deeper eye structures (Goldenring, 2004d; Zhao & Enzenauer, 2004).

## Signs and Symptoms

Ophthalmia neonatorum is characterized by watery, bloody drainage from the infant's eyes. The drainage may contain thick pus. The eyelids of the infant are inflamed.

## Treatment

In the United States, hospitals routinely use antibiotic drops, such as erythromycin, in newborns' eyes to prevent disease. Although it was once commonly used, silver nitrate is used less often and has been replaced by antibiotic eyedrops. In cases of infection, opical antibiotic eyedrops and ointments, oral antibiotics, and intravenous antibiotics are all used depending on the severity of the infection.

## Testing

Tests used to diagnose ophthalmia neonatorum include a standard ophthalmologic examination, slit-lamp examination, and culture of the drainage.

## OPISTHORCHIASIS

### Description

Opisthorchiasis is caused by the Southeast Asian liver fluke *Opisthorchis viverrini* and the cat liver fluke *Opisthorchis felineus*. *O. viverrini* is found mainly in northeast Thailand, Laos, and Kampuchea; *O. felineus* is found mainly in Europe and Asia. Humans contract opisthorchiasis by ingesting raw freshwater fish. The adult flukes reside in the biliary and pancreatic ducts of the digestive system, where they attach to the mucosal tissues (*Opisthorchiasis*, 2004).

### Signs and Symptoms

Although most infections are asymptomatic, in mild cases, the infected person may experience indigestion, abdominal pain, diarrhea, or constipation. In more prolonged illness, symptoms may include enlarged liver and malnutrition. In rare cases, cholangitis, cholecystitis, and cholangiocarcinoma may develop. Infections due to *O. felineus* may include an acute phase characterized by fever, facial swelling, lymphadenopathy, arthralgias, and a rash.

### Treatment

Opisthorchiasis is treated with the drug praziquantel.

### Testing

Diagnosis of opisthorchiasis is based on identification of eggs in stool specimens.

## ORCHITIS

### Description

Orchitis is an acute inflammatory reaction in the testicle, occurring in boys under the age of 10, as a result of the mumps virus. Orchitis can, however, be caused by other microbial infections. Orchitis currently occurs in approximately 20 percent of boys who contract mumps, and it normally develops between four and seven days after mumps virus infection (Gilbert, 2004b; Kang, 2002). Orchitis of one testicle rarely results in sterility or increased risk of tumors in later life.

## Signs and Symptoms

The onset of orchitis is typically acute, often causing initial symptoms within hours. Orchitis is characterized by severe pain in the testicle and groin, fatigue, muscle pain, fever, chills, nausea, and headache. The scrotum swells, there is pain upon urination, there is pain with ejaculation during intercourse, and blood in the semen.

## Treatment

In cases of orchitis that is caused by bacteria, antibiotics are prescribed. Pain medications and anti-inflammatory medications are also prescribed. Bed rest, with elevation of the scrotum and ice packs applied to the area, is recommended. With treatment of bacterially caused orchitis, normal function of the testicle is usually preserved. Mumps orchitis cannot be treated, and the outcome is unpredictable. Sterility may follow mumps orchitis.

## Testing

Orchitis is primarily diagnosed through a physical exam, but diagnosis may include urinalysis, a clean catch urine culture, a urethral smear, CBCs, doppler ultrasound to rule out testicular torsion and to detect scrotal abcesses, and a nuclear medicine testicular scan.

## OSGOOD-SCHLATTER DISEASE

### Description

Osgood-Schlatter disease is an inflammation of the anterior tibial tubercle, which is located on the front of the upper tibia just below the knee. Osgood-Schlatter disease is probably caused by a minor injury due to repetitive overuse, prior to the complete maturity of the anterior tibial tubercle attachment. Running, jumping, and climbing stairs cause discomfort, and symptoms may occur in either or both legs. Osgood-Schlatter disease primarily occurs in active, athletic boys (A. Chen, 2003c).

### Signs and Symptoms

Osgood-Schlatter disease is characterized by leg pain or knee pain in one or both knees. The pain worsens with activity, especially running, jumping, or climbing. Pain also worsens when pressure is applied to the area. As with all inflammatory disorders, the symptoms of redness, swelling, heat, and loss of function of the inflamed area are common.

### Treatment

Treatment of Osgood-Schlatter disease includes rest, ice, and nonsteroidal anti-inflammatory medications. In many cases, the condition will disappear with rest, pain medication, and the reduction of sports or exercise. Rarely, surgery may be needed. Most cases of Osgood-Schlatter disease resolve spontaneously within a few months.

### Testing

Diagnosis of Osgood-Schlatter disease is based on a physical exam. X-rays, CT scans, or MRI scans of the leg may be used to confirm diagnosis.

## OSLER-WEBER-RENDU SYNDROME

### Description

Osler-Weber-Rendu syndrome is an inherited disorder of the blood vessels that causes excessive bleeding. The genes affected include mutations of endoglin genes and *ALK-1* genes. Osler-Weber-Rendu syndrome is also known as hereditary hemorrhagic telangiectasia. Affected children develop reddish-purple spiderlike bumps of blood vessels called telangiectases. Telangiectases occur on the lips, tongue, nasal mucosa, brain, lungs, throat, gastrointestinal tract, liver, bladder, and vagina. The telangiectases bleed easily, and brain hemorrhage and stroke may cause seizures. If severe, this brain hemorrhage may be fatal (Balevicience & Schwartz, 2005; Stewart, 2003l).

### Signs and Symptoms

Osler-Weber-Rendu syndrome is characterized by frequent nosebleeds, gastrointestinal bleeding, bloody urine, seizures, strokes, coughing up blood, bloody stool, difficulty breathing, and the appearance of telangiectases during late childhood on the tongue, lips, eyes, ears, fingertips, nail beds, and skin. Some patients only discover that they have Osler-Weber-Rendu syndrome when they cough up blood and a chest X-ray shows an arterio-venous malformation.

### Treatment

Osler-Weber-Rendu syndrome is treated by surgically correcting bleeding in vital areas. Nosebleed may be treated with electrocautery or laser surgery. Some patients respond to estrogen therapy. The prognosis for patients with Osler-Weber-Rendu syndrome is good, barring a fatal intracranial hemorrhage.

### Testing

Tests used in the diagnosis of Osler-Weber-Rendu syndrome include chest X-rays, echocardiograms, liver function tests, blood tests for anemia, endoscopy, and genetic testing for mutations in the endoglin or ALKI genes.

## OSTEITIS FIBROSA

### Description

Osteitis fibrosa is a complication of the excess production of parathryroid hormone. Bones become softened, become deformed, and may develop cysts (Sidhaye, 2004b). The parathyroid glands are in the neck and they produce parathyroid hormone, which helps control calcium levels in the body. Osteitis fibrosa may be caused by overproduction of parathyroid hormone or by parathyroid cancer.

### Signs and Symptoms

Osteitis fibrosa cystica is characterized by bone pain or tenderness. There may be fractures or bowing of the bones. Hyperparathyroidism itself may cause kidney stones, nausea, constipation, or fatigue.

## Treatment

Treatment for hyperparathyroidism may require surgery to remove the abnormal parathyroid glands. Radioactive tracers and rapid parathyroid hormone blood tests may make the surgery quicker and easier. Drugs may also be used to lower calcium levels. The bone problems of osteitis fibrosa cystica are usually reversible with surgery, except for the fluid-filled cysts.

## Testing

Tests used in the diagnosis and treatment of osteitis fibrosa cystica may include blood tests, and imaging exams of the bones and teeth.

# OSTEOARTHRITIS

## Description

Osteoarthritis, or degenerative joint disease, is caused by the deterioration of joint cartilage, which causes bones to rub against each other, resulting in pain, inflammation, and loss of movement. Osteoarthritis affects the hands and weight-bearing joints such as the knees, hips, feet, and the back. People with joint injuries due to sports, work-related activity, or accidents may be at increased risk of developing osteoarthritis, and people who are obese may develop osteoarthritis of the knees. Osteoarthritis may first appear without symptoms between 30 and 40 years of age and is present in almost everyone by the age of 70 (A. Chen, 2004b).

## Signs and Symptoms

Osteoarthritis is characterized by a gradually progressive onset of deep, aching joint pain. The cartilage of the affected joint is roughened and becomes worn down, until bones rub on articulating bones. Bony spurs usually develop around the joint. The joints of the hands and fingers, hips, knees, big toe, and cervical and lumbar spine are commonly affected. Symptoms of osteoarthritis may also include joint swelling, loss of function of the joint, morning stiffness, grating of the bones with motion, and variations in joint pain with changes in the weather.

## Treatment

There is no cure for osteoarthritis. Treatment depends upon the affected joints, but medications commonly used may include a variety of nonsteroidal anti-inflammatory drugs, steroids, glucosamine, and chondroitin. COX 2 inhibitors (e.g., Celebrex, Vioxx, Bextra) have been prescribed in place of NSAIDS because they are less likely to cause stomach upset; however, the use of Vioxx and Bextra has come into question. Artificial joint fluid (e.g., Synvisc, Hyalgan) can be injected into the joint and leads to temporary relief of pain for up to six months. Surgical treatment to replace or repair damaged joints is indicated in severe, debilitating disease. Surgical options include arthroplasty, arthroscopic surgery, and arthrodesis.

## Testing

Tests used in the diagnosis of osteoarthritis may include a variety of imaging tests (e.g., X-rays, MRI scans, CT scans, PET scans), and blood tests to rule out other causes of arthritis.

## OSTEOMALACIA

### Description

Osteomalacia involves softening of the bones caused by a deficiency or failure to metabolize vitamin D (Sidhaye, 2004c). In children, the condition is called rickets and is usually caused by a deficiency of vitamin D. Conditions that may lead to osteomalacia include inadequate dietary intake of vitamin D; inadequate exposure to sunlight (ultraviolet radiation), which produces vitamin D in the body; and malabsorption of vitamin D by the intestines. Other conditions that can cause osteomalacia include hereditary or acquired disorders of vitamin D metabolism; kidney failure and acidosis; phosphate depletion associated with low dietary intake of phosphates; kidney disease or cancer (rare), and side effects of medications used to treat seizures. Use of strong sunscreen, limited exposure of the body to sunlight, short days of sunlight, and smog are factors that decrease formation of vitamin D within the body.

### Signs and Symptoms

Osteomalacia is characterized by diffuse bone pain, especially in the hips. It is accompanied by muscle weakness and bone fractures with minimal trauma. Figure 2-55 illustrates different types of fractures.

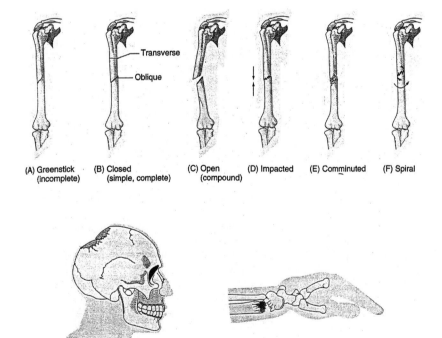

(A) Greenstick (incomplete)    (B) Closed (simple, complete)    (C) Open (compound)    (D) Impacted    (E) Comminuted    (F) Spiral

(G) Depressed    (H) Colles

**Figure 2-55** Types of fractures

Symtpoms of low calcium levels include numbness around the mouth, numbness of the extremities, spasms of the hands or feet, and abnormal heart rhythms.

## Treatment

Ostoemalacia is treated with supplements of vitamin D, calcium, and phosphorus, depending on the underlying cause of the disorder. Complete healing with treatment takes place in about six months.

## Testing

Tests used in the diagnosis and treatment of osteomalacia may include bone biopsy, serum vitamin D levels, serum calcium levels, serum phosphate levels, bone X-rays, a bone mineral density scan (DEXA), PTH, ionized calcium tests, and a test for alkaline phosphatase (ALP) isoenzyme.

## OSTEOMYELITIS

### Description

Osteomyelitis is an inflammatory disorder of the bone marrow resulting from pus-causing bacteria (King, 2002; Levy, 2004a). Hematogenous osteomyelitis is an infection caused by bacteria that migrate from the blood into the bone, primarily in children. Rapidly growing bones contain many blood vessels. Where the blood vessels make sharp angles at the ends of the bones, the blood flow slows, predisposing these sites to blood clot formation. The slowed blood combined with the clots can result in necrosis of the bone and the promotion of bacterial growth. Direct inoculation osteomyelitis is caused by contact of the tissue and bacteria during trauma or surgery. Any trauma forcing bacteria into the tissues can result in a focal infection. The focal infection may then spread to the bone, causing direct inoculation osteomyelitis.

### Signs and Symptoms

Osteomyelitis is characterized by acute high fever, fatigue, irritability, restriction of movement, localized swelling, redness, tenderness, nonhealing ulcers, and late-stage sinus drainage due to infection.

### Treatment

Osteomyelitis is treated with antibiotics, surgical removal of dead bone tissue, and surgical removal of infected prostheses. The outcome for acute osteomyelitis is good, but it is worse for chronic osteomyelitis, even with surgery. Resistant or extensive chronic osteomyelitis may result in amputation, especially in diabetics or other patients with poor blood circulation.

### Testing

Tests used in the diagnosis and treatment of osteomyelitis may include bone scans, CBC, ESR levels, blood cultures, MRI and needle aspiration of the area, bone lesion biopsy, and skin lesion biopsy.

## OSTEOPOROSIS

### Description

Osteoporosis is loss of bone mass. Healthy bone constantly remodels itself by taking up structure elements from one area and patching others. In osteoporosis, more bone is resorbed than laid down, and the skeleton loses some of its strength. Type I osteoporosis occurs as a result of the loss of the protective effects of estrogen on bone. Osteoporosis is associated with an increased demand for calcium in women's bodies after menopause. This disorder has a long, slow onset, and it is characterized by loss of bone tissue, causing weak, brittle bones. Type II osteoporosis, which used to be known as senile osteoporosis, is caused by aging. Women over 60 are more prone to osteoporosis because they may have an inadequate intake of calcium and vitamin D in their diets. They are also less likely to participate in weight-bearing exercise such as walking, which strengthens bones (Cooper, 2004).

### Signs and Symptoms

Fractures of the bones of the hip, spine, and wrist are common among persons with osteoporosis, and the individual's body weight may cause enough force to result in bone fracture. Often, when elderly persons fall and break a hip, it is likely that their hip broke culminating in a fall. One characteristic of advanced osteoporosis is severe curvature of the spine. This curvature of the spine is depicted in Figure 2-56.

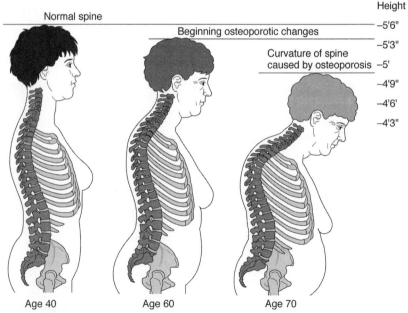

Height
−5'6"
Normal spine
Beginning osteoporotic changes
−5'3"
Curvature of spine
caused by osteoporosis −5'
−4'9"
−4'6'
−4'3"

Age 40          Age 60          Age 70

**Figure 2-56** Osteoporosis

## Treatment

There are several different kinds of drugs used to treat osteoporosis (e.g., alendronate, risedronate, calcitonin, and raloxifene). Hormone therapy may also be used to treat osteoporosis. Vertebroplasty can be used to treat minor fractures in the spinal column.

## Testing

Tests used in the diagnosis and treatment of osteoporosis include bone mineral density tests (DEXA), a spine CT scan, hip X-rays, urinalysis for calcium levels and measurement of urinary *N*-telopeptides.

## OSTEOSARCOMAS

## Description

Osteosarcoma is an aggressive, rapid growing tumor that often spreads to the lungs in its early stages. The cells that cause osteosarcoma produce bone matrix in a similar fashion to healthy osteoblasts, with the exception that the malignant bone tissue of an osteosarcoma is not as strong as normal bones. Osteosarcomas can spread to other nearby tissues, and cells from osteosarcoma may fragment from the main tumor and metastasize through the bloodstream to the rest of the body. In 80 percent of osteosarcomas, the tumor is located in the bones of the knee. The second most common site is in the shoulder (Blackman, 2004g; Enneking, 1995).

## Signs and Symptoms

Osteosarcoma appears as a hard, white tissue with scattered areas of fleshlike tissue that bleeds. Osteosarcomas are painful, enlarging masses that can invade joints by growing along the path of surrounding ligaments.

## Treatment

Chemotherapy is responsible for a dramatic increase in survival rates and a decrease in the need for amputation. When the tumor is not responsive to chemotherapy, amputation is necessary to contain the spread of this cancer of the bone. In the absence of pulmonary metastasis, long-term survival may reach 70 percent. If the cancer has spread, permanent cure is less likely.

## Testing

Tests used in the diagnosis of osteosarcoma include X-rays, CT scans, blood tests, open biopsy, and bone scans.

## OTITIS MEDIA

## Description

Otitis media is often caused by the bacterium *Streptococcus pneumoniae*, although other microorganisms such as *Haemophilus influenzae* and *Staphylococcus aureus* are also known causes. Otitis media is an infection of the fluids of the middle ear, and it is often a complication of the common cold and infections of the nose and throat. *S. pneumoniae* may be spread through contact with contaminated water found in swimming pools, through eardrum puncture, and through skull fractures. This pustulant infection causes pressure behind the eardrum resulting in earaches.

## Signs and Symptoms

Otitis media is an acute ear infection characterized by an earache. In infants, the clearest sign is often irritability and inconsolable crying. Many infants and children develop a fever or have trouble sleeping. Parents often think that tugging on the ear is a symptom of an ear infection, but studies have shown that children tug on the ear whether or not the ear is infected. Other possible symptoms include fullness in the ear, vomiting, diarrhea, and hearing loss (Greene, 2004b).

## Treatment

As a result of the narrow diameter of a child's ear (i.e., eustachian) tubes, these passages become easily blocked by bacterial colonies. When this occurs frequently, tubes may be implanted to help keep the eustachian tube open. Otitis media is treated with antibiotics like penicillin.

## Testing

Otitis media is diagnosed based on a physical examination with an otoscope. A hearing test may be recommended if your child has had persistent ear infections.

## OTOSCLEROSIS

## Description

Otosclerosis, which is also known as otospongiosis, is an abnormal bone growth in the middle ear causing hearing loss due to a genetic disorder. This abnormal bone growth prevents the stapes from vibrating in response to sound waves, thus leading to progressive hearing loss. Otosclerosis affects about 10 percent of the population of the United States (Fung, 2004). Otosclerosis usually affects both ears and is most commonly seen in women because they are more likely than men to report hearing loss (Roland, 2004).

## Signs and Symptoms

Otosclerosis is characterized by slow, progressive hearing loss, ringing in the ears, and occasionally dizziness.

## Treatment

Otosclerosis may be treated with supplements that stabilize hearing loss (e.g., fluoride, calcium, or vitamin D). A hearing aid may be required. Most patients elect surgery to remove the stapes and replace it with a prosthesis.

## Testing

In addition to hearing tests, the diagnosis and treatment of otosclerosis may require a head CT scan or head X-ray to rule out other causes of hearing loss.

## OVARIAN CYSTS

### Description

Ovarian cysts are sacs filled with fluids that develop on or within the ovary, as illustrated in Figure 2-57. Ovarian cysts may be present at birth, or they may occur late in women's lives. Most ovarian cysts occur during women's childbearing years, and although they are usually benign, they may mask the presence of other conditions, such as cancer, ectopic pregnancy, or appendicitis. Ovarian cysts occur in 30 percent of women with regular menstrual cycles and 50 percent of women with irregular menstrual cycles.

### Signs and Symptoms

Ovarian cysts occur and resolve without treatment during women's menstrual cycle. When these cysts rupture, they can lead to sharp, severe abdominal pain, which is experienced by 25 percent of menstruating women. Ovarian cysts may also become inflamed and cause spontaneous bleeding. Sometimes, ovarian cysts can lead to more complicated cyst formation, which can result in infection, blood clots in the ovarian vessels, emboli in the lungs, blood poisoning, and death. Ovarian cysts also may be associated with infertility and irregular menstrual bleeding. In infants, ovarian cysts can cause fluid in the abdomen and insufficient development of the lungs and kidneys.

### Treatment

Although they are not malignant, ovarian cysts may have to be removed surgically because of twisting of part of the ovary, which may lead to gangrene. Another reason to remove ovarian cysts is the pressure they may exert on surrounding tissues as they grow.

### Testing

According to P. Chen (2004c), tests used in the diagnosis of ovarian cysts include a pelvic exam, a pregnancy test, an ultrasound or CT scan, a test

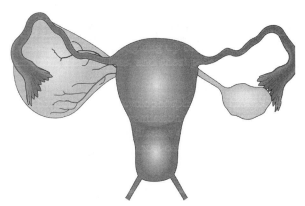

**Figure 2-57** Fibroid tumors

of hormone levels in the blood, and a Ca-125 test. The Ca-125 test identifies the presence of an ovarian cancer marker that may help identify cancerous cysts in older women.

## PAGET'S DISEASE

### Description

Paget's disease is an excessive growth, in the form of hyperplasia, of the bones of the elderly, causing chronic inflammation, thickening, and softening of the bones. Bowing of long bones may also be present. This idiopathic disease is also known as osteitis deformans and is more common in men than women. The progression of Paget's disease includes bone tissue being reabsorbed and synthesis of new bone at abnormally high rates. The new growth of bone tissue may cause compression of the spinal and cranial nerves leading to disability and death. The increased number of blood vessels in the bone leads to increased cardiac output, which may culminate in cardiac failure.

### Signs and Symptoms

Paget's disease is characterized by deafness, increased head size, headaches, heart failure, and pain in the back, hips, and pelvis. Most patients with Paget's disease have no symptoms.

### Treatment

Paget's disease is treated with several classes of medications that inhibit bone resorption (e.g., bisphosphonates, calcitonin, and plicamycin). Localized Paget's disease requires no treatment, if there are no symptoms and no evidence of active disease. Orthopedic surgery may be required to correct deformities in severe cases. Malignant changes of bone occur in less than 1 percent of the cases of Paget's disease (Jain, 2004b).

### Testing

According to Jain (2004b), tests that may indicate Paget's disease include bone X-rays, bone scans, elevated serum alkaline phosphatase, serum calcium tests, alkaline phosphatase (ALP) isoenzyme tests, and elevated markers of bone breakdown (e.g., N-telopeptide).

## PANCREATITIS

### Description

Pancreatitis is an inflammatory process in which the pancreas is digested by its own enzymes. Although the pancreas may heal without any anatomical or physiological impairment, permanent damage may also occur. The location of the pancreas in the retroperitoneal space, combined with its lack of an outer capsule, results in the easy spread of both infection and inflammation. The primary causes of pancreatitis are a history of binge alcohol consumption and gallstones. If the gallstones become lodged in the pancreatic duct or the papilla of Vater, the flow of pancreatic fluids becomes blocked and the autolytic enzymes in the pancreatic fluids digest the pancreas (Khoury & Deeba, 2001).

## Signs and Symptoms

Pancreatitis is characterized by nausea, vomiting, jaundice, fever, bruising of the abdominal flanks, and upper abdominal pain that radiates to the back. Pancreatitis is also characterized by the presence of swelling in the retroperitoneum and necrosis of the peripancreatic fat. In necrotizing pancreatitis, the tissue death extends from the peripancreatic fat into the pancreas itself, and it is accompanied by hemorrhage and pancreas dysfunction. Pancreatic abscesses and cysts then form as a result of pancreatic juices being walled off by necrotic and bleeding tissue. Necrotizing pancreatitis can cause vasodilatation, increased vascular permeability, pain, and accumulation of white blood cells in the walls of blood vessels. Breathing difficulties and muscular spasms may also occur.

## Treatment

If no kidney or lung complications occur, acute pancreatitis usually improves on its own. If pancreatic pseudocysts occur, they may be drained or surgically removed. Pancreatic enzymes may be administered. Insulin may be needed to control blood glucose levels. In some cases, the pancreas may need to be removed.

## Testing

Tests used in the diagnosis of pancreatitis may include abdominal X-rays, endoscopic retrograde cholangiopancreatography (ERCP), CT scans, and blood tests evaluating levels of pancreatic enzymes.

## PAPILLOMAS

### Description

Papillomas are wartlike tumors caused by the human papillomavirus, which can cause abnormal tissue changes on the feet, hands, vocal cords, face, and genitals (see Color Plate 44). Papilloma lesions of the larynx can grow large enough to interfere with breathing and be fatal. Genital warts are growths found on the external sex organs as illustrated in Figure 2-58. They are usually painless, but they may cause itching, burning, or slight bleeding. Warts can also be found around the urethra and anus. Inside the vagina and on the cervix, warts are usually flat and can be identified by a Pap smear. There are two kinds of abnormal tissue caused by human papillomavirus; condyloma (warts) and dysplasia (precancer) (Human papilloma virus, 1997; Papilloma, 2002).

### Signs and Symptoms

Warts are characterized by raised, flesh-colored lesions with a cauliflower-like appearance. Genital warts are accompanied by increased dampness in the area, itching, vaginal discharge, and vaginal bleeding after sexual intercourse (see Color Plate 45).

### Treatment

The main treatment for laryngeal papilloma is surgical removal. Because the tumors are confined to the surface of the vocal folds, patients often retain their voice after surgery. Surgical treatments of genital warts

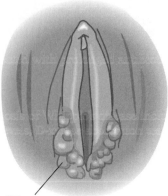

Warts caused by
human papillomavirus (HPV)

**Figure 2-58** Genital warts

include cryosurgery, electrocauterization, laser therapy, or excision. Genital warts should not be treated with over-the-counter remedies meant for other kinds of warts (Hart, 2004b). With proper treatment, genital wart outbreaks usually can be controlled.

### Testing
Tests used in the diagnosis of genital warts include a Pap smear and a tissue biopsy.

## PARAGONIMIASIS

### Description
Paragonimiasis is an infection of both human and nonhuman animals caused by the oriental lung fluke *Paragonimus westermani*, although more than 30 other species of *Paragonimus* may also cause paragonimiasis. Infection is by eating contaminated crab or crawfish that have been undercooked or pickled. The immature flukes penetrate the intestines and travel to the lungs, where they develop into adult flukes. Infections may last as long as 20 years, and it may be 65 to 90 days before systemic illness develops. Animals such as pigs, dogs, and cats can also harbor *Paragonimus*, which is found in the Far East, both North and South America, and Africa (*Paragonimiasis*, 2004).

### Signs and Symptoms
The acute phase of paragonimiasis is characterized by diarrhea, abdominal pain, fever, cough, hives, enlarged liver and spleen, and pulmonary abnormalities. During the chronic phase, pulmonary manifestations include cough, expectoration of discolored sputum, and coughing up blood.

### Treatment
Paragonimiasis is treated with praziquantel.

**Testing**

Paragonimiasis is diagnosed by examination of microbes found in stool or sputum samples, and through tests used to identify specific antibodies in the blood.

## PARINAUD'S SYNDROME

### Description

Parinaud's syndrome, which is also known as oculoglandular syndrome, is an eye problem similar to conjunctivitis (Levy, 2004r). It usually affects only one eye and is accompanied by swollen lymph nodes and fever. Parinaud's syndrome may be caused by a variety of infectious microorganisms. The most common causes are tularemia, which is also known as rabbit fever, and catscratch disease.

### Signs and Symptoms

Parinaud's syndrome is characterized by inflammation of the eye with an increased amount of tears. There may be swelling of the lymph glands nearby, often in front of the ear. A fever and generalized illness may be present.

### Treatment

Parinaud's syndrome is treated with antibiotics and/or surgery to remove infected tissues. With treatment, the outcome of Parinaud's syndrome is positive.

### Testing

For many of the infections that cause Parinaud's syndrome, blood tests to check antibody levels are the main methods used to make a diagnosis. Sometimes, culture of the eye, lymph node, or blood or biopsy of the lymph node may be required.

## PARKINSON'S DISEASE

### Description

Parkinson's disease is a chronic nervous disease characterized by a fine, slowly spreading tremor, muscular weakness and rigidity, and a peculiar gait (Figure 2-59). Persons with Parkinson's disease have diminished levels of dopamine, a neurotransmitter, in their brains, which causes them to exhibit signs of a fine tremor of the hands or feet that spreads to other parts of the body (Campellone, 2004l; Parkinson's disease backgrounder, 2001).

### Signs and Symptoms

In advanced cases of Parkinson's, individuals have an expressionless face and a speech impairment. In addition, they have a bowed head, a forward bend to their body, and thumbs that are turned in toward their palms. Parkinson's causes flexed arms as the muscles become rigid. An examination may show jerky, stiff movements, known as cogwheel rigidity and difficulty initiating or completing voluntary movements. Reflexes are essentially normal.

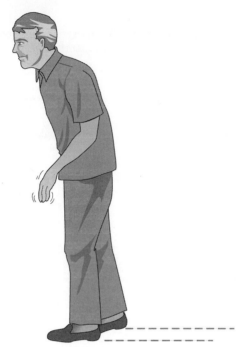

**Figure 2-59** Parkinson's disease

## Treatment

There is no known cure for Parkinson's disease. Medications increase the levels of dopamine in the brain. Deprenyl may provide some improvement. Amantadine or anticholinergic medications may be used to reduce early or mild tremors. Levodopa is a medication that the body converts to dopamine, which may improve movement and balance. Carbidopa is a medication that reduces the side effects of levodopa. Additional medications include antihistamines, antidepressants, dopamine agonists, and monoamine oxidase inhibitors. Untreated, Parkinson's progresses to total disability and an early death.

## Testing

There is no specific test for Parkinson's.

## PARONYCHIA

### Description

Paronychia is a superficial infection of the skin around the nails, most commonly caused by staphylococcus bacteria or fungi (Lehrer, 2003e). Fungal paronychia frequently accompanies cases of diabetes and among people who have their hands in water for long periods of time. It may also be caused by removing hangnails or trimming the cuticles.

## Signs and Symptoms

Paronychia is characterized by skin lesions located around the nail, often at the cuticle or at the site of a hangnail or other injury. Other symptoms include pain, swelling, redness, pustules, nail changes, discolorations, distorted shape of the finger and nail, and nail detachment.

## Treatment

In bacterial paronychia, hot water soaks may reduce inflammation and pain. Topical or oral antibiotics may be prescribed. In severe cases, the lesion may need to be excised and drained by a physician. Fungal paronychia may be treated with topical or oral antifungals. Paronychia is superficial and responds well to treatment.

## Testing

Diagnosis of paronychia is based primarily on the physical examination of the skin lesions, but aspiration and culture of inflammatory exudates may be used to isolate the organism causing the infection.

## PAROXYSMAL NOCTURNAL HEMOGLOBINURIA

### Description

Paroxysmal nocturnal hemoglobinuria is a rare disorder in which red blood cells rupture prematurely, releasing hemoglobin into the urine (Besa & Woermann, 2002; Cutler, 2003). Paroxysmal nocturnal hemoglobinuria is caused by a defect in a red blood cell surface protein anchor called GP1 and in the gene *PIGA*. Paroxysmal nocturnal hemoglobinuria may arise in relation to aplastic anemia, and may progress to acute myelogenous leukemia.

### Signs and Symptoms

Paroxysmal nocturnal hemoglobinuria is characterized by bloody urine, abdominal pain, back pain, skin nodules, headache, difficulty breathing, easy bruising, absent bowel sounds, and bleeding in the skin.

### Treatment

Paroxysmal nocturnal hemoglobinuria is treated with steroids, bone marrow transplant, blood transfusions, and anticoagulation therapy. With treatment, most people survive approximately 10 years following diagnosis, but the disease can be fatal. Drugs that may be used include oxymetholone, stanozdo, donazol, and Atgam.

### Testing

Tests used in the diagnosis of paroxysmal nocturnal hemoglobinuria include CBC, sucrose hemolysis tests, Ham's acid hemolysin test, flow cytometry, urinalysis, and serum hemoglobin.

## PARROT FEVER

### Description

Parrot fever, which is also known as psittacosis or as ornithosis, is a disease caused by *Chlamydia psittaci*, which is a gram-negative, obligate intracellular bacterium. The disease receives its name from its association with psittacine birds, such as parakeets and parrots. It can also be contracted from pigeons, chickens, ducks, and turkeys. *C. psittaci* is spread to humans by inhaling the aerosolized microbes from bird droppings. People who work with birds are most at risk for this disorder, although those who work in buildings that provide nesting sites for birds may become infected from breathing the microbes. These bacteria enter buildings through ventilation systems, and courthouses and city buildings with ledges near the roof are excellent candidates for nesting (Psittacosis, 2003).

## Signs and Symptoms
Parrot fever is characterized by fever and chills, muscle aches, headache, fatigue, cough, difficulty breathing, rales, and coughing up blood.

## Treatment
Parrot fever is treated with antibiotics (e.g., tetracycline, doxycycline, erythromycin, azithromycin). Full recovery is expected.

## Testing
Tests used in the diagnosis of parrot fever include chest X-rays, CT scans of the chest, sputum culture, blood culture, and antibody titers (Hart, 2004m).

## PELVIC INFLAMMATORY DISEASE

### Description
Most cases of pelvic inflammatory disease occur in two stages. During the first stage, a vaginal or cervical infection develops, and during the second stage, the infection spreads to the upper genital tract. Table 2-6 lists some of the most common inflammatory conditions of the female reproductive system, which is illustrated in Figure 2-60. Many cases of pelvic inflammatory disease are asymptomatic, and the only characteristic of symptomatic cases may be lower abdominal pain.

### Signs and Symptoms
Salpingitis is characterized by vaginal discharge, abdominal pain, fever, chills, irregular menstrual bleeding, pain during sexual intercourse,

**Table 2-6** Inflammatory Conditions of the Female Reproductive System

| | |
|---|---|
| Endometritis | inflammation of the lining of the uterus due to bacterial infection |
| Endocervicitis | inflammation of the uterus and the cervix |
| Salpingitis | inflammation of the fallopian (uterine) tube |
| Oophoritis | inflammation of the ovary |
| Vaginitis | inflammation of the vagina |

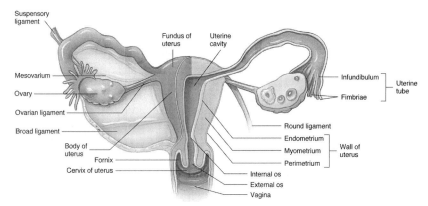

**Figure 2-60** Female reproductive system

bleeding after intercourse, back pain, fatigue, loss of appetite, nausea, frequent urination, and painful urination.

## Treatment

PID is treated with antibiotics. Surgery may be considered for complicated, persistent cases that do not respond to adequate antibiotic treatment. In 15 percent of cases, the initial antibiotic therapy fails, and 20 percent experience a recurrence of PID (Hecht, 2004).

## Testing

Tests used in the diagnosis of PID include CBC, erythrocyte sedimentation rate, cultures, pregnancy tests, pelvic ultrasound or CT scan, and laparoscopy.

## PEMPHIGUS

### Description

Pemphigus is a rare autoimmune disorder characterized by blistering of the skin and mucous membranes (Chan, 2003; Kantor, 2004c, Zeina, 2003). In cases of pemphigus, antibodies produce a reaction that leads to a separation of epidermal cells in the skin. The exact cause of the development of antibodies is unknown. Pemphigus may be a side effect of ACE inhibitors or chelating agents. About one half of the cases of pemphigus vulgaris begin with blisters in the mouth, followed by skin blisters. The lesions spread, and complications develop rapidly. Pemphigus may be debilitating or fatal.

### Signs and Symptoms

Pemphigus is characterized by recurrent blisters of the skin and mucous membranes of the mouth. These lesions may drain, ooze, or crust. The may also be located on the scalp and trunk. The superficial skin peels and detaches easily.

## Treatment

Severe cases of pemphigus are treated similarly to severe burns. Intravenous fluids, electrolytes, and proteins may be required. Antibiotics and antifungal medications may be appropriate to prevent infections. Other treatments include corticosteroids, medications containing gold, or medications that suppress the immune system (e.g., azathioprine, methotrexate). Plasmapheresis may be used to reduce the amount of antibodies in the bloodstream. If not treated, pemphigus vulgaris is usually fatal due to generalized infection.

## Testing

Tests used in the diagnosis of pemphigus include skin lesion biopsy, examination of biopsied tissue with immunofluorescence, and a Tzanck test of a smear from the base of a blister indicating acantholysis. Pemphigus also results in a positive positive Nikolsky's sign. This occurs when the surface of uninvolved skin is rubbed with a cotton swab or finger, and the skin separates easily.

## PEPTIC ULCERS

## Description

Peptic ulcers occur in the stomach and duodenum of the small intestine (Figure 2-61). In the stomach, they are known as gastric ulcers, and in the duodenum they are known as duodenal ulcers. An ulcer is a localized area

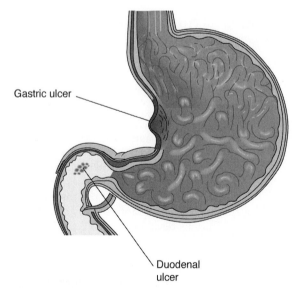

Gastric ulcer

Duodenal ulcer

**Figure 2-61** Peptic ulcers

of dead tissue that can slough off, eventually leaving behind a hole in the damaged area of tissue known as a perforation. This allows the contents of the digestive tract to pass through the ulcer into the abdominal cavity where microorganisms can cause peritonitis, which can be fatal. If peptic ulcers occur in the pyloric region of the stomach, scar tissue may form and narrow the opening through which the food passes into the small intestine. The bacteria that cause most peptic ulcers are *Helicobacter pylori* (Hart, 2003h). A rare cause of peptic ulcers may be Zollinger-Ellison syndrome, in which the presence of a tumor in the pancreas causes peptic ulcers in the stomach and duodenum (Radebold, 2003).

## Signs and Symptoms

Peptic ulcers are characterized by abdominal pain, especially occurring two to three hours after eating or after skipping a meal. The pain may abate with the use of antacids or by drinking milk. Other symptoms of peptic ulcers include nausea, vomiting, weight loss, fatigue, heartburn, indigestion, belching, chest pain, vomiting blood, or blood in the feces.

## Treatment

Treatment of peptic ulcers often involves a combination of medications to kill the *Helicobacter pylori* bacteria, reduce acid levels, and protect the GI tract. The medications may include antibiotics, acid blockers (e.g., cimetidine, ranitidine, famotidine), proton pump inhibitors (e.g., omeprazole), medications that protect the tissue lining (e.g., sucralfate), and bismuth, which may help protect the lining and kill the bacteria (Hart, 2003h). Peptic ulcers tend to recur if untreated.

## Testing

Tests used in the diagnosis of peptic ulcers may include an upper GI, tissue biopsies, and an esophagogastroduodenoscopy.

## PERICARDITIS

## Description

Pericarditis is an inflammation of the pericardium, which is the sac that surrounds the heart. Two common causes of pericarditis include infections and blunt force trauma, such as that resulting from the chest striking the steering wheel during an automobile collision. There is a small amount of fluid normally present between the two layers of the pericardium. If, during the inflammatory process, an excessive amount of fluid accumulates within the pericardial sac, a fatal condition known as cardiac tamponade may occur. The excess fluid results in a disturbance of the electrolyte and protein balance in the pericardial sac, and the pressure inside the pericardial sac increases as the fluid accumulates. The result of these changes is that the heart is unable to expand fully and has less force when it contracts, so it cannot pump as much blood. The blood pressure drops, and more fluid accumulates around the heart (Hart, 2004j; Valley & Fly, 2002).

## Signs and Symptoms

Pericarditis is characterized by chest pain that is usually relieved with sitting, a sharp pain known as pleuritis, increased deep breathing, breathing difficulty when lying down that is relieved when seated or standing, bending over and holding the chest while breathing, cough, difficulty swallowing, hiccups, anxiety, and fever.

## Treatment

Pericarditis is treated with analgesics, antibiotics, antifungal agents, nonsteroidal anti-inflammatories, diuretics, and corticosteroids. Pericardial fluid may be drained through pericardiocentesis, which may be either percutaneous by using an echocardiogram to guide a needle to the pericardium, or through minor surgery. In severe cases, a pericardiectomy may need to be performed in which part of the pericardium is removed. Although pericarditis can be fatal, most people recover in a few months.

## Testing

Tests used in the diagnosis of pericarditis may include chest X-rays, echocardiograms, chest MRI scans, heart MRI or CT scans, radionuclide scanning, electrocardiogram, and tests for serial cardiac marker levels (CL-MB and troponin I). Other laboratory tests may include blood culture, CBC, C-reactive protein, erythrocyte sedimentation rate, and pericardiocentesis with chemical analysis and pericardial fluid culture.

## PERITONITIS

### Description

Peritonitis is an inflammation of the peritoneum, which is the membrane that lines the wall of the abdomen and covers the abdominal organs (Molmenti, 2004). Primary peritonitis occurs when an infection is present in the abdomen without obvious organ rupture. Primary peritonitis is the result of cirrhosis and fluid in the abdomen, especially in cases of tuberculosis related to AIDS and in dialysis patients. Secondary peritonitis occurs when an organ is ruptured by the infection. Secondary peritonitis is usually the result of a ruptured appendix, perforated ulcer, abdominal trauma, or Crohn's disease. The air, acid, fecal material, and bacteria in the ruptured organ spill into the abdomen, resulting in infection.

### Signs and Symptoms

Peritonitis is characterized by abdominal pain, abdominal distention, fever, low urine output, thirst, fluid in the abdomen, inability to pass feces or gas, nausea, vomiting, shaking chills, and signs of shock. If the patient is undergoing peritoneal dialysis, the dialysis fluid will become cloudy.

### Treatment

The cause of peritonitis must be identified and treated promptly. Typically, treatment involves surgery and antibiotics. The outcome for peritonitis is often good, but sometimes the outcome is poor, even with prompt and adequate treatment.

## Testing

Tests used in the diagnosis of peritonitis may include blood tests, X-rays, and CT scans.

# PERNICIOUS ANEMIA

## Description

Pernicious anemia is caused by a failure of the body to produce enough intrinsic factor, an intestinal chemical, to absorb vitamin $B_{12}$ in the intestine. Vitamin $B_{12}$ is required for the process of absorbing iron in the diet. Eating more iron-containing foods does not resolve cases of pernicious anemia (Hart, 2004k).

## Signs and Symptoms

Pernicious anemia is characterized by difficulty breathing, fatigue, pallor, rapid heart rate, loss of appetite, diarrhea, tingling and numbness of the hands and feet, sore mouth, unsteady gait, tongue problems, impaired smell, bleeding gums, loss of deep tendon reflexes, and personality changes. Patients with pernicious anemia also exhibit a positive Babinski's reflex, which indicates a diminished Achilles tendon reflex.

## Treatment

Pernicious anemia is treated with vitamin $B_{12}$ injections. The outcome is usually excellent with treatment.

## Testing

Tests used in the diagnosis and treatment of pernicious anemia include CBC, reticulocyte count, bone marrow examination, serum LDH, serum vitamin $B_{12}$ levels, Schilling test, serum holotranscobalamin II levels, and methylmalonic acid levels.

# PERTUSSIS

## Description

Whooping cough, which is also known as pertussis, is caused by the bacterium *Bordetella pertussis*. Whooping cough is one of the most highly communicable childhood diseases, infecting over 90 percent of susceptible households. Even in immunized populations like the United States, outbreaks of pertussis still occur every few years and isolated cases occur continuously. Adults appear to carry bacteria without symptoms, but they transmit the disease to children, especially when immunization rates decrease (Bordetella pertussis, 2001; Goldenring, 2004e).

## Signs and Symptoms

The initial infection in whooping cough takes about one to two weeks to develop into a mild respiratory infection resembling the common cold. At this stage, the disease is highly communicable, and the immune system is affected by bacterial toxins. About one to two weeks after the initial stage, *B. pertussis* impedes the tiny hairlike cilia of the respiratory tract, resulting in the accumulation of mucus. The infected individual makes a whooping sound while gasping for air between violent coughs. These spells of coughing may occur many times a day, followed by vomiting. Less common but more severe complications associated with pertussis are subcutaneous emphysema, bleeding in the eyes and nose, umbilical and inguinal hernias, and rupture of the diaphragm. In infants and young children the rectal lining may prolapse through the anus.

## Treatment

Erythromycin, an antibiotic, may shorten the duration of the symptoms of pertussis somewhat, if initiated early enough. Most patients are only diagnosed after antibiotics are effective. Intravenous fluid may be indicated if coughing spells are severe. Cough expectorants and suppressants are not helpful. The prognosis is generally good (Goldenring, 2004f).

## Testing

Tests used in the diagnosis of pertussis may include a culture of secretions from the nose and mouth, a throat swab culture, CBC, serologic tests for *Bordetella pertussis,* and immunologic tests.

## PHAEOHYPHOMYCOSIS

### Description

Phaeohyphomycosis consists of a group of fungal infections. Many infections of the eyes and skin by black fungi are classified as phaeohyphomycosis. The fungi have melanin in their cell walls. The primary fungi causing phaeohyphomycosis include *Cladophialophora bantiana, Curvularia, Bipolaris, Exserohilum, Exophiala jeanselmei, Scedosporium prolificans, Ochroconis gallopava, Coniothyrium fuckelii, Phialophora parasitica, Phialophora repens, Wangiella dermatitidis,* and *Lasiodiplodia theobromae* (Phaeohyphomycosis, 2004).

### Signs and Symptoms

Clinical forms of phaeohyphomycosis range from localized superficial infections of the skin, to subcutaneous cysts, to invasion of the brain.

### Treatment

Phaeohyphomycosis is treated by surgical excision and chemotherapy. Amphotericin B and 5-fluorocytosine or itraconazole are the drugs of choice. The prognosis for phaeohyphomycosis is good with treatment, but invasion of the brain or bone can be fatal.

### Testing

The diagnosis of phaeohyphomycosis is based on the identification of fungi in cultures of tissue and pus. Standardized testing procedures are not available.

## PHARYNGITIS

### Description
Pharyngitis is an inflammatory condition of the pharynx that is most commonly caused by a virus, although it can be bacterial in nature. Group A streptococci are the most commonly encountered etiological agent of bacterial pharyngitis (Hurtado, 2003).

### Signs and Symptoms
Pharyngitis is characterized by sore throat and flulike symptoms. The presence of exudates in the pharynx, fever, or lack of a cough suggest pharyngitis caused by *Streptococcus pygenes* (i.e., strep throat).

### Treatment
Pharyngitis is treated with antibiotics.

### Testing
Laboratory diagnosis of pharyngitis is determined by direct microscopic examination, culture, latex agglutination, coagglutination tests, and enzyme immunoassays.

## PHENYLKETONURIA

### Description
Phenylketonuria (PKU) is an inherited condition in which the amino acid phenylalanine is not properly metabolized (Arnold, 2003). Phenylalanine is one of the eight essential amino acids found in protein-containing foods. In PKU, a missing enzyme prevents the use of phenylalanine. Subsequently, toxic levels of phenylalanine and phenylalanine derivatives build up in the body.

### Signs and Symptoms
PKU can cause severe mental retardation if not treated in infants. Older children may develop eczema, seizures, tremors, spasticity, and hyperactivity. Because phenylalanine is involved indirectly in the production of melanin, children with phenylketonuria often have light complexions. There is a characteristic odor that results from the accumulation of phenylacetic acid that may be detected on their breath, skin, and urine.

### Treatment
Treatment for PKU includes a diet devoid of phenylalanine. Phenylalanine is present in many foods (e.g., milk, eggs), and in Nutrasweet (aspartame). Lofenalac is formula made for infants with PKU.

### Testing
PKU is a treatable disease that can be easily detected by simple blood tests. Prenatal diagnosis is possible through a chorionic villus sample. Parents

can be detected as carriers through an enzyme assay. A heelstick blood sample from an infant is mandatory in most states for PKU screening.

## PHEOCHROMOCYTOMA

### Description
Pheochromocytoma is a rare tumor of the adrenal gland that causes high blood pressure due to the release of epinephrine and norepinephrine. Pheochromocytoma may occur as a single tumor or as multiple growths. Normally, pheochromocytoma develops in the adrenal medulla. Less than 10 percent of pheochromocytomas are malignant. Pheochromocytoma may occur at any age, but they are most common in young-adult to mid-adult life. These tumors are twice as common in men (Brose, 2004c; Vuguin & Perez, 2002).

### Signs and Symptoms
Pheochromocytoma is characterized by paroxysms, which are attacks that occur at unpredictable intervals. Paroxysms include severe headache, rapid heart rate, sweating, chest pain, abdominal pain, changes in appetite, difficulty sleeping, hand tremor, and wide fluctuations in blood pressure.

### Treatment
Pheochromocytomas are treated by surgical removal, which is high-risk surgery may cause the condition to worsen due to manipulation of the tumor. Radiation therapy and chemotherapy have not been effective in curing pheochromocytoma. For patients who have noncancerous tumors that are removed with surgery, the five-year survival rate is 95 percent, with recurrence in less than 10 percent of patients. For patients who have malignant tumors, the five-year survival rate after surgery is less than 50 percent.

### Testing
Tests used in the diagnosis of pheochromocytoma include adrenal biopsy, MIBG scintiscan, abdominal MRI scan, abdominal CT scan, urinalysis for levels fo metanephrine and catecholamines, blood glucose level tests, and tests for abnormal levels of catecholamines in the blood.

## PHLEBITIS

### Description
Phlebitis is an inflammatory condition of the veins of the legs, in which blood clots form along the walls and valves of the veins. The valves within the veins help prevent gravity from causing the blood to reverse its flow, as illustrated in Figure 2-62. Phlebitis can be caused by changes in the blood's ability to form clots, pooling of the blood in the veins of the legs due to pregnancy or immobility, or even cancer.

Blood flow toward the heart

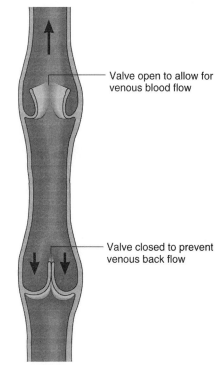

Valve open to allow for
venous blood flow

Valve closed to prevent
venous back flow

**Figure 2-62** Valves of the veins

## Signs and Symptoms

The most common characteristic of phlebitis is pain and redness along the involved veins of the lower leg. Most cases of phlebitis occur in the calf muscle region, and the clots that form there can travel to the lungs blocking the pulmonary artery causing cardiac failure. Chronic phlebitis may cause ulcers in the skin, usually by the ankles and lower shin bones, that are slow to heal due to the pooling of nutrient-depleted venous blood. The lower legs often swell, and the skin becomes hard and thick.

## Treatment

Phlebitis is treated with analgesics, anticoagulants, blood thinners, thrombolytics, nonsteroidal anti-inflammatories, and antibiotics. Support stockings and wraps may be used to reduce discomfort. Surgical removal, stripping, or bypass of the vein is rarely needed but may be recommended in some situations. Phlebitis usually responds to prompt medical treatment (Burke, 2004).

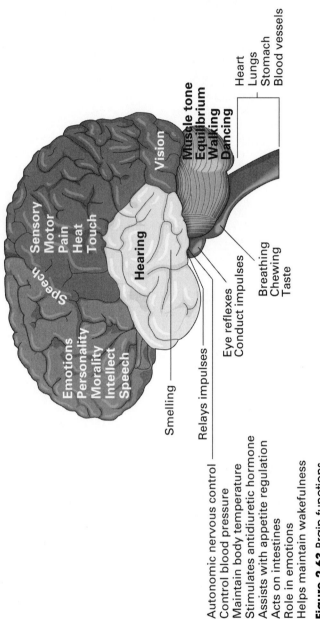

**Figure 2-63** Brain functions

Speech

Emotions
Personality
Morality
Intellect
Speech

Sensory
Motor
Pain
Heat
Touch

Hearing

Vision

Muscle tone
Equilibrium
Walking
Dancing

Heart
Lungs
Stomach
Blood vessels

Breathing
Chewing
Taste

Eye reflexes
Conduct impulses

Relays impulses

Smelling

Autonomic nervous control
Control blood pressure
Maintain body temperature
Stimulates antidiuretic hormone
Assists with appetite regulation
Acts on intestines
Role in emotions
Helps maintain wakefulness

## Testing

If the cause of the phlebitis is not readily identifiable, Doppler ultrasound, extremity arteriography, and blood coagulation studies may be performed to determine the cause.

## PICK'S DISEASE

### Description

Pick's disease is a disease of the brain in which abnormal brain cells known as Pick's bodies cause a deterioration of tissues in specific parts of the brain. The functions of various regions of the brain are illustrated in Figure 2-63. Pick's bodies are tangles of tau protein, and their presence causes symptoms similar to those found in Alzheimer's patients. Unlike Alzheimer's, Pick's disease does not affect the entire brain. Pick's disease also differs from Alzheimer's in that Pick's disease only lasts about six years before death occurs. Typically, Pick's disease only affects the frontal and temporal lobes (Barret, 2004).

### Signs and Symptoms

Pick's disease is characterized by progressive loss of mental function and neurological impairments.

### Treatment

There is no cure for Pick's disease, and treatment is aimed at relief of symptoms.

### Testing

Tests used in the diagnosis of Pick's disease begin with psychological studies, neurological assessments, imaging exams of the brain, and brain biopsy.

## PICKWICKIAN SYNDROME

### Description

Pickwickian syndrome, which is also known as obesity hypoventilation syndrome, is a condition related to sleep apnea among obese persons. The cause of Pickwickian syndrome is unknown, but it is likely due to a combination of central nervous system dysfunction and the effects of obesity on the chest wall. The excess weight of massive obesity can cause the muscles of the chest wall to not expand enough for the proper exchange of air (Blaivas, 2003a).

### Signs and Symptoms

Pickwickian syndrome is characterized by sleep deprivation, which causes excessive daytime sleepiness and falling asleep at inappropriate times. In addition, symptoms may include difficulty breathing or fatigue after minimal physical effort. Signs of Pickwickian Syndrome may also include cyanosis and heart failure.

## Treatment

Treatment of Pickwickian syndrome involves weight loss and aids to ventilation. This may be accomplished through a mask that fits tightly over the nose or nose and mouth, or by tracheostomy. The prognosis for Pickwickian syndrome is good when treated, but it can lead to death.

## Testing

Tests used in the diagnosis of Pickwickian syndrome include arterial blood gas levels, sleep studies, and tests of pulmonary function.

## PINTA

### Description

Pinta is an endemic infection caused by *Treponema carateum*. Pinta is characterized by chronic skin lesions that occur primarily in young adults. Pinta does not occur in the United States (Fine, 2002; Klein, 2004).

### Signs and Symptoms

Pinta is classified into an early and late stage. The early stage comprises the initial lesion and the secondary lesions; the late stage comprises the latent phase and tertiary stage. After an incubation period of approximately three weeks, the initial lesion appears on the legs, dorsum of the foot, forearm, or hands. The lesion enlarges, becomes pigmented, and the regional lymph glands swell. Disseminated lesions, referred to as pintids, are similar to the primary lesion and may appear three to nine months after infection. These secondary lesions vary in size and location and become pigmented with age. Late or tertiary pinta is characterized by a mottled appearance of the skin. Lesions may be red, white, blue, violet, and brown.

### Treatment

After penicillin therapy, lesions become noninfectious in 24 hours. Alternatives to penicillin include tetracycline or erythromycin.

### Testing

Pinta is diagnosed during a physical exam. Diagnosis is confirmed by serologic tests for syphilis. Darkfield examination of exudates from early lesions indicates the presence of treponemes, and they are identifiable in the primary and secondary lesions using silver stain. Treponemes are absent in later lesions. Findings of pinta and yaws are similar, but no ulcer formation occurs in pinta.

## PINWORM INFECTION

### Description

Pinworm is the most common worm infection in the United States, affecting school-age children and then preschoolers with the highest frequency of infection (Levy, 2003b; *Pinworm infection*, 1999). In some groups nearly 50 percent of children are infected, and infection often occurs in more than one family member. Pinworm infection is caused by a small, white intestinal worm *Enterobius vermicularis,* which is approximately the length of a staple and resides in the human rectum. While an infected person sleeps, female pinworms leave the rectum through the anus and deposit eggs on the surrounding skin. Pinworm eggs can survive up to two weeks on clothing and bedding, and they are spread through ingesting infective eggs after contact with contaminated surfaces.

## Signs and Symptoms
Pinworm infection is characterized by itching around the anus, disturbed sleep, loss of appetite, and irritability. Most pinworm infections are mild or asymptomatic. At night, the adult worms can sometimes be seen directly in bedclothes or around the anal area.

## Treatment
Pinworm infection is treated with antiparasitic medication (e.g., pyrantel pamoate, mebendazole albendazole). Treatment of the entire household is recommended and repeated after two weeks. The prognosis for pinworm is excellent, if treated.

## Testing
A piece of cellophane tape is pressed against the skin around the anus, preferably in the morning before bathing or using the toilet. Then the tape is removed and stuck to a microscope slide for the observation of eggs.

## PITYRIASIS ROSEA

## Description
Pityriasis rosea is a common skin rash of young adults (Lehrer, 2003f). It is believed to be a viral infection, and it is most frequent in the fall and spring. Pityriasis rosea is not thought to be highly contagious. Attacks generally last one or two months, and symptoms may not be present after the first month.

## Signs and Symptoms
Pityriasis rosea is characterized by a skin lesion or rash (see Color Plate 46). The disease begins with a single, herald lesion followed several days later by more lesions. The rash may follow cleavage lines or appear in a christmas tree pattern. The rash contains oval lesions with a sharp border that form plaque, bumps, and macules. The rash itches, and its centers have a cigarette paper appearance. The surrounding skin is inflamed.

## Treatment
Mild cases of pityriasis rosea are often not treated. Gentle bathing, mild lubricants or creams, or mild hydrocortisone creams may be used to soothe inflammation. Oral antihistamines may reduce itching. Sun exposure or ultraviolet light may help as well. Pityriasis rosea is self-resolving within three months, and recurrences are unusual.

## Testing

Pityriasis rosea is diagnosed based on the appearance of the rash. A blood test and skin biopsy may be used to rule out secondary syphilis.

# PLACENTA PREVIA

## Description

Placenta previa literally means "afterbirth" first, and it is a condition that may occur during pregnancy when the placenta implants in the lower part of the uterus and obstructs the cervical opening to the vagina. Possible causes of placenta previa include a scarred endometrium, digital examination, a large placenta, an abnormal uterus, sexual intercourse, or abnormal formation of the placenta. The incidence of placenta previa is approximately 1 out of 200 births but increases with each pregnancy. Women who have had six or more deliveries may be at risk in as many as 1 in 20 births (Gaudier, 2003; Joy & Lyon, 2004).

## Signs and Symptoms

Placenta previa is characterized by painless vaginal bleeding that may be profuse during the third trimester. Bleeding may not occur until after labor starts in some cases, and the bleeding may signal labor. Fetal distress is not usually present unless vaginal blood loss has been heavy enough to induce maternal shock or placenta abruptio.

## Treatment

Treatment depends on a variety of factors, including the stage of pregnancy, the cause of disease, the degree of disease, and the development of the fetus. Treatment may include blood transfusions, medications to time delivery, and cesarean section delivery. With proper treatment, the prognosis is excellent for both mother and baby.

## Testing

In cases of placenta previa, an abdominal ultrasound performed during the second trimester indicates low positioning of the placenta. Transvaginal or transperineal ultrasound are also used to determine the position of a low-lying placenta.

# PLAGUE

## Description

Over one-fourth of the population of Europe was killed in the Middle Ages due to the spread of *Yersinia pestis* from infected rats to fleas and then to humans (Levy, 2003g; Plague, 2001). *Yersinia pestis* is the causative pathogen of bubonic plague. It is a gram-negative, short, plump rod that has a safety-pin appearance. There are approximately 10 to 15 cases of plague in the United States each year, and the World Health Organization reports 1,000 to 3,000 cases globally per year. Also known as the Black Death, the plague receives this name from the dark hemorrhagenic areas present on the body. *Y. pestis* has been isolated in rats, wild rodents, ground squirrels, prairie dogs, and chipmunks. Infection results from contact with infected animals, which can occur from scratches, skinning the animal, or similar contact.

## Signs and Symptoms

Plague spreads through the blood and lymph causing growths of the lymph nodes known as buboes (see Color Plate 47). Death occurs in untreated cases of plague in less than a week after the appearance of symptoms. There is also a pneumonic form of plague in which the infection is found in the respiratory system. Pneumonic plague can be transmitted from person to person, and it is often a result of bubonic plague.

## Treatment

Immediate treatment with antibiotics (e.g., streptomycin, chloramphenicol, tetracycline) is required to treat plague. Half of bubonic plague cases result in death if not treated, and almost all victims of pneumonic plague die if not treated. Treatment reduces the death rate to 5 percent.

## Testing

Tests used in the diagnosis of plague include bubo culture, sputum culture, blood culture, and lymph node culture.

## PLANTAR FASCIITIS

### Description

The plantar fascia is a thick band of tissue that covers the bones on the bottom of the foot. In cases of plantar fasciitis, this fascia becomes inflamed and painful, making walking more difficult. Plantar fasciitis is referred to as heal spurs, although this is a misnomer. Some risk factors for development of this problem include foot arch problems, obesity, and trauma caused by running. Typical onset occurs in an active male between the ages of 40 and 70 (A. Chen, 2004c; Young, 2002).

### Signs and Symptoms

The most common complaint is heal pain that is worst in the morning and improves throughout the day.

### Treatment

Treatment of plantar fasciitis may last anywhere from several months to years, although about 90 percent of patients will be better in nine months. Initial treatment usually consists of heel stretching exercises, shoe inserts, night splints, and anti-inflammatory medications. If these fail, casting the foot is often successful. Steroid injections, which are painful and not for everyone, may provide relief in about 50 percent of people. In some cases, surgery is necessary.

### Testing

There is no specific test used to diagnose plantar fasciitis, but X-rays may be taken to rule out other disorders.

## PLEURISY

### Description

Pleurisy is an inflammatory condition of the membranes that surround the lungs (Figure 2-64). Pleurisy is associated with lung infections, rheumatic diseases, chest trauma, certain cancers, and asbestos-related disease. The normally smooth pleural surfaces become inflamed and rub together with each breath, producing a rough, grating sound called a friction rub (Blaivas, 2004c). The fluid that develops between the pleura may contain pus, causing a condition known as empyema. Pleurisy may also involve the development of fibrous materials, causing the pleura to adhere to the diaphragm or the chest wall. A condition known as hemorrhagic pleurisy also exists, wherein blood is found in the pleural space.

### Signs and Symptoms

Pleurisy is characterized by stabbing pain, worsening pain upon deep inhalation, chills, fever, coughing, pallor, anxiety, and guarding the affected side or lying on the affected side.

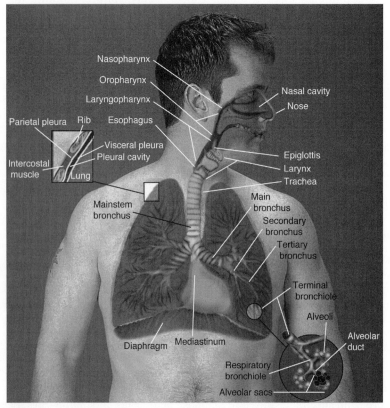

**Figure 2-64** Respiratory tract

## Treatment

Bacterial infections are treated with appropriate antibiotics, but tuberculosis requires special treatment. Viral infections do not usually require medications. The pain of pleurisy can often be controlled with acetominophen or anti-inflammatories. Recovery from infections of all types is expected with treatment.

## Testing

Tests used in the diagnosis of pleurisy include CBC, chest X-rays, chest ultrasound, and thoracentesis, which is the collection of fluid from the pleural cavity.

## PLUMMER-VINSON SYNDROME

### Description

Plummer-Vinson syndrome is an idiopathic disorder. It is associated with severe, long-term iron deficiency. There is a weblike membrane of tissue growing in the throat that makes swallowing difficult. Plummer-Vinson syndrome may be related to esophageal cancer.

### Signs and Symptoms

Plummer-Vinson syndrome is characterized by difficulty swallowing, weakness, and spooning of the nails. A weblike membrane is present in the throat.

### Treatment

Plummer-Vinson syndrome is treated with iron supplements and upper endoscopy.

### Testing

An upper GI series or upper endoscopy reveals the web of tissue in the throat. Anemia is diagnosed with blood tests for iron levels.

## PNEUMOCOCCAL MENINGITIS

### Description

Pneumococcal meningitis is an infection of the membranes covering the brain and spinal cord caused by *Streptococcus pneumoniae,* which is also known as pneumococcus. Half the cases of pneumococcal meningitis occur in children under four, and typically follow other infections with *S. pneumoniae* such as otitis media and pneumonia. *S. pneumoniae* is found in the nose and throat. Figure 2-65 depicts the highly virulent capsule surrounding *S. pneumoniae*. About 15,000 cases occur in the United States each year (Incesu & Khosla, 2004; Levy, 2004n).

### Signs and Symptoms

Pneumococcal meningitis is characterized by high fever, severe headache, rapid heart rate, stiff neck, nausea, vomiting, sensitivity to light, and mental status changes.

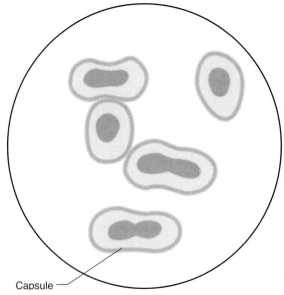

Capsule

**Figure 2-65** *Streptococcus pneumoniae* bacteria

## Treatment

Pneumococcal meningitis is treated with antibiotics (e.g., ceftriaxone, penicillin, vancomycin, rifampin) and corticosteroids. Even with treatment, the mortality rate of pneumococcal meningitis is high (20 percent), and 50 percent will have serious long-term complications. A vaccine for pneumococcal meningitis is available.

## Testing

Tests used in the diagnosis of pneumococcal meningitis include a spinal tap to test for elevated protein and low glucose levels in the cerebrospinal fluid, Gram stain of the cerebrospinal fluid for the presence of pneumococcus bacteria, and blood cultures.

## PNEUMOCONIOSIS

## Description

Pneumoconiosis is an inflammatory disorder of the respiratory system caused by the inhalation of mineral dusts. Some experts include the inhalation of certain organic compounds and chemical fumes and vapors as causes of pneumoconiosis. The four most common pneumoconioses result from the inhalation of coal dust, silica, asbestos, and beryllium. Although pneumoconioses were once thought to be strictly occupational disorders among individuals who worked with these minerals, the increased frequency of cancers in family members extends the potential of these irritants to cause disease outside the workplace.

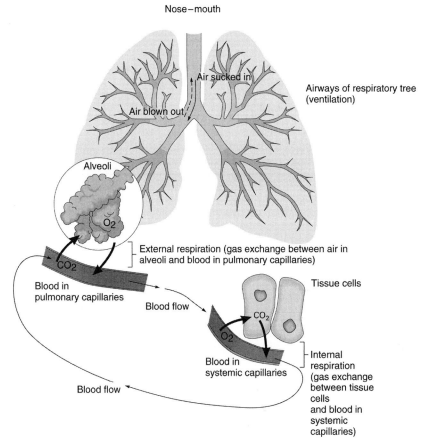

**Figure 2-66** Respiration

## Signs and Symptoms

The reaction of the lung to mineral dusts depends on the size, shape, solubility, and reactivity of the dust particles. Large particles do not reach the distal airway, whereas extremely small pieces enter the alveoli and the blood (Figure 2-66). Coal dust is relatively inert and usually requires a fairly large amount of dust to accumulate before a disease reaction occurs in the body; however, silica, asbestos, and beryllium are more reactive than coal and cause disease at lower concentrations. Smoking tobacco worsens the effects of all inhaled mineral dusts, but it is especially harmful in the case of asbestos exposure. Pneumoconiosis is typically associated with other respiratory disorders, heart failure, and cancer.

## Treatment

There is no specific treatment for pneumoconiosis, other than treatment of complications. The outcome for the simple form of pneumoconiosis is usually good, but the complicated form may become a disabling illness that is ultimately fatal.

## Testing

Tests used in the diagnosis of pneumoconiosis include chest X-rays and pulmonary function tests.

## PNEUMOCYSTIS PNEUMONIA

### Description

*Pneumocystis carinii* is a primary opportunistic pathogen in infections among the immunosuppressed (Wener, 2004i). Pneumocystis pneumonia (PCP), which is also known as pneumocystosis, not only occurs in the immunosuppressed, but was originally observed prior to world war II among malnourished infants and children in orphanages. At one time, *P. carinii* was categorized as a yeast, then it was later believed to be a protozoan, and it is currently being reevaluated for classification as a fungus (*Pneumocystis carinii* pneumonia, 2003). The lifecycle of *P. carinii* is illustrated in Figure 2-67.

   *P. carinii* has a cell wall that increases its virulence against antimicrobial agents, which is why PCP is considered a multidrug-resistant disease. The fungus is widespread among animals, including dogs, cats, horses, and rodents, persisting in their lungs. *P. carinii* has been isolated among hospitalized patients, malnourished infants, and elderly residents of nursing homes, suggesting that it is spread through airborne transmission.

### Signs and Symptoms

Symptoms of *P. carinii* infection include fever, cough, and shortness of breath. As the disease progresses, a dusky discoloration appears on the skin and mucous membranes, which is due to the gradual loss of oxygen in the tissues. Respiratory failure is the result of the fungus entering the alveoli of the lungs, where they multiply until the alveoli fill with inflammatory fluid, macrophages, and the fungus.

### Treatment

Pneumocystis pneumonia is treated with antimicrobial therapy. Trimethoprim-sulfamethoxazole is the drug of choice. Corticosteroids are frequently used as well. Other drugs include pentamidine, trimethoprim-dapsone, clindamycin, primaquine, and atovaquone. The progressive respiratory failure associated with PCP is ultimately fatal. Although PCP was once a leading cause of death among AIDS patients, early detection and treatment has resulted in increased prevention prior to the appearance of symptoms.

### Testing

Tests used in the diagnosis of pneumocystis pneumonia include chest X-rays and bronchoscopy. Rarely, a lung biopsy may also be needed.

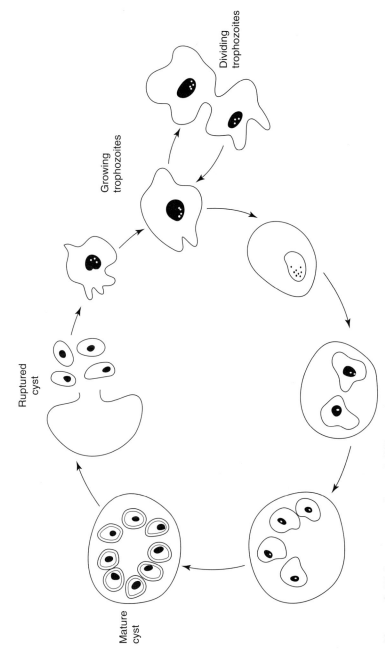

**Figure 2-67** *Pneumocystis carinii* life cycle

Dividing trophozoites

Growing trophozoites

Ruptured cyst

Mature cyst

287

## PNEUMONIA

### Description

The majority of cases of pneumonia are due to a bacterial infection, although viruses and fungi also cause pneumonia. Bacterial pneumonias tend to be the most serious, and in adults, the most common cause is *Streptococcus pneumoniae*. Respiratory viruses are the most common causes of pneumonia in young children. Pneumonias are categorized by the site of the infection and by the causative agent. Lobar pneumonia affects a single lobe of the lung; bronchial pneumonia affects smaller lung areas in several lobes. Pneumonia is a common illness that affects millions of people each year in the United States.

### Signs and Symptoms

Pneumonia is characterized by a cough with greenish or yellow mucus, coughing up blood, fever and shaking chills, sharp chest pain that worsens upon deep inhalation, rapid and shallow breathing, difficulty breathing, headache, excessive sweating, loss of appetite, and fatigue.

### Treatment

Pneumonia is treated with antibiotics if the cause is bacterial. Respiratory treatments to remove secretions may be necessary. Occasionally, steroid medications may be used to reduce wheezing. With treatment, most patients will improve within two weeks, although elderly or debilitated patients may die from respiratory failure.

### Testing

Tests used in the diagnosis of pneumonia include chest X-rays, Gram stain and culture of sputum, CBC, thoracic CT scan, pulmonary ventilation/ perfusion scan, and pleural fluid culture (Hart, 2003i).

## POLIO

### Description

Poliomyelitis, or polio, is a neurotropic, viral infection caused by the poliovirus. Humans are the only known host for the poliovirus, and infected populations shed the virus in their feces. The virus is usually transmitted through contaminated water supplies. The poliovirus multiplies first in the throat and small intestine, then it travels to the lymph nodes of the neck and ileum. The virus spreads to the blood, at which point the infection has run its course in the majority of cases. If the disease spreads past this stage to the central nervous system, it migrates toward the anterior horn cells of the motor nerves of the spinal cord (Poliomyelitis, n/d). Color Plate 48 pictures a child displaying a deformity of her right leg due to poliovirus infection.

### Signs and Symptoms

Approximately 95 percent of polio cases are subclinical. Persons with subclinical polio infections may experience slight fever, headache, fatigue, sore throat, and vomiting. Nonparylitic polio is characterized by moderate fever, headache, vomiting, diarrhea, fatigue, irritability, neck pain and stiffness, backache, calf muscle pain, arm pain, abdominal pain, and skin rash. Paralytic poliomyelitis is chacterized by fever, headache, stiff neck and back, asymetric muscle weakness that progresses to paralysis, abnormal sensations without loss of sensation in the affected area, difficulty beginning to urinate, drooling, difficulty breathing, constipation, bloating, difficulty swallowing, muscle pain, and muscle spasms of the calf, neck, and back.

## Treatment

Lifesaving measures, particularly assistance with breathing, may be necessary in severe cases of polio. Antibiotics may be used to treat urinary tract infections. Bethanechol may reduce urinary retention. Pain killers are used to reduce headache, muscle pain, and spasms. Narcotics are not usually given because they increase the risk of breathing difficulty. If the spinal cord and brain are not affected, which is the case over 90 percent of the time, complete recovery is likely. There are two common vaccines for polio, the Salk vaccine, which is a series of injections, and the Sabin vaccine, which is taken orally. Polio has been eradicated from most of the world.

## Testing

Tests used in the diagnosis of polio include viral cultures of throat washings, stools, or cerebrospinal fluid. Routine cerebrospinal fluid examination may be normal or show slight increase in pressure, protein, and white blood cells. Polio patients also exhibit a positive Babinski's reflex.

## POLYCYSTIC KIDNEY DISEASE

### Description

Polycystic kidney disease is an inherited disorder due to multiple cysts on the kidneys. Figure 2-68 illustrates how the presence of these cysts can greatly enlarge the size of the kidneys externally, thereby compressing the nephrons inside. This compression eventually disrupts the filtration of the blood as well as the production of urine. Figure 2-69 illustrates the healthy nephron. Cysts in the kidneys can cause aneurysms in the brain, diverticula of the colon, and cysts in the liver, pancreas, and testes.

### Signs and Symptoms

Symptoms include bloody urine, excessive urination at night, abdominal pain, nail abnormalities, painful menstruation, arthritis, and high blood pressure.

### Treatment

There is no treatment that can prevent cysts from forming or enlarging in cases of polycystic kidney disease. Treatment of symptoms may include antihypertensive and diuretic medications and a low-salt diet. Infections are treated with antibiotics. Surgical or radiologic drainage of cysts may be necessary. Removal is not feasible due to the number of cysts. Surgical

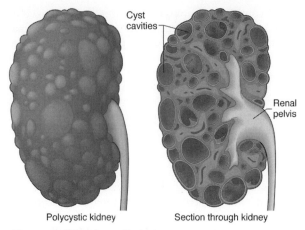

Cyst
cavities

Renal
pelvis

Polycystic kidney      Section through kidney

**Figure 2-68** Polycystic kidney

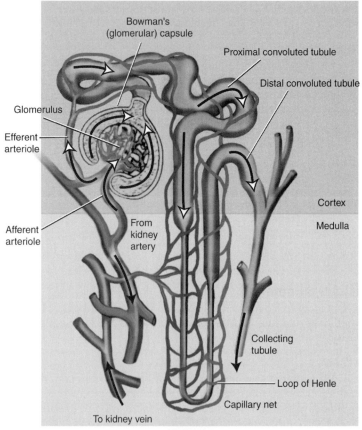

Bowman's
(glomerular) capsule

Proximal convoluted tubule

Distal convoluted tubule

Glomerulus

Efferent
arteriole

Afferent
arteriole

From
kidney
artery

Cortex

Medulla

Collecting
tubule

Loop of Henle

Capillary net

To kidney vein

Henle's loop

**Figure 2-69** Nephron of the kidney

removal of the kidneys may also be necessary. Dialysis or kidney transplantation may be eventual end-stage kidney failure may occur.

## Testing

Tests used in the diagnosis of polycystic kidney disease include urinalysis, CBC, and cerebral angiography indicating the presence of aneurysms. Imaging exams may include abdominal ultrasounds, CT scans, MRI scans, and an IVP. Genetic linkage tests can be performed to determine whether a person carries the gene for autosomal dominant polycystic kidney disease (Agha, 2003e).

## POLYCYTHEMIA VERA

### Description

Polycythemia vera, which is also known as erythrocytosis, is an idiopathic disorder of the blood. Polycythemia vera is a chronic disorder involving bone marrow. In addition to a high red blood cell count, which increases the viscosity of the blood causing clotting, there is an increase in the concentration of hemoglobin in the blood. Polycythemia vera is a rare disease (Hart, 2004l).

### Signs and Symptoms

Polycythemia vera is characterized by fatigue, dizziness, ringing in the ears, irritability, enlarged spleen, congestion of the face, difficulty breathing, itching, bruising of the skin, coma, and stroke.

### Treatment

Phlebotomy is used to reduce blood viscosity. In phlebotomy, 1 unit (pint) of blood is removed weekly until the hematocrit is less than 45. Drugs are used to suppress the activity of the bone marrow. Allopurinol is given for gout.

### Testing

Tests used in the diagnosis of polycythemia vera may include CBC with differential, bone marrow biopsy, vitamin $B_{12}$ levels, a chemistry panel, tests for lactate dehydrogenase, urinalysis, serum uric acid, total white blood cell count (TWBC), platelet aggregation tests, leukocyte alkaline phosphatase, hemoglobin, ESR, and levels of erythropoietin.

## POLYPS

### Description

Polyps are benign tumors of vascular organs that contain a stem that attaches the tumor to its surrounding tissue. Polyps are typically found in vascular organs such as the nose, uterus, and rectum. Polyps can be found on the lining of the intestinal tract, trachea, esophagus, stomach, small intestine, or colon. Polyps can range in size from a few millimeters to several centimeters in diameter. Inflammatory polyps occur with acute or chronic inflammation and are present by the dozen in cases of chronic ulcerative colitis. Some polyps are precancerous, meaning that they have a potential to develop into cancers over time (Stone, 2004d).

## Signs and Symptoms

Polyps usually cause no symptoms, although rectal bleeding, bloody stool, and fatigue may occur.

## Treatment

Polyps are surgically removed if they are malignant or if they occlude the organ. Polyps often require removal due to bleeding or blockage of the bowel.

## Testing

Tests used in the diagnosis of polyps include sigmoidoscopy, colonoscopy, barium enema, stool guaiac, and CBCs.

## PONTIAC DISEASE

### Description

Pontiac disease is a form of bacterial infection caused by *Legionella*. Unlike Legionnaires' disease, there is no pneumonia present in cases of Pontiac fever (Legionellosis, 2001).

### Signs and Symptoms

The incubation period is about two days. Patients complain of fever, headache, and muscle pain for two to five days. Then symptoms suddenly subside.

### Treatment

When infections are diagnosed early, they can usually be treated successfully with erythromycin and rifampin. Alternative drugs include newer macrolides (azithromycin, clarithromycin), fluoroquinolones (ciprofloxacin, doxycycline), and trimethoprim-sulfamethoxazole.

### Testing

Direct examination, culture, and antigen and antigody detection are used to detect *Legionella*.

## PRADER-WILLI SYNDROME

### Description

Prader-Willi syndrome is a congenital disease characterized by obesity, decreased muscle tone, decreased mental capacity, and hypogonadism (Scheimann, 2003). Prader-Willi is caused by the deletion of a gene on chromosome 15. In approximately 70 percent of cases, the deletion occurs in the father's DNA, and the other 30 percent usually have two copies of the mother's chromosome 15. Because the mother's chromosome 15 is turned off in everyone, the deletion of the father's DNA leaves the patient with only the inactive, maternal copy.

## Signs and Symptoms

Signs of Prader-Willi may be seen at birth. Infants are small and lack muscle tone, causing them to be floppy. Male infants may have undescended testicles. The growing child exhibits slow mental and delayed motor development, almond-shaped eyes, a bifrontal skull, limb abnormalities, and characteristically small hands and feet. Rapid weight gain may occur during the first few years because the patient develops uncontrollable hunger that leads to morbid obesity. Mental development is slow, and the IQ seldom exceeds 80. Morbid obesity may lead to respiratory failure with hypoxia, right-sided heart failure, and death (Scheimann, 2003).

## Treatment

There is no cure for Prader-Willi syndrome, and obesity represents the greatest problem. Growth hormone treatment causes accelerated growth, improved physical strength, and decreased percent body fat. Hormone therapy may also be needed (Blackman, 2004d).

## Testing

Prader-Willi is diagnosed by physical exam and confirmed by genetic testing.

# PRESBYCUSIS

## Description

Presbycusis, or age-related hearing loss, is a progressive loss of the ability to hear high frequencies, which occurs as people get older (Angelo, 2002; Marcincuk, 2004). Presbycusis begins with the loss of high-frequency sounds such as speech. Presbycusis appears to be inherited.

## Signs and Symptoms

Presbycusis is characterized by progressive hearing loss. Patients experience difficulty understanding sounds in noisy environments.

## Treatment

There is no known cure for this form of hearing loss. Hearing aids, lip reading, and using visual cues may aid in communication. These skills may be difficult for elderly patients to learn. Age-related hearing loss may eventually lead to deafness.

## Testing

Audiology tests determine the extent of hearing loss.

# PRIMARY AMEBIC MENINGOENCEPHALITIS

## Description

Primary amebic meningoencephalitis is caused by *Naegleria fowleri*. Likely places to find *Naegleria fowleri* include lakes, rivers, hot springs, unchlorinated swimming pools, and in warm water discharge pools from industrial plants. Although infections are rare, the amoebas enter the body through the nose while swimming or diving. The amoebas then migrate to the central nervous system. Primary amebic meningoencephalitis is not communicable. To avoid infection, swimming pools need to be properly cleaned, maintained, and chlorinated (*Naegleria infection,* 2004).

## Signs and Symptoms

Primary amebic meningoencephalitis is characterized by headache, fever, nausea, vomiting, stiff neck, confusion, lack of attention to people and surroundings, loss of balance and bodily control, seizures, and hallucinations.

## Treatment

Primary amebic meningoencephalitis is treated with high-dose amphotericin B. If not diagnosed and treated, primary amebic meningoencephalitis is fatal and usually results in death within a week.

## Testing

Diagnosis of primary amebic meningoencephalitis requires a culture and an indirect fluorescent antibody test.

## PRIMARY ATYPICAL PNEUMONIA

### Description

*Mycoplasma pneumoniae* causes primary atypical pneumonia, which is better known as walking pneumonia (Levy, 2004a). About half of the cases of pneumonia in the military and about 20 percent of the cases of pneumonia in the general population are caused by *M. pneumoniae.* Other groups living in close contact, like college students and prisoners, are also at a higher risk of contracting walking pneumonia. *M. pneumoniae* is a slowly growing, aerobic organism. Figure 2-70 illustrates the characteristic fried-egg appearances of *M. pneumoniae* colonies. *M. pneumoniae* are not removed by the passage of mucous secretions. The microbes are spread by coughing (*Mycoplasma pneumoniae,* 2002).

### Signs and Symptoms

Primary atypical pneumonia is characterized by headache, low-grade fever, loss of appetite, sore throat, dry cough, earache, cardiovascular complications, central nervous sytem involvement, and gastrointestinal disorders.

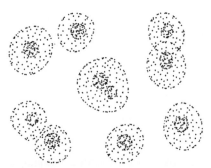

**Figure 2-70** Fried-egg appearance of mycoplasma

## Treatment

Primary atypical pneumonia is treated with antibiotics. Mycoplasmas are resistant to penicillin and similar antibiotics because they do not posses a cell wall. Respiratory treatments to remove secretions may be necessary. Occasionally, steroid medications may be used to reduce wheezing. With treatment, most patients will improve, although elderly or debilitated patients may die from respiratory failure.

## Testing

Crackles and other abnormal breathing sounds are heard through a stethoscope or via chest percussion. Other tests used in the diagnosis of walking pneumonia include chest X-rays, Gram stain and culture of sputum, CBC, thoracic CT scan, pulmonary ventilation/perfusion scan, and pleural fluid culture.

## PROSTATE CANCER

### Description

Prostate cancer is a tumor of the prostate gland. The incidence of the diagnosis of prostate cancer has increased dramatically in the 1990s due to the availability of the prostate-specific antigen (PSA) blood test. Although prostate cancer may have many causes, it is a hormone (i.e., testosterone)-sensitive tumor. Prostate cancer affects African-American men more than Caucasians, Asian Americans, or Native Americans.

### Signs and Symptoms

Early prostate cancer often does not cause symptoms, but prostate cancer can cause a need to urinate frequently at night, difficulty starting urination, incontinence, inability to urinate, painful urination, impotence, bloody urine, blood in semen, and pain or stiffness in the lower back, hips, or upper thighs.

### Treatment

Treatment options vary based on the stage of the tumor, and the appropriate treatment of prostate cancer is often controversial. In the early stages, prostatectomy and radiation therapy may be used to eradicate the tumor. Metastatic cancer of the prostate may be treated by hormonal manipulation or chemotherapy. The outcome varies greatly, primarily because the disease is found in older men who may have a variety of other complicating diseases or conditions. Prostate cancer can be fatal.

### Testing

Prostate cancer may be initially detected by a digital rectal exam, during which the health-care professional inserts a lubricated, gloved finger into the rectum and feels the prostate through the rectal wall to check for lumps. There is also a blood test that measures prostate-specific antigen. Other tests may include urinalysis, prostatic fluid cytology, and imaging exams to rule out metastasis (e.g., CT scans, bone scan, chest X-rays). x-methylacyl-CoA racemase (AMACR) testing, which detects a gene related to prostate cancer, is more sensitive for determining the presence of prostate cancer than the prostate-specific antigen test and may become more widely used to diagnose disease (Brose, 2004d).

## PROSTATITIS

### Description

Prostatitis is inflammation of the prostate gland. The difference in acute and chronic prostatitis is that in cases of chronic prostatitis, the infection settles into the prostate gland due to a defect in the prostate gland. Chronic prostatitis is also known as chronic pelvic pain syndrome. Asymptomatic inflammatory prostatitis is a condition that does not have noticeable symptoms.

### Signs and Symptoms

Prostatistis is characterized by symptoms of chills, fever, frequent urination, urgency in urination, burning urination, and lower back or genital pain. Chronic prostatitis may or may not be accompanied by inflammation of the prostate. Asymptomatic inflammatory prostatitis is not accompanied by pain or discomfort (Prostatitis, 2003).

### Treatment

Treatment options for prostatitis include a combination of medication, surgery, and lifestyle changes. Antibiotics used in the treatment of prostatitis include trimethoprim-sulfamethoxazole (Bactrim), ciprofloxacin (Cipro), tetracycline, carbenicillin, erythromycin, and nitrofurantoin. Most antibiotics are not able to adequately penetrate the prostate tissue, and infectious organisms persist despite long periods of treatment. Recurrence of symptoms is common. Transurethral resection of the prostate may be necessary if antibiotic therapy is unsuccessful or recurrence is frequent.

### Testing

Tests used in the diagnosis of prostatitis include urinalysis, urine culture, semen analysis, and culture of prostatic secretions (Gilbert, 2004c).

## PSORIASIS

### Description

Psoriasis is a chronic, inflammatory skin disease. Although the cause of psoriasis is unknown, it is believed that an abnormality in the functioning of white blood cells triggers an immune system response that causes the skin cells to shed prematurely. This is accompanied by excessive growth of the skin, which causes psoriatic plaques to form. Normally, it takes about a month for new skin cells to move up from the lower layers to the surface. In psoriasis, this process takes only a few days, resulting in a buildup of dead skin cells and formation of thick scales. Psoriasis is exacerbated by trauma to the skin such as cuts or sunburns. Psoriasis also may be activated by certain drugs or by infections such as strep throat. Flare-ups are common during dry winter months, when the skin is exposed to less sunlight. Psoriasis of the nails may cause the nail to fall from the nail bed.

## Signs and Symptoms

Psoriasis is characterized by frequent episodes of redness, itching, and thick, dry, silvery scales on the skin (see Color Plate 49). The skin may crack and become infected. There also may be small scaling dots present on the skin. Joint pain may be caused by psoriatic arthritis. Nail abnormalities, genital lesions in males, and eye inflamation may also occur in cases of psoriasis.

## Treatment

There is no cure for psoriasis. Treatments may include steroids, scalp treatments with coal tar or cortisone, application of a synthetic form of vitamin D (e.g., calcipotriene), topical retinoid creams, ultraviolet light therapy, anticancer drugs (e.g., methotrexate), and drugs that inhibit rejection after organ transplant (e.g., cyclosporine).

## Testing

The diagnosis of psoriasis is based on the appearance of the skin. A skin biopsy, skin scraping, and skin lesion culture may be needed to rule out other disorders. An X-ray may be used to check for psoriatic arthritis if joint pain is present and persistent.

## PUBIC LICE

### Description

Crabs is the common term for pubic lice, which are parasitic insects found in the genital area. Infection is common and worldwide, but should not be confused with head lice, which are a different type of insect. Pubic lice are most commonly spread sexually, although sharing linens or bedclothes with an infected person may spread the lice. The three stages in the life of a pubic louse are the nit, the nymph, and the adult. Nits are pubic lice eggs, and they are hard to see and are found firmly attached to the hair shaft. Nits are oval and usually yellowish-white, and take about one week to hatch. The nit hatches into a nymph, which looks like an adult pubic louse, but is smaller. Nymphs mature into adults about seven days after hatching (*Pubic lice infestation*, 2004).

### Signs and Symptoms

Adult pubic lice resemble tiny crabs when viewed through a strong magnifying glass. They have six legs, but their two front legs resemble the pincher claws of a crab. Pubic lice are tan to grayish-white in color. Without human blood, pubic lice die within 48 hours. Although pubic lice are frequently found in pubic hair, they can infest other coarse body hair on the legs, axillae, or face. Pubic lice cause itching in the area of infestation.

### Treatment

Pubic lice are treated with special shampoos and a physical regimine to remove sources of reinfestation such as contaminated underwear, bedclothes, and linens.

## Testing
Pubic lice are diagnosed based on physical exam.

## PYELONEPHRITIS

### Description
Pyelonephritis is commonly known as a kidney infection, and it involves both the renal pelvis and the remainder of the kidney. Many microorganisms, especially bacteria, can invade the body by traveling through the urethra to the bladder and then up the ureters to the kidneys, and pyelonephritis may migrate from the bladder. The healthy urinary system is illustrated in Figure 2-71. Chronic pyelonephritis occurs almost exclusively in persons with major anatomic anomalies such as urinary tract obstructions, kidney stones, or structural birth defects of the kidneys (Gowda & Nzerue, 2003).

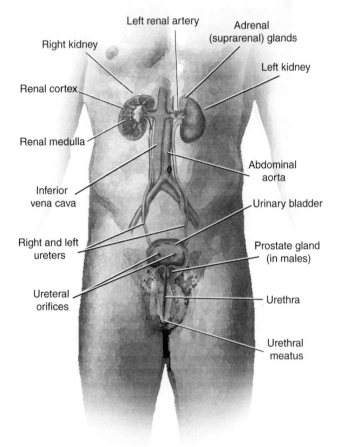

**Figure 2-71** Urinary system

## Signs and Symptoms

Pyelonephritis is characterized by fever, nausea, vomiting, flank pain, abdominal pain, hypertension, and insufficient urine production. Mental changes and confusion may be the only symptoms of urinary tract infections in elderly patients.

## Treatment

Pylonephritis is treated with antibiotics including sulfa drugs (e.g., sulfisoxazole and trimethoprim), amoxicillin, cephalosporins, levofloxacin, and ciprofloxacin. Acute symptoms usually resolve within 72 hours after treatment; however, there is a high mortality rate in the elderly population.

## Testing

Tests used in the diagnosis of pyelonephritis include urinalysis, a clean catch urine culture, a catheterized specimen urine culture, blood culture, a CT scan of the abdomen, and an intravenous pyelogram (IVP). Other tests may include voiding cystourethrogram, renal ultrasound, renal scan, and renal biopsy.

# Q FEVER

## Description

Q fever is caused by the pathogen *Coxiella burnetii* (Levy, 2004i; Q Fever, 2003). The disease gets its name from the word query, which refers to something that is unknown. The cause of an outbreak of the disease in Queensland, Australia, during the 1930s was unknown, so the disease was named Q fever. *C. burnetii* is resistant enough to survive airborne transmission, although most *Rickettsia* are not. It is passed from animal to animal via tick bite after ticks feed on infected cattle. Humans, however, become infected by ingesting contaminated milk or inhaling aerosols of the microbe in dairy barns, especially from placental material at calving time. Handling infected animals such as goats, cattle, and sheep places workers at a higher risk of infection. Other sources of infection include meat- and hide-processing plants.

## Signs and Symptoms

Unlike other rickettsial infections, no rash is present in cases of Q fever. The disease usually resolves without treatment in humans after about two weeks. A fatal inflammation of the lining of the heart may occur up to 20 years after infection in a small percentage of cases. Chest pain is present in about one-third of cases in addition to fever, headache, muscle pain, nausea, and vomiting. Other symptoms may include difficulty breathing, pneumonia, hepatitis, jaundice, clay-colored stools, night sweats, and chills.

## Treatment

The cornerstone of treatment for Q fever is antibiotic therapy (e.g., doxycycline and hydroxychloroquine). The prognosis for Q fever is good if treated early, but it can be a chronic disease that can be ultimately fatal.

## Testing

The primary test used to diagnose Q fever is a blood serology antibody test because it is difficult to grow the causative bacteria in culture.

## RABIES

### Description

Rabies is an acute, neurotropic, infectious disease caused by a rhabdovirus known as the rabies virus (Levy, 2004t). The rabies virus is shaped like a bullet. Rabies is contracted through bite of animals like raccoons, foxes, bats, skunks, and dogs. Figure 2-72 is a close-up of a dog's face during late-stage dumb paralytic rabies. The rabies virus travels along a peripheral nerve to the spinal cord and brain where it causes encephalitis. Eventually, both nonhuman animals and humans with rabies become completely paralyzed. There are an estimated 15,000 cases of rabies worldwide each year, but there are few cases in the United States due to extensive animal vaccination programs (Rabies, 2001).

### Signs and Symptoms

Rabies is characterized by alternating periods of calm and agitation. Infected persons present with spasms of the mouth and pharynx that cause the common sign of foaming at the mouth. The sight or thought of water can trigger these spasms. Because of this reaction to water, the

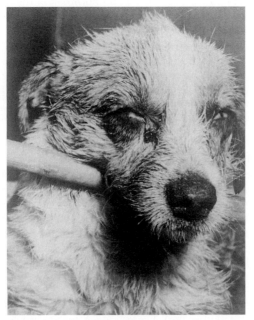

**Figure 2-72** Dog with rabies (Courtesy of the CDC)

disease was once well known as hydrophobia, which means fear of water. Death occurs within a few days after the final stage of the disease.

## Treatment

Because lymph does not circulate in the brain and spinal cord, the immune system cannot suppress the infection once it reaches the central nervous system (CNS). Because of its relatively long incubation period, a vaccine can be given that is quite effective in controlling the spread of the virus to the CNS. The vaccine is administered in a series of five or six injections at intervals during a 28-day period. Unlike previous treatments that included injections in the abdomen, the current treatment includes painless injections in the arm similar to a flu or tetanus vaccine.

## Testing

Several tests are necessary to diagnose rabies. Saliva can be tested by virus isolation or reverse transcription followed by polymerase chain reaction (RT-PCR). Serum and spinal fluid are tested for antibodies to rabies virus. Skin biopsy specimens are examined for rabies antigen in the cutaneous nerves at the base of hair follicles.

## RAYNAUD'S DISEASE

### Description

In Raynaud's disease, which is also known as Raynaud's phenomenon, exposure to the cold or strong emotions triggers blood vessel spasms that result in interruption of blood flow to the fingers, toes, ears, and nose (Shields, 2002). Raynaud's can occur without associated disease. Raynaud's phenomenon can be associated with Buerger's disease, athero-sclerosis, rheumatoid arthritis, scleroderma, and systemic lupus erythe-matosus. It can also follow repeated trauma, particularly vibrations such as those caused by typing or playing the piano. An overdose of ergot com-pounds or methysergide, which are both used to control migranes, may also cause Raynaud's phenomenon.

### Signs and Symptoms

Strong emotion or exposure to the cold causes the fingers, toes, ears, or nose to become pale, due to a lack of blood flow in the area. Cyanosis occurs as the capillaries dilate to allow more blood to remain in the tis-sues. There is tingling, swelling, and painful throbbing. The attacks last from minutes to hours. If blood flow becomes permanently decreased to the fingers, they may become thin and tapered. The skin will be smooth, shiny, and with slow growing nails. Blocked arteries can cause gangrene or ulceration of the skin.

### Treatment

Medications to relax the walls of the blood vessels may be prescribed, but treatment of the underlying condition is key. Smoking further constricts the blood vessels and should, therefore, be avoided. The prognosis for Raynaud's syndrome varies depending on severity.

## Testing

A physical examination of the affected parts reveals typical changes, and blood flow studies and cold stimulation tests may be used to confirm diagnosis (Clowse, 2003b).

## REITER'S SYNDROME

### Description

Reiter's syndrome is an idiopathic disorder associated with a group of symptoms consisting of arthritis, urethritis, conjunctivitis, and lesions of the skin and mucous membranes. Reiter's syndrome may follow an infection with *Chlamydia, Campylobacter, Salmonella,* or *Yersinia,* and it may have a genetic predisposition (Scoggins, 2004).

### Signs and Symptoms

Reiter's syndrome is characterized by urinary urgency, urethral discharge, burning urination, eye inflammation, hip pain, knee pain, ankle pain, low back pain, heel pain, Achilles tendon pain, penis pain, genital lesions, and skin lesions and inflammation of the palms and soles resembling psoriasis. Small, painless ulcers in the mouth, tongue, and glans penis may also be present. The symptoms of urethritis usually appear within days or weeks of infection followed by a low-grade fever, conjunctivitis, and arthritis.

### Treatment

The conjunctivitis and skin lesions resolve on their own. Antibiotics are used to treat underlying infections; however, this has not been shown to affect the course of the arthritis, which is treated with nonsteroidal anti-inflammatories, analgesics, and corticosteroids. Reiter's syndrome may resolve in about four months, but up to half of those affected experience recurrences over a period of years (Clowse, 2003b).

### Testing

Reiter's syndrome is diagnosed on the basis of symptoms. Tests may include joint X-rays, urinalysis, and HLA-B27 antigen tests.

## RENAL CELL CARCINOMA

### Description

Renal cell carcinoma is a form of kidney cancer that affects about 3 in 10,000 people, resulting in about 31,000 new cases in the United States per year. Approxmiately 12,000 people in the United States die from renal cell carcinoma annually. Originally, it was believed that renal cell carcinoma was derived from the adrenal glands, hence its alternate name of hypernephroma. Renal cell carcinoma typically originates in the epithelium of the proximal renal tubule, which is located in the medulla (Figure 2-73). Renal cell carcinoma is the sixth leading cause of cancer death in the United States, and it is more common among persons of European descent than Asian or African descent. Renal cell carcinoma

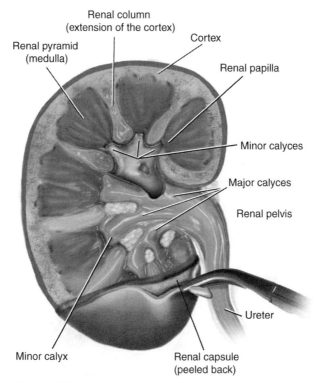

**Figure 2-73** Structures of the kidney

is also twice as prevalent in men as it is in women. Renal cell carcinoma frequently metastasizes to the lung, soft tissues, bone, liver, and brain (Konety & Pirtskhalaishvili, 2002).

## Signs and Symptoms

Renal cell carcinoma is characterized by bloody urine, enlargement of one testicle, flank pain, cold intolerance, an abdominal mass, vision abnormalities, weight loss, loss of appetite, fever, hypertension, and night sweats.

## Treatment

Renal cell carcinoma is characterized by a lack of early warning signs, diverse clinical manifestations, and resistance to both radiation and chemotherapy. The combination of its rapid metastasis and its resistance to conventional treatments explains its high mortality. Surgical removal of all or part of the kidney is usually required. The five-year survival rate is around 60 to 75 percent if the tumor is in the early stages and has not spread outside the kidney. If it has metastasized to other organs, the five-year survival is less than 5 percent (Brose, 2004e).

## Testing

Tests used in the diagnosis of renal cell carcinoma may include CBC, urinalysis, serum calcium levels, elevation of SGPT and alkaline phosphatase, urine cytology for carcinoma cells, liver function tests, abdominal ultrasound, kidney X-rays, IVP, renal arteriography.

## RENAL FAILURE

### Description

The loss of function of the kidneys is known as renal failure. There are two forms of renal failure: acute and chronic. Acute renal failure results from a sudden drop in blood pressure brought on by trauma, complications in surgery, septic shock, hemorrhage, burns, or dehydration. Acute renal failure may also occur as a result of blockage or narrowing of the renal artery. Infections such as acute pyelonephritis or septicemia may also cause acute renal failure.

Unlike acute renal failure with its sudden reversible failure of kidney function, chronic renal failure is slowly progressive and rarely reversible, progressing to a fatal stage. Chronic renal failure results from other diseases (e.g., glomerulonephritis, diabetes, polycystic kidney disease, kidney stones, chronic infections). Chronic renal failure results in the accumulation of fluid and waste products in the body, causing uremia, which is the buildup of nitrogenous waste products in the blood.

### Signs and Symptoms

Acute renal failure is characterized by decreased urine output, decreased urine volume, coma, swelling of the lower extremities, bruising, hallucinations, nosebleed, bloody vomit, and seizures. Chronic renal failure is characterized by weight loss, nausea, vomiting, headache, hiccups, generalized itching, changes in urine output, bruising, bloody urine, bloody stool, delirium, coma, muscle twitching and cramps, seizures, and depositis of white crystals in and on the skin.

### Treatment

Antibiotics may be used to treat infection. Diuretics may be used to remove fluid from the kidney, and medications may be used to control the level of potassium in the blood. These may include intravenous calcium, glucose or insulin, and administration of potassium exchange resin (Kayexalate). Dialysis and kidney transplant may also be required. Acute renal failure usually reverses within a few months after the underlying cause has been treated. Chronic renal failure and end-stage renal disease are fatal if they do not respond to treatment.

### Testing

Tests used in the diagnosis and treatment of renal failure include urinalysis, serum creatinine, blood urea nitrogen (BUN), serum potassium, blood chemistries, abdominal imaging tests, and renal arteriography (Koren, 2001a).

## RESPIRATORY SYNCYTIAL VIRUS INFECTION

### Description
Respiratory syncytial virus is the most common cause of bronchiolitis and pneumonia among infants and children younger than one year of age. Between 25 and 40 percent of infants and young children develop bronchiolitis or pneumonia during their first infection with respiratory syncytial virus. The majority of the 0.5 to 2 percent of infants requiring hospitalization are under the age of six months, and most recover within two weeks. Respiratory syncytial virus is spread through respiratory secretions, close contact with infected persons, and contact with contaminated surfaces (Respiratory syncytial virus, 2003 and 1997).

### Signs and Symptoms
Respiratory syncytial virus infection is characterized by fever, runny nose, cough, and sometimes wheezing. Respiratory syncytial virus causes repeated infections throughout life, and although most are mild coldlike symptoms, severe lower respiratory tract disease may also occur at any age, especially among the immunocompromised.

### Treatment
In most cases of respiratory syncytial virus infection, no treatment is necessary. Severe cases may require ribavirin aerosol, oxygen therapy, and sometimes mechanical ventilation.

### Testing
Respiratory syncytial is diagnosed by cultures of respiratory secretions.

## RETINITIS PIGMENTOSA

### Description
Retinitis pigmentosa is a progressive degeneration of the retina of the eye affecting night vision and peripheral vision. Retinitis pigmentosa is caused by defects in a number of recently identified genes (De Beus, 2004).

### Signs and Symptoms
The hallmark of retinitis pigmentosa is the presence of dark pigmented spots in the retina. As the disease progresses, peripheral vision is gradually lost. The condition may eventually lead to blindness, but usually not complete blindness. Signs and symptoms often first appear in childhood, but severe visual problems do not usually develop until early adulthood.

### Treatment
There is no effective treatment for retinitis pigmentosa, but complete blindness is rare (Brooks, 2004).

### Testing
Tests used in the diagnosis of retinitis pigmentosa include tests of visual acuity, refraction tests, color defectiveness determination, pupillary reflex

response, slit lamp examination, intraocular pressure determination, retinal exam by ophthalmoscopy, ultrasound of the eye, rentinal photography, fluorescein angiography, and an electroretinogram.

## RETINOBLASTOMA

### Description

Retinoblastoma is a malignant tumor of the eye that generally affects children under the age of six (Aventura, 2002). Retinoblastoma occurs when a cell of the growing retina develops a mutation in the RB gene, which suppresses tumors. One or both eyes may be affected, and a visible whiteness is present in the pupil. Blindness can occur, and the eyes may be crossed. The tumor can spread to the eye socket and the brain.

### Signs and Symptoms

Retinoblastoma may cause a white glow in the eye that is often seen in photographs taken with a flash, instead of the typical red eye in healthy eyes. Retinoblastoma may also cause the eyes to be crossed, white spots in the pupils, eye inflammation, and poor vision. The iris may be a different color in each eye.

### Treatment

Laser surgery, radiation therapy, and chemotherapy may be options. The eye may need to be removed if the tumor does not respond to other treatments. If the cancer has spread beyond the eye, the likelihood of a cure is much lower and depends on which organs are affected. Retinoblastoma can be fatal.

### Testing

Tests used in the diagnosis of retinoblastoma may include a CT or MRI study of the head to evaluate the degree of metastasis and an echoencephalogram (Blackman, 2004e).

## REYE'S SYNDROME

### Description

Reye's syndrome is associated with the use of aspirin in children, and it involves liver damage and brain damage, in the form of encephalopathy. Although the most common age of appearance is six, Reye's syndrome is seen in children as old as 12. It is often associated with giving children who are given aspirin-containing medicines while they have either chickenpox or the flu.

### Signs and Symptoms

The illness has a rapid onset. Typically, Reye's syndrome follows an upper respiratory infection or chickenpox by about a week. It begins with vomiting, which is persistent over many hours. The vomiting is rapidly followed by irritable and combative behavior. As the condition progresses, the child may become semiconscious or stuporous. Ultimately, seizures and coma develop, which can quickly lead to death.

## Treatment

There is no specific treatment for Reye's syndrome, but intensive, supportive care is needed. Steroids reduce brain swelling, and intravenous fluids are given to provide electrolytes and glucose. During a coma, a mechanical ventilator may be needed. The fatality rate for Reye's syndrome is about 40 percent, but the prognosis for those who survive the acute episode is good (Goldenring, 2004g; Weiner, 2001).

## Testing

Tests used in the diagnosis of Reye's syndrome include blood chemistry tests, liver function tests, liver biopsy, spinal tap and cerebrospinal fluid analysis, neurological exam, and imaging tests of the head.

## RHABDOMYOSARCOMA

## Description

Rhabdomyosarcoma is a rare, fast-growing cancer of voluntary muscle, which accounts for over half of the soft tissue sarcomas in children. Although it also affects adolescents between the ages of 13 and 15, it is more common among children ages 1 to 5. The most common sites of rhabdomyosarcomas are the head, neck, urogenital tract, and the extremities (Rhabdomyosarcoma, 2002).

## Signs and Symptoms

Rhabdomyosarcoma often causes a noticeable lump on a child's body, but other signs may also be present. For example, tumors in the nose or throat may cause bleeding, congestion, swallowing problems, or neurological problems if they extend into the brain.

## Treatment

Surgery and radiation therapy are used to treat the primary site of the tumor; chemotherapy is used to treat the spread of rhabdomyosarcoma. The mortality rate of this form of cancer is high, with only 50 percent of children surviving five years.

## Testing

Diagnosis of rhabdomyosarcoma is often delayed due to a lack of symptoms, and it is usually diagnosed during examinations associated with other injuries. Tests used to diagnose rhabdomyosarcoma include tumor biopsy, CT and MRI scans of the tumor site, bone scan for metastases, bone marrow biopsy, and possible spinal tap for brain metastases (Blackman, 2004f).

## RHEUMATIC FEVER

## Description

Rheumatic fever is an inflammatory disease that may develop after an infection with streptococcus bacteria and can involve the heart, joints, skin, and brain (Wener, 2003). Rheumatic fever occurs mainly between the ages of 4 and 18, where it develops as a type of arthritis noted by nodules at the joints. This septic infection may lead to inflammation of the heart valves, where it is known as rheumatic heart disease. Rheumatic heart disease is characterized by lesions of the heart valves, which prevents the valves from properly closing, allowing the blood flow to reverse. In the early 1980s, it was believed that rheumatic fever was being eradicated, but within a decade, cases began to appear with increasing regularity.

## Signs and Symptoms

Rheumatic fever is characterized by fever, joint pain, migratory arthritis, abdominal pain, skin rash with eruptions that are ring-shaped or snake-like in appearance, skin nodules, nosebleed, and cardiac involvment. Sydenham's chorea, or St. Vitus' dance, may also develop. St. Vitus' dance is characterized by purposeless, involuntary movements during waking hours. Self-injury may occur from flailing arms and legs.

## Treatment

Rheumatic fever is treated with antiobiotics. It is important that antibiotic treatment be continued even after the symptoms of bacterial infections cease. It is possible for bacterial infections to remain dormant in the body for many years, only to surface at a later date causing severe disease. In many cases, St. Vitus' dance disappears in a few months without treatment, but the underlying infection may still be present.

## Testing

Given the different manifestations of this disease, there is no specific test that can definitively establish a diagnosis. Some tests used in the diagnosis of rheumatic fever include tests for recurrent strep infection (e.g., ASO or antiDNAse B), CBCs, and ESR. As part of the cardiac evaluation, an electrocardiogram may also be done.

## RHEUMATOID ARTHRITIS

### Description

Rheumatoid arthritis is an inflammation of the lining of the joints or internal organs (Peng, 2004b). Rheumatoid arthritis is chronic, affecting many different joints with periodic flare-ups and remissions. This systemic disease affects the entire body and is one of the most common forms of arthritis. The direct cause of rheumatoid arthritis is unknown, but it is an autoimmune disease.

### Signs and Symptoms

Rheumatoid arthritis is characterized by inflammation of the synovial membrane and the cardinal signs of inflammation (i.e., pain, loss of function, heat, redness, and swelling). The inflammatory cells release enzymes that digest bones and cartilage resulting in severe deformities, as represented in Figure 2-74.

### Treatment

Disease-modifying antirheumatic drugs such as methotrexate and gold, in the form of myochrysine, solganal, and auranofin, are used to treat

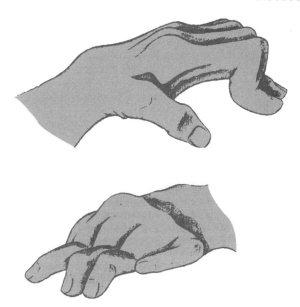

**Figure 2-74** Joint damage due to arthritis

rheumatoid arthritis. Nonsteroidal anti-inflammatories are used to control pain and inflammation. COX-2 inhibitors cause less gastrointestinal upset than nonsteroidal anti-inflammatories, but due to their side effects, many have been removed from the market. Antimalarial medications (e.g., hydroxychloroquine and sulfasalazine) and corticosteroids also may be prescribed. Inhibitors of tumor necrosis factor (e.g., etanercept, infliximab, adalimumab), medications that block the inflammatory protein interleukin-1 (e.g., anakinra), and drugs that inhibit the metabolism of nucleotides required for DNA synthesis in lymphocytes (e.g., leflunomide) show great promise in treating rheumatoid arthritis. Drugs that suppress the immune system (e.g., azathioprine and cyclophosphamide) are used when other therapies fail.

A recent treatment for nonresponsive cases of rheumatoid arthritis is the Prosorba column, which works by removing inflammatory antibodies from the blood. The blood is removed through a small catheter and then passed through a column that binds the antibodies and removes them from the blood. The procedure takes three hours, and must be done once a week for 12 weeks. Side effects include anemia, fatigue, fever, low blood pressure, and nausea. Some people have developed an infection from the catheter. Often there is a flare-up of joint pain for several days after the treatment. Currently, patients with severe forms of rheumatoid arthritis may die up to 15 years earlier than expected.

### Testing

Tests used in the diagnosis, treatment, and monitoring of rheumatoid arthritis include joint X-rays, rheumatoid factor tests, ESR, CBC, and synovial fluid analysis.

## RHINITIS

### Description

Rhinitis is a term describing the symptoms produced by nasal irritation or inflammation. Either infections or chemical irritants can cause rhinitis, but chronic rhinitis is usually due to an allergy commonly referred to as hay fever (Rhinitis, 2000).

### Signs and Symptoms

Rhinitis is characterized by runny nose, itching, sneezing, and stuffy nose due to blockage or congestion. Itching of the eyes is also commonly associated with both rhinitis and sinusitis. The normal process of trapping small particles such as dust, pollen, and microorganisms in the mucus of the nose results in mucus flowing from the nose and draining into the throat. This drainage causes runny nose and coughing in many people.

### Treatment

Rhinitis may be treated with short-acting antihistamines (e.g., Claritin), long-acting antihistamines (e.g., Allegra and Zyrtec), nasal corticosteroid sprays (e.g., Flonase, Nasonex, Nasacort), decongestants, and cromolyn sodium in the form of nasal sprays (e.g., Nasalcrom) and eyedrops. Allergy shots are occasionally recommended if the allergen cannot be avoided and if symptoms are hard to control.

### Testing

Tests used in the diagnosis of rhinitis may include cultures of the material from the nose and skin testing. This may include intradermal, scratch, patch, or other tests. In individuals who cannot undergo skin testing, the radioallergosorbent test (RAST), which tests for blood levels of IgE, is a blood test may be used to identify specific allergen sensitivity.

## RICKETS

### Description

Rickets is a deficiency disease of the bone affecting infants and young children. Deficiencies in calcium and phosphate in the bone's matrix cause softening of the bone. These deficiencies are typically due to deficiencies in vitamin D in the diet, which is necessary for proper calcification of bone tissue. In its active form, vitamin D acts as a hormone to regulate calcium absorption from the intestine and to regulate levels of calcium and phosphate in the bones. Other conditions that can cause rickets include hereditary or acquired disorders of vitamin D metabolism, kidney failure, low dietary intake of phosphates, cancer, and medications used to treat seizures. Children are at an increased risk for rickets when they do not get enough sunlight, and when they do not intake enough milk products, which may result from lactose intolerance.

## Signs and Symptoms

Rickets is characterized by diffuse bone pain in the hips, muscle weakness, bone fractures with minimal trauma, numbness around the mouth, numbness of extremities, spasms of hands or feet, and abnormal heartbeat. Rickets also results in impaired growth, short stature, deformities of the teeth, bowlegs, pigeon chest, bumps in the rib cage known as rachitic rosary, abnormally shaped skull, spinal deformities, and pelvic deformities.

## Treatment

The replacement of deficient calcium, phosphorus, or vitamin D will eliminate most symptoms of rickets. Exposure to moderate amounts of sunlight is encouraged. Bracing may be used to reduce or prevent deformities, and some skeletal deformities require surgery.

## Testing

Tests used in the diagnosis and treatment of rickets may include serum calcium levels, serum phosphorus levels, PTH, urine calcium levels, ionized calcium levels, alkaline phosphatase (ALP) isoenzyme levels, serum alkaline phosphatase levels, bone X-rays, and bone biopsy (Goldenring, 2004h).

## RIFT VALLEY FEVER

### Description

Rift Valley fever is an acute, fever-causing, viral disease of humans and domestic animals (e.g., cattle, buffalo, sheep, goats, and camels) that causes mosquito-borne epidemics during years of unusually heavy rainfall in certain regions of eastern and southern Africa, although it has also been found in other parts of the world (e.g., Madagascar, Saudi Arabia, Yemen). Rift Valley fever is caused by the Rift Valley Fever virus, which is a member of the genus *Phlebovirus* in the family Bunyaviridae. During years of heavy rainfall and localized flooding, infected mosquitos lay eggs in the water. It is believed that other insects that feed on infected animals can spread the virus. Humans also can become infected by handling infected blood or body fluids of infected domestic animals during slaughter or preparation of food (*Rift valley fever*, 2004).

### Signs and Symptoms

Rift Valley fever is characterized by fever, liver dysfunction, hemorrhagic fever, encephalitis, and ocular disease.

### Treatment

The fatality rate for humans is approximately 1 percent, but in most cases the disease is mild and recovery occurs within one week. There is no established course of treatment for patients infected with Rift Valley fever virus.

### Testing

Blood culture are used to diagnose Rift Valley fever.

## RILEY-DAY SYNDROME

### Description

Riley-Day syndrome, which is also known as familial dysautonomia, is an inherited disorder that affects the function of the nervous system. The disease is caused by mutation of the *IKBKAP* gene on chromosome 9. It is rare in the general population, but not amongst Ashkenazi Jews, where the incidence is estimated to be 1 in 3,700 people (Akroush, 1997).

### Signs and Symptoms

Riley-Day syndrome is characterized in infants by feeding problems and pneumonia caused by aspirating formula and food. Vomiting and sweating spells begin as the infant matures. Young children may also have breath-holding spells that produce unconsciousness, because they can hold their breath for long enough to pass out without feeling discomfort. A hallmark of Riley-Day syndrome is insensitivity to pain, which leads to injuries. Seizures occur in half of affected children, and acute problems with high and low blood pressure occur. Children also exhibit severe scoliosis and an unusually smooth tongue due to the absence of fungiform papillae, and they may have problems regulating their body temperature.

### Treatment

There is no specific treatment or cure for Riley-Day sundrome. Protection from injury is critical, and symptoms are treated as they occur. Life expectancy is shortened, with half not surviving past 20 and most dying by the age of 40.

### Testing

Genetic testing may be used to diagnose Riley-Day syndrome, but case history and physical exam are the primary basis of diagnosis.

## RINGWORM

### Description

There are a wide variety of fungi that can infect the integumentary system. These infectious fungi are known as dermatophytes. The infections they cause are dermatomycoses or ringworms. Dermatophytes grow in the keratin of the skin, hair, and nails, causing infections called ringworms (tineas). Ringworm of the scalp is known as tinea capitis, which begins as an infection of the hair follicle that spreads to the scalp (see Color Plate 50). Tinea cruris is a ringworm of the groin that is commonly referred to as jock itch. Tinea pedis is a fungal infection of the foot that is commonly known as athlete's foot (see Color Plate 51). Dermatomycoses are caused by three genera of fungi: *Trichophyton*, *Microsporum*, and *Epidermophyton*. Recurrence of fungal infections of the skin are common, and many are chronic, especially those infecting the nail beds.

## Signs and Symptoms

The symptoms of ringworm include itchy, red, raised, scaly patches that may blister and ooze. The patches often have sharply defined edges, and are often redder around the outside with normal skin tone in the center creating the appearance of a ring. The skin may also appear unusually dark or light. Infections of the scalp or beard result in bald patches. Infected nails are discolored, thick, and brittle to the point of crumbling.

## Treatment

Ringworm responds within about a month to antifungal agents (e.g., miconazole, clotrimazole, ketoconazole). Antibiotics may be needed to treat related bacterial infections (Hart, 2003j).

## Testing

Diagnosis of ringworm is primarily based on the appearance of the skin. Tests may include a Wood's lamp exam, in which the fungus may appear florescent when the skin is examined with a blue light in a dark room. A definitive diagnosis is made by examination of a skin scraping.

## ROCKY MOUNTAIN SPOTTED FEVER

## Description

Rocky Mountain spotted fever is the most severe rickettsial infection, and it is caused by *Rickettsia rickettsii* (Levy, 2003h). Rocky Mountain spotted fever is most prevalent in the Southeastern United States and in Appalachia, although it was first reported in the Rocky Mountains. *Rickettsia rickettsii* is a parasite found in a variety of ticks. It is passed from one generation of ticks to another through their eggs (Rocky Mountain spotted fever, 2000).

## Signs and Symptoms

A rash similar to measles is present in cases of Rocky Mountain spotted fever, with the exception that it is found on the soles of the feet and the palms of the hands. The rash begins on the extremities, usually around the ankles and wrists, and then spreads centripetally toward the trunk of the body (see Color Plate 52). The rash is not normally present on the neck or face. Other characteristics of Rocky Mountain spotted fever include headache, nausea, fever, vomiting, and muscle pain.

## Treatment

Rocky Mountain spotted fever is treated by carefully removing the tick from the skin and using antibiotics (e.g., doxycycline, tetracycline, chloramphenicol) to eliminate the infection. Treatment usually cures the infection, but rare complications can include paralysis, hearing loss, and nerve damage. Death occurs in approximately 5 percent of the reported cases of Rocky Mountain spotted fever from kidney and heart failure, although the mortality rate can be as high as 20 percent in untreated cases.

### Testing

Tests used in the diagnosis of Rocky Mountain spotted fever include CBC, creatinine levels, blood clotting tests, urine cultures, antibody titer by complement fixation or immunofluorescence, and biopsy of the rash.

## ROSEOLA

### Description

Roseola is an acute disease of infants and young children characterized by a high fever and skin rash. The disease is common in children under four years old, most commonly in those between six months and one year. It is caused by human herpesvirus 6, although similar syndromes are possible with other viruses.

### Signs and Symptoms

Roseola is characterized by the abrupt onset of high fever and irritability. Between the second and fourth day of illness, the fever falls dramatically, and a rash appears on the trunk that spreads to the limbs, neck, and face. The rash lasts from a few hours to two days. Febrile convulsions may occur when the fever is high.

### Treatment

There is no specific treatment for roseola. The disease usually resolves without complications (Graham, 2004).

### Testing

Roseola is usually diagnosed based on the appearance of the rash and the presence of swollen lymph nodes on the back of the scalp, which are referred to as occipital nodes.

## ROTAVIRUS DISEASE

### Description

Rotavirus is the most common cause of severe diarrhea among children. The incubation period for rotavirus disease is approximately two days. Rotavirus disease is spread through the fecal-oral route, although transmission may also occur through contaminated food, water, or contaminated surfaces (*Rotavirus*, 2003).

### Signs and Symptoms

Rotavirus disease is characterized by vomiting and watery diarrhea, fever, and abdominal pain.

### Treatment

In most cases, rotavirus disease is self-limiting and lasts only a few days. In 1998, a live virus vaccine known as Rotashield was approved for use in children. Rotashield is no longer recommended for infants due to a strong association between Rotashield and intussusception, which is a telescoping of the intestine, among vaccinated infants.

## Testing

Rotavirus is stable in the environment and has a characteristic wheel-like appearance when viewed by electron microscopy. Rotaviruses are nonenveloped, double-shelled viruses. Diagnosis may be made by rapid antigen detection of rotavirus in stool specimens. Strains may be further characterized by enzyme immunoassay or reverse transcriptase polymerase chain reaction, but such testing is not commonly done.

## RUBINSTEIN-TAYBI SYNDROME

### Description

Rubinstein-Taybi syndrome affects about 1 in 125,000 people (Stewart, 2003g). In 1995, a gene mutation in the CREB-binding protein (CREBBP) was identified as the cause of Rubinstein-Taybi syndrome.

### Signs and Symptoms

The classic feature of Rubinstein-Taybi syndrome is broad thumbs and great toes. There is also short stature, an unusual face, low-set ears, portwine stain, undescended testicles, mental deficiencies, and a downward slant of the eyes. About 40 percent of patients have heart defects with some requiring surgery (Stewart, 2003m).

### Treatment

There is no treatment for Rubinstein-Taybi syndrome.

### Testing

Genetic or mutation testing, including deletion testing, is used to see if the CREBBP gene is missing in cases of Rubinstein-Taybi syndrome.

## RUSSELL-SILVER SYNDROME

### Description

Russell-Silver syndrome is a congenital disease characterized by short stature and asymmetry in the size of the two halves or other parts of the body. Russell-Silver syndrome is believed to be genetic (Stewart, 2003n).

### Signs and Symptoms

Children with Russell-Silver syndrome are born small. Side-to-side asymmetry may occur. Other characteristics include excessive sweating, a small triangular face that makes the skull look large by comparison, inward curving fifth fingers, and colored spots on the skin called café-au-lait spots on the skin. Intelligence is normal.

### Treatment

There is no specific treatment for Russell-Silver syndrome.

### Testing

Tests used in the diagnosis of Russell-Silver syndrome include a glucose tolerance test, skeletal X-rays, and a karyotpe, which is a microscopic examination of chromosomes.

## SALMONELLOSIS

### Description

*Salmonella* gastroenteritis, or salmonellosis, is a type of food infection caused by *S. enteritidis* (Smith, 2003f). Symptoms appear approximately 8 to 36 hours after ingestion. Meat products, especially poultry, are commonly contaminated with *Salmonella* bacteria. To slow the transmission of *Salmonella* in the food preparation area, food handlers should thoroughly wash their hands after dealing with any meats or eggs. In addition, any items used in food preparation, such as cutting boards and mixing bowls, should be washed with soap and water after they have been in contact with raw meats or eggs. Eggs cooked to allow the yolk to remain liquid may still be contaminated. Foods containing raw eggs, such as hollandaise sauce, salad dressings, and eggnog, may also be contaminated.

### Signs and Symptoms

Complications of salmonellosis include fever, chills, nausea, vomiting, muscle pain, abdominal pain, and watery diarrhea. A rash of pink spots may accompany salmonellosis.

### Treatment

The objective of treatment in cases of salmonellosis is to replace fluids and electrolytes lost by diarrhea. Antidiarrheal medications are generally not given because they may prolong the infectious process. Antibiotic therapy may be indicated for those with severe symptoms. The prognosis for salmonellosis is usually good, with symptoms subsiding within a week. In severe cases, salmonellosis can be fatal.

### Testing

The primary test used in diagnosis of salmonellosis is a stool culture.

## SARCOIDOSIS

### Description

Sarcoidosis is an idiopathic disease in which inflammation occurs primarily in the lymph nodes, lungs, liver, eyes, and skin. Tissue samples from affected organs show clusters of immune cells (e.g, macrophages, lymphocytes, multinucleated giant cells) called granuloms. The healthy composition of blood cells is illustrated in Figure 2-75. Sarcoidosis is probably due to an allergic response to some factor in the environment, a genetic predisposition, or an extreme immune response to infection. The disease is most common among African Americans and Northern European Caucasians. The onset of sarcoidosis usually occurs in people between 30 and 50 years old (Kaufman, 2003; Yakobi, 2001).

### Signs and Symptoms

Although there may be no symptoms in cases of sarcoidosis, symptoms may include fever, difficulty breathing, cough, rash, headache, vision difficulties, neurological changes, enlarged axillary lymph nodes, enlarged liver, enlarged spleen, dry mouth, fatigue, weight loss, decreased tearing,

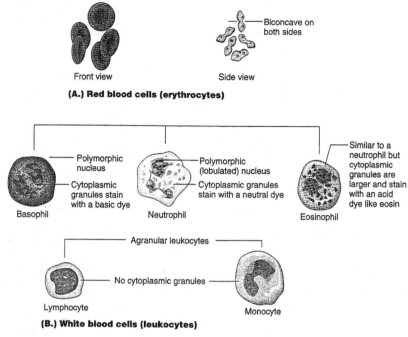

**Figure 2-75** Blood cells

seizures, nosebleed, joint stiffness, hair loss, and rales or other abnormal breathing sounds. The eyes may burn, itch, or exhibit a discharge.

## Treatment

Sarcoidosis symptoms often gradually resolve on their own without treatment. Severe cases may require treatment with corticosteroids and immunosuppressive agents (e.g., methotrexate, azathioprine, cyclophosphamide). Rarely, some individuals require organ transplantation. Thirty to 50 percent of cases resolve without treatment in three years. About 20 percent of those with lung involvement will develop residual lung damage. Death from sarcoidosis is rare.

## Testing

Tests used to diagnose sarcoidosis may include CBC, chem-7 or chem-20, ACE levels, chest X-rays, lymph node biopsy, skin lesion biopsy, bronchoscopy, open lung biopsy, liver biopsy, kidney biopsy, and EKG.

## SARS

### Description

Severe acute respiratory syndrome (SARS) is a serious form of pneumonia, resulting in acute respiratory distress and sometimes death. SARS has recently been reported in Asia, North America, and Europe. SARS appears to spread by close person-to-person contact and respiratory droplet inhalation. Most cases of SARS have involved people who cared for or lived with someone with SARS, or had direct contact with infectious material (e.g., respiratory secretions). Currently, there is no evidence that SARS is spreading in the United States. Scientists have detected a previously unrecognized coronavirus in patients with SARS. The new coronavirus is the leading hypothesis for the cause of SARS, although little is known about this new disease. According to the CDC, SARS was first described on February 26, 2003, by Dr. Carlo Urbani, who died of SARS just one month later on March 29, 2003, at the age of 46 (SARS, 2003).

### Signs and Symptoms

In general, SARS begins with a fever greater than 100.4°F. Other symptoms may include headache, an overall feeling of discomfort, and body aches. Some people also experience mild respiratory symptoms. After two to seven days, a dry cough and trouble breathing may develop. Complications may include respiratory failure, liver failure, heart failure, and nervous system failures.

### Treatment

People with SARS should be isolated immediately. Antibiotics are sometimes given in an attempt to treat bacterial causes of atypical pneumonia. Antiviral medications have also been used. High doses of steroids have been employed to reduce lung inflammation. In some serious cases, serum from people who have already gotten well from SARS has been given. Evidence of the general benefit of these treatments has been inconclusive. As the first wave of SARS began to subside, the death rate was about 15 percent.

### Testing

In most people with SARS, progressive chest X-ray changes or chest CT changes demonstrate the presence of pneumonia or respiratory distress syndrome. Tests used in the diagnosis of SARS include CBC, blood clotting tests, and blood chemistries. Specific tests for the SARS virus include the PCR test for SARS virus, antibody tests to SARS (e.g., ELISA or IFA), and direct SARS virus isolation. All current tests have some limitations.

## SCABIES

### Description

Scabies is a contagious skin disease caused by a small mite (see Color Plate 53). Scabies is spread by direct contact with infected individuals. The mites dig into the skin and deposit their eggs. The burrow resembles a pencil mark. Eggs mature in 21 days. In infants, the mites cause pimples over the trunk or small blisters over the palms and soles. In young children, the head, neck, shoulders, palms, and soles are involved. In older children and adults, hands, wrists, genitals, and abdomen are involved (Kantor, 2004d).

### Signs and Symptoms

Scabies is characterized by itching at night, pencil-mark lines on the skin, rashes, and abrasions of the skin caused by scratching.

## Treatment
The most commonly used cream is permethrin. Ivermectin may be used in severe cases.

## Testing
Diagnosis is based on physical exam and confirmed by skin scrapings.

## SCARLET FEVER

### Description
Scarlet fever is a bacterial disease of the upper respiratory system caused by *Streptococcus pyogenes*. It is known as scarlet fever because of the reddening toxin produced by the bacteria, which results in inflammation of the throat. Scarlet fever is a communicable disease spread by inhalation of droplet spray. Scarlet fever does not have the high mortality rate that it once had in the United States due to the effectiveness of antibiotics in treating streptococcal infections.

### Signs and Symptoms
Scarlet fever typically begins with a fever and sore throat. It may be accompanied by chills, vomiting, abdominal pain, and malaise. The toxin associated with scarlet fever causes a pinkish-red skin rash (see Color Plate 54) and high fever. The rash is described as sandpapery in quality. The tongue is spotted with a strawberry-like appearance (see Color Plate 55), after which it loses its upper membrane and becomes red and enlarged. The affected skin peels off the body in a process known as desquamation. Pastia's lines, which have a bright red color and are present in the axillae and groin, are characteristic of scarlet fever.

### Treatment
The treatment for scarlet fever is antibiotic therapy. The symptoms of scarlet fever resolve quickly with treatment, though the rash can last for up to three weeks (Goldenring, 2003b).

### Testing
In addition to a physical exam, tests used to diagnose scarlet fever include a throat swab for rapid antigen detection and culture for Group A Strep.

## SCHISTOSOMIASIS

### Description
Schistosomiasis, which is also known as bilharzia, is caused by parasitic worms (e.g., *Schistosoma mansoni*, *S. haematobium*, and *S. japonicum*). Over 200 million people are infected worldwide with schistosomiasis, although it is not found in the United States (Levy, 2004aa). Most cases of schistosomiasis occur in Africa, South America, the Middle East, southern China, the Carribean, and Southeast Asia. Schistosomiasis is transmitted when skin comes in contact with fresh water contaminated with schistosomes by infected snails. Within several weeks, worms grow inside the blood vessels of the body, producing eggs that migrate to the bladder or

intestines and are eventually passed in the urine or feces (Levy, 2004v; *Schistosomiasis*, 2004).

## Signs and Symptoms

During the early phase of infection, most people are asymptomatic. Schistosomiasis is characterized by a rash that appears within days after infection, which progresses to fever, chills, cough, and myalgia within two months of infection. In rare cases, eggs may be found in the central nervous system, where they cause seizures, paralysis, or spinal cord inflammation.

## Treatment

The treatment for schistosomiasis is praziquantel (Cooper, 2002).

## Testing

Tests used in the diagnosis of schistosomiasis include tests for schistosome eggs in the urine and feces, tissue biopsy, antibiody tests, and CBC.

## SCLERITIS

### Description

Scleritis is an inflammation of the sclera, which is the white of the eye. Inflammation of the sclera is usually associated with infections, chemical injuries, or autoimmune diseases such as rheumatoid arthritis and systemic lupus erythematosis. Scleritis occurs most often in people between the ages of 30 and 60 and is rare in children (Douglas, 2002).

### Signs and Symptoms

Scleritis is characterized by severe eye pain, red patches on the sclera, blurred vision, painful sensitivity to light, and tearing of the eye.

### Treatment

Scleritis is treated with oral corticosteroid or by corticosteroid eyedrops. If scleritis is caused by an underlying disease, treatment of that disease is necessary. Although scleritis may recur, it usually responds to treatment. The underlying disorder causing the scleritis may be serious, and the outcome depends upon the specific disorder.

### Testing

Scleritis is diagnosed based on eye examinations and confirmed by blood tests to rule out other underlying causes.

## SCLERODERMA

### Description

Scleroderma is a connective tissue disease characterized by changes in the skin, blood vessels, skeletal muscles, and internal organs (Koening, 2002). Scleroderma is an idiopathic disease that may produce local or systemic symptoms. Excess collagen deposits in the skin and other organs produce the symptoms. In the skin, ulceration, calcification, and changes in pigmentation may occur. Systemic disease may include fibrosis and degeneration of the heart, lungs, kidneys and gastrointestinal tract. The disease usually affects people 30 to 50 years old. Women are affected more often than men. Risk factors are occupational exposure to silica dust and polyvinyl chloride.

## Signs and Symptoms

Scleroderma is characterized by Raynaud's syndrome, skin thickening, shiny hands and forearms, hardening of the skin, tight and masklike facial skin, ulcerations on fingertips and toes, esophageal reflux, difficulty swallowing, bloating, weight loss, diarrhea, constipation, and difficulty breathing. Associated symptoms may include wrist pain, wheezing, abnormally dark or light skin, joint pain, hair loss, and eye inflammation.

## Treatment

There is no specific treatment for scleroderma, except to treat the symptoms.

## Testing

Tests used in the diagnosis of scleroderma may include ESR, rheumatoid factor, antinuclear antibodies, urinalysis, chest X-rays, pulmonary function tests, and skin biopsy.

## SCOLIOSIS

### Description

Scoliosis is a developmental disorder of the spine, in which the spinal column exhibits a lateral curvature. Scoliosis is often discovered at about the age of eight, when signs become apparent. The cause of scoliosis is unknown, but many theories have been proposed implicating connective tissue disorders, hormone imbalance, and nervous system disorders. Scoliosis runs in families and may be hereditary. Girls are more likely than boys to have scoliosis, and girls with scoliosis grow faster and begin puberty earlier than girls without scoliosis (A. Chen, 2004d; Scoliosis, 2002).

### Signs and Symptoms

Figure 2-76 compares scoliosis to two other spinal deformities. In cases of kyphosis, the abnormal curvature is in a posterior direction, while in cases of lordosis, the lumbar vertebra curve abnormally toward the anterior of the body. Scoliosis may cause deformities of the shoulders, shoulder blades, waist, hips, and leaning to one side.

### Treatment

Treatment consists of casts, braces, traction, electrical stimulation, or surgery.

### Testing

Tests used to confirm diagnosis of scoleosis may include spine X-rays, scoliometer measurements, and MRI scans (Chen, 2004d).

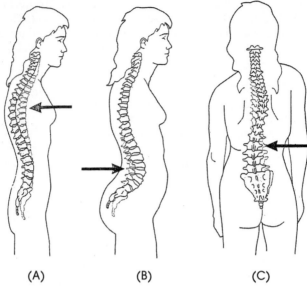

**(A)**          **(B)**          **(C)**

**Figure 2-76** (A) Kyphosis, (B) lordosis, (C) scoliosis

## SCROFULA

### Description

Tuberculosis is the oldest documented disease, and it was once believed that the touch of a king could cure it. Scrofula is a tuberculous infection of the skin of the neck, most often caused by *Mycobacterium tuberculosis* in adults. In children, it is usually caused by *Mycobacterium scrofulaceum* or *Mycobacterium avium*. Infection with mycobacteria is usually contracted through the air. Rubbery enlargement of the lymph nodes in the neck occurs. The lymph nodes eventually become ulcerated, producing draining sores (Levy, 2004x; Lewis & McClay, 2004).

### Signs and Symptoms

Scrofula is characterized by painless swelling of the cervical lymph nodes and enlargement of the lymph nodes. Other symptoms include fever, chills, sweats, and weight loss.

### Treatment

Several antibiotics are administered simultaneously due to the antibiotic-resistance of scrofula. Common antibiotics used to treat scrofula include isoniazid (INH), rifampin, pyrazinamide, and ethambutol. Other therapy usually involves antibiotics such as rifampin, ethambutol, and clarithromycin. Recovery is usually complete, and surgery is rarely needed.

### Testing

Tests used to diagnose scrofula include microscopic examination of specimens positive for granulomas, positive acid-fast bacillus (AFB) staining, positive tuberculin (TB) tine tests, positive purified protein derivative (PPD) tests, and cultures of lymph node specimines that are positive for mycobacteria.

## SEBACEOUS CYSTS

### Description
A sebaceous cyst is a closed sac found just under the skin containing a cheeselike material formed from skin secretions. Sebaceous cysts, which are also known as epidermal cysts, keratin cysts, or epidermoid cysts, are the product of swollen hair follicles or trauma to the skin. A sac of cells is created when a protein known as keratin is secreted from sebaceous sweat glands.

### Signs and Symptoms
Sebaceous cysts are commonly found on the face, neck, and trunk of the body. Color Plate 56 is a photograph of an epidermoid cyst in the urethra of the penis. They are usually slow-growing, painless, lumps under the skin; however, they may become inflamed and painful. They may be accompanied by redness and a grayish-white, cheesy, foul-smelling material that drains from the cyst.

### Treatment
Typically, sebaceous cysts do not require treatment, although they may be excised if they form an abscess. It is not uncommon for sebaceous cysts to return after they are surgically removed.

### Testing
In most cases, sebacious cysts are diagnosed based on appearance. Occasionally, a biopsy may be needed to rule out other conditions with a similar appearance.

## SEBORRHEIC DERMATITIS

### Description
Seborrheic dermatitis, which is also known as seborrhea, is a disorder of the sebaceous glands of the scalp, face, and trunk (Kantor, 2004e; Seldon, 2001). In addition to sebum, this skin disorder has been linked to a fungus (*Pityrosporum ovale*) and immune system abnormalities. The symptoms of seborrhea are aggravated by humidity, scratching, change in seasons, and emotional stress. Seborrhea may be as mild as dandruff or as severe as thick crust formation over the scalp, which is known as cradle cap. Seborrheic dermatitis may appear in combination with systemic disorders like Parkinson's disease or AIDS. Seborrhea is common on the scalp of infants, which is believed to be the result of hormones in the uterus. Among the elderly, cradle cap is due to a fungal infection. The scalp and hair are quite fragile in cases of seborrhea, which is pictured in Color Plate 57.

### Signs and Symptoms
Cradle cap appears as thick, crusty, yellow or brown scales over the child's scalp. Similar scales may also be found on the eyelids, on the ear, around

the nose, and in the groin. Cradle cap may be seen in newborns and small children up to the age of three years and is a harmless, temporary condition. Cradle cap is not contagious, nor is it caused by poor hygiene.

## Treatment

Flaking and dryness may be reduced by use of over-the-counter medicated shampoo, with active ingredients of salicylic acid, coal tar, zinc, resorcin, or selenium. Shampoos containing selenium, ketoconazole, or corticosteroids may be prescribed for severe cases of seborrheic dermatitis. There is no cure for seborrheic dermatitis.

## Testing

The diagnosis is based on the appearance and location of the skin lesions. Biopsy and tissue culture may be conducted to rule out other disorders, but this is rare.

## SHEEHAN'S SYNDROME

### Description

Sheehan's syndrome occurs due to severe uterine hemorrhage during childbirth. Severe blood loss causes tissue death in the mother's pituitary gland and leads to hypopituitarism following the birth. Sheehan's syndrome is rare in the United States due to access to good obstetrical care. Conditions that increase the risk of an obstetric hemorrhage and Sheehan's syndrome include multiple pregnancies (twins or triplets) and abnormalities of the placenta increase the risk for this disease (P. Chen, 2004d).

### Signs and Symptoms

A deficiency in pituitary hormones results in inability to breast feed, fatigue, loss of pubic and axillary hair, lack of menstrual bleeding, and low blood pressure.

### Treatment

The treatment for pituitary insufficiency is lifelong hormone substitute medication, including estrogen, progesterone, thyroid, and adrenal hormones. Sheehan's syndrome can be fatal if not treated, but it has an excellent prognosis with treatment.

### Testing

Tests to measure hormone levels in the blood and CT scans or MRI scans of the head to rule out other disorders of the pitutitary gland (e.g., tumors) are used to diagnose Sheehan's syndrome.

## SHINGLES

### Description

Like all herpesviruses, the varicella-zoster virus can remain latent in the body (Levy, 2004n). After recovery from chickenpox, the varicella-zoster virus remains indefinitely in the dorsal root ganglia of the spinal cord.

Later, under periods of stress or compromised immunity, the virus is reactivated causing skin lesions in the form of shingles.

## Signs and Symptoms

The blisters are found around the waist, and on the face, chest, and back (see Color Plate 58). The vesicles follow the affected cutaneous sensory nerve and usually affect only one side of the body. Shingles is a painful disorder that may lead to nerve impairment and paralysis.

## Treatment

Herpes zoster usually resolves spontaneously and may not require treatment except for symptomatic relief, such as pain medication. Acyclovir, desciclovir, famciclovir, valacyclovir, and penciclovir may be used in the treatment of shingles. Shingles is fatal in approximately 17 percent of the reported cases in the United States.

## Testing

Diagnosis is based on the appearance of the skin lesions, and tests are rarely necessary, but they may include culture of skin lesions, Tzanck test of skin lesions, CBC, and specific antibody tests.

## SICKLE CELL ANEMIA

## Description

Sickle cell anemia is a hereditary, chronic anemia, characterized by the presence of a large number of crescent- or sickle-shaped red blood cells. To inherit sickle cell anemia, both parents must have possessed the recessive gene for hemoglobin S. Inheriting the trait for hemoglobin S from only one parent results in other forms of sickle cell anemia (e.g., sickle cell-b0 thalassemia, hemoglobin SC disease, or sickle cell-b + thalassemia). Figure 2-77 describes the chain of events associated with malformed red blood cells, and the disorders sickle cell anemia can cause.

The alteration in the hemoglobin of these deformed red blood cells is due to a single amino acid substitution in one of the chains of amino acids from which hemoglobin is produced, resulting in hemoglobin S. Because people with sickle trait were more likely to survive malaria outbreaks in Africa than those with normal hemoglobin, it is believed that hemoglobin S is a genetic alteration that evolved as a protection against malaria. Around the world, sickle cell anemia occurs almost exclusively among blacks.

## Signs and Symptoms

Sickle cell anemia is usually present after about six months of age. It continues throughout life with sudden exacerbated episodes known as crises. The most serious crises involve severe pain emanating from damaged bone marrow, which leads to necrosis of the bone marrow. Fat emboli can spread from the necrotic bone marrow, causing sudden death by stroke or heart failure.

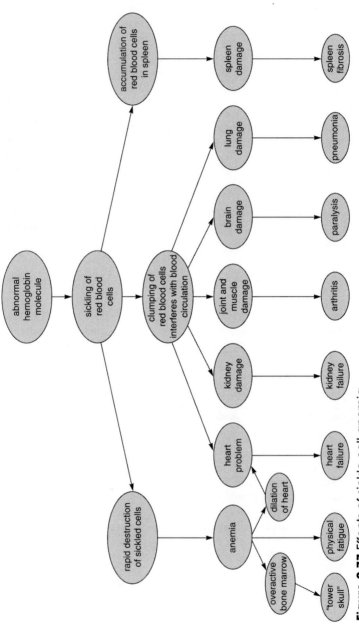

**Figure 2-77** Effects of sickle cell anemia

## Treatment

Patients with sickle cell disease need treatment even when not experiencing a crisis. Folic acid, an essential element in producing cells, is required due to rapid red blood cell turnover. Bacterial infections are treated with antibiotics and vaccines, and routine eye exams are necessary due to the risk of damage to the retina. Treatment during crises may include antibiotics, partial exchange transfusion for acute chest syndrome, partial exchange transfusions or surgery for neurological events (e.g., strokes, dialysis), kidney transplant, irrigation or surgery for priapism, surgery for eye problems, hip replacement for avascular necrosis of the hip, gallbladder removal, and zinc oxide or surgery for leg ulcers (A. Levy, 2002; Cohen, 2003c).

Hydroxyurea was found to help some patients, but there has been some concern about the possibility of hydroxyurea causing leukemia. As yet, there are no definitive data that hydroxyurea causes leukemia in sickle cell patients. Newer drugs are being developed to manage sickle cell anemia by inducing the body to produce more fetal hemoglobin, thereby decreasing the amount of sickling, or by increasing the binding of oxygen to sickle cells. But as yet, there are no other widely used drugs that are available for treatment. Bone marrow transplants are currently the only potential cure for sickle cell anemia. However, it is difficult to find the right bone marrow donor, and the drugs needed to make the transplant possible are highly toxic. Persons with sickle cell anemia may die due to organ failure and infection in their 50s.

## Testing

Tests used in the diagnosis and treatment of sickle cell anemia include CBC, hemoglobin electrophoresis, and a sickle cell test.

## SIDS (SUDDEN INFANT DEATH SYNDROME)

## Description

According to the Center for Disease Control and Prevention (SIDS, 2001), Sudden Infant Death Syndrome (SIDS) is the diagnosis given for the sudden death of an infant under one year of age that remains unexplained after a thorough case investigation. SIDS is also known as cot death or crib death. Most SIDS deaths occur between the ages of two and four months, and approximately 3,000 SIDS deaths occur in the United States annually. Death occurs during sleep without any apparent struggle. Although the cause of SIDS is unknown, there are certain risk factors associated with SIDS (Goldenring, 2004i):

- babies who sleep on their belly
- babies whose mothers smoked during pregnancy
- babies born to mothers less than 20 years old
- babies born to mothers who had inadequate prenatal care
- babies born to mothers who abused drugs during pregnancy

- babies who are premature or of low birth weight
- babies who sleep on soft surfaces (e.g., soft mattresses, sofas, cushions, water beds, sheepskins)
- babies who sleep on fluffy or loose bedding (e.g, pillows, quilts, stuffed toys)
- babies who are male
- babies who are African American or Native American

## Signs and Symptoms

Evidence suggests that some SIDS babies are born with abnormalities in the brain stem, which controls breathing during sleep by regulating carbon dioxide and oxygen levels. A large number of babies who die from SIDS have respiratory or gastrointestinal infections prior to their deaths. Other SIDS babies have excess immune system cells and proteins that interact with the brain to alter heart rate, slow breathing during sleep, or induce deep sleep. Some scientists believe that SIDS is a manifestation of an inborn error of fatty acid metabolism associated with a deficiency of an enzyme known as acetyl coenzyme A.

## Testing

SIDS is diagnosed after a postmortem case investigation and autopsy.

## SILICOSIS

### Description

Silicosis is the inhalation of crystalline silica, which primarily occurs as a result of occupational exposure. Some of the occupations that are at high risk of silica exposure include sandblasting, quarry mining, drilling, tunneling, and stone cutting. Crystalline forms of silica include quartz, cristobalite, and tridymite. These crystals are used in artwork, watches, lenses, ceramics, plastics, and products such as bricks, chalk, and gypsum board.

### Signs and Symptoms

Silicosis is characterized by chronic cough, difficulty breathing, fever, and the presence of progressive, massive fibrosis. People with silicosis are at high risk for developing tuberculosis (TB). Silica is believed to interfere with the body's immune response to the bacteria that causes TB.

### Treatment

There is no specific treatment for silicosis. Removal of the source of silica exposure is important to prevent further worsening of the disease. Supportive treatment includes cough suppression medications, bronchodilators, and oxygen if needed. Antibiotics are prescribed for respiratory infections as needed. Yearly skin testing to check for exposure to TB is recommended. Treatment with anti-TB drugs is recommended for people with a positive skin test. Any change in the appearance of the chest X-ray may indicate TB. Silicosis is a chronic condition that can be fatal.

## Testing

Silicosis is primarily diagnosed through case history of exposure to silica and a physical exam. Diagnostic tests to confirm the diagnosis and exclude other diseases include chest X-rays, pulmonary function tests, and purified protein derivative (PPD) skin test for tuberculosis (Blaivas, 2003b).

## SINUSITIS

### Description

Sinusitis refers to inflammation of the sinuses, generally caused by a viral, bacterial, or fungal infection. The sinuses are air-filled spaces around the forehead, cheeks, and eyes that are lined with mucus membranes and are open to allow the mucus to drain and air to circulate (Figure 2-78). When inflamed, the sinuses become blocked with mucus. Each year, over 30 million adults and children develop sinusitis (Sharma, 2004b).

### Signs and Symptoms

Acute sinusitis is characterized by the onset of symptoms following a cold that does not improve or worsens after a week. Symptoms include nasal congestion and discharge, sore throat and postnasal drip, headache, cough, fever, bad breath, loss of smell, and fatigue. The symptoms worsen at night and when lying down. Symptoms of chronic sinusitis are the same as acute sinusitis, but tend to be milder and last longer than eight weeks.

### Treatment

Treatment of sinusitis may include nasal corticosteroid sprays (e.g., Flonase, Nasonex, Nasacort) and antibiotics (e.g., ampicillin, amoxicillin,

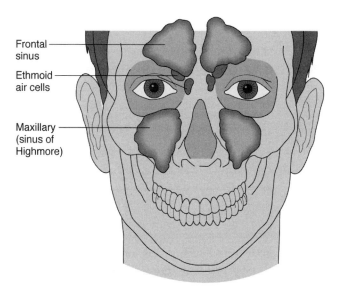

Frontal sinus

Ethmoid air cells

Maxillary (sinus of Highmore)

**Figure 2-78** Sinuses

trimethoprim with sulfamethoxazole, augmentin, cefuroxime, cefprozil). Surgery to clean and drain the sinuses may also be necessary, especially for fungal sinus infections.

### Testing

A variety of tests may be used to diagnose sinusitis, but the most accurate are a CT scan of the sinuses and, if the sinusitis is presumed to involve tumors or fungal infection, an MRI of the sinuses (Hart, 2003k).

## SJÖGREN'S SYNDROME

### Description

Sjögren's syndrome is a systemic inflammatory disorder characterized by dry mouth, decreased tearing, and other dry mucous membranes. The cause of Sjögren's syndrome is unknown. Sjögren's syndrome is rare in children, and occurs most often in women 40 to 50 years old (Jung, 2004). Children usually present with another autoimmune disorder before developing the signs of Sjögren's syndrome. Sjögren's syndrome affects 3 percent of the population. Sjögren's syndrome may be associated with rheumatoid arthritis, systemic lupus erythematosus, scleroderma, polymyositis, and other diseases.

### Signs and Symptoms

Dryness of the eyes and mouth are the most common symptoms of Sjögren's syndrome. Symptoms may occur alone or in concetion with connective tissue diseases. There may be an associated enlargement of the salivary glands. Other symptoms may include loss of taste, dental cavities, hoarseness, fatigue, joint pain and swelling, and clouding of the cornea.

### Treatment

There is no cure for Sjögren's syndrome. Dry eyes may be treated with artificial tears, and dry mouth may be treated with drugs (e.g., pilocarpine) that increase the flow of saliva. Arthritis symptoms are treated with nonsteroidal anti-inflammatory medications.

### Testing

Tests used to diagnose Sjögren's syndrome include antinuclear antibodies (ANA) tests, salivary gland biopsy, rheumatoid factor, tear tests, and slit lamp examination with rose bengal dye (Clowse, 2003d).

## SMALLPOX

### Description

Variola is the poxvirus that causes smallpox (Levy, 2003i; Smallpox, 2002). During the Middle Ages, much of Europe contracted smallpox. The disease ravaged Native Americans who had no previous exposure to it when it was brought to the Americas by European explorers. By the time the characteristic pox lesions form on the skin, many organs are infected. The smallpox virus enters the body through the respiratory system. Smallpox has been eradicated through vaccination programs, although two samples of the virus have been stored in Russia and the United States. Smallpox virus may be available for use as a biological weapon in certain countries. Smallpox is highly contagious from one person to another.

## Signs and Symptoms

Smallpox is characterized by high fever, fatigue, severe headache, backache, delirium, vomiting, diarrhea, and bleeding. The rash associated with smallpox is pink with raised areas. It starts centrally and spreads outward beginning in the mouth and throat, then the face, forearms, trunk, and legs. The rash turns into pustular lesions that crust on approximately the eighth day.

## Treatment

If the smallpox vaccination is given within four days of exposure, symptoms may be prevented or lessened. There is no specific treatment for smallpox once symptoms present. Antibiotics are given for secondary infections, and vaccinia immune globulin may shorten the disease. In the past, smallpox was fatal up to 30 percent of the time.

## Testing

Tests used in the diagnosis of smallpox include virus identification by electron microscope and by culture, CBC, a positive disseminated intravascular coagulation (DIC) panel, and positive antibody tests (Levy, 2003i).

## SPINA BIFIDA

## Description

Spina bifida is a structural abnormality that results in the failure of the fetus's spine to close properly during the first month of gestation (Newmark, 2003b; NINDS spina bifida, 2001). The opening is typically located in the lumbar vertebrae, forming a tumor in a condition known as spina bifida cystica. This is accompanied by developmental insufficiencies of the brain, spinal cord, or meninges. Even if the opening can be surgically repaired, the nerve damage is usually permanent and results in paralysis. In cases of spina bifida with no opening of the spinal cord, there may be absent or structurally damaged vertebrae and nerve damage.

## Signs and Symptoms

In addition to the obvious physical challenges, most children with spina bifida also exhibit mental disability. Bowel and bladder complications often accompany spina bifida, and infants with spina bifida may have a condition known as hydrocephalus, in which excessive amounts of cerebrospinal fluid accumulate in the brain. The three most common types of spina bifida and their characteristics are listed in Table 2-7.

## Treatment

There is no cure for spina bifida, and the prognosis for spina bifida depends on severity. Possible treatments may include surgery, medication, and physical therapy. Currently, there are centers attempting experimental in utero surgical repair of spina bifida. Although the prognosis is poorest

**Table 2-7** Types of Spina Bifida

| | |
|---|---|
| Myelomeningocele | The most severe form of spina bifida and is character-ized by the protrusion from an opening in the spine of both the malformed spinal cord and the meninges. |
| Meningocele | Occurs when the spinal cord develops normally but the meninges protrude from a spinal opening. |
| Occulta | The least severe form, in which one or more vertebrae are malformed and covered by a layer of skin. |

for infants with complete paralysis, with proper care, most children with spina bifida will live well into adulthood.

## Testing

During the first trimester, pregnant women can have a blood test called a triple screen for spina bifida, Down syndrome, and other congenital diseases in the baby. Eighty-five percent of women carrying a fetus with spina bifida will show elevated maternal serum alpha fetoprotein, which is one of the three proteins measured in the triple screen. The triple screen has a high false positive rate, so if it is positive, further testing is required to confirm the diagnosis. A prenatal ultrasound is then done and is usually a reliable test for spina bifida. After birth, tests may include spinal X-rays, spinal ultrasound, spine CT scan, and spine MRI scan.

## SPLENOMEGALY

### Description

Splenomegaly is an enlargement of the spleen beyond its normal size. The spleen is involved in the production of red blood cells, white blood cells, and functions in the lymphatic and immune systems. Rupture of the enlarged spleen is possible in cases of infectious mononucleosis, and appropriate limitations on activity may help prevent trauma that might cause the spleen to rupture. Common causes of splenomegaly include viral, parasitic, and bacterial infections, cirrhosis of the liver, inflammation of the gall bladder, cystic fibrosis, anemia, leukemia, lymphomas, and sickle cell anemia.

### Signs and Symptoms

Splenomegaly is characterized by pain in the upper left quadrant of the abdomen, especially after eating.

### Treatment

Splenomegaly is treated based on the underlying cause of illness. If the spleen is surgically removed, the procedure is known as a splenectomy.

### Testing

Tests used in the diagnosis of enlarged spleen include a CBC, tests for suspected causes, and imaging exams of the abdomen and spleen (Hart, 2004k).

## SPOROTRICHOSIS

### Description

Sporotrichosis is a fungal infection of the skin caused by *Sporothrix schenckii* (Levy, 2004y). The fungus is found on some thorny plants, sphagnum moss, and baled hay. Outbreaks have occurred among nursery workers handling sphagnum moss topiaries and among children playing on baled hay. *Sporothrix schenckii* enters the skin through small cuts or punctures from thorns, barbs, pine needles, or wires and does not spread from person-to-person (*Sporotrichosis*, 2004).

### Signs and Symptoms

The first symptom of infection is the appearance of a painless redish-purple nodule resembling an insect bite on the fingers, hand, or arm where the fungus first enters through a break on the skin. Additional nodules then appear that open and resemble boils, eventually developing into slow-healing ulcerations that may spread to other areas of the body. The first nodule typically appears within 12 weeks after exposure to the fungus, and the ulcerations become visible within three weeks after infection. The ulcers spread in a line away from the initial ulcer.

### Treatment

Sporotrichosis is treated with potassium iodide. Itraconazole (Sporanox) is also used for treatment, but experience with this drug is still limited. Treatment may require a number of weeks, until the skin lesions are completely healed. With treatment, full recovery can be expected. Disseminated sporotrichosis can be life-threatening for the immunocompromised.

### Testing

Sporotrichosis is diagnosed by a physical examination revealing the typical lesions. A culture of biopsied tissue confirms diagnosis.

## SQUAMOUS CELL CARCINOMAS

### Description

Squamous cell carcinoma is the second most common skin cancer (Grund, 2004e). It arises from the epidermis and resembles the squamous cells in the outer layers of the skin (see Color Plate 59). Although squamous cell carcinomas may remain isolated in the epidermis, they will eventually penetrate the underlying tissues if not treated. Squamous cell carcinoma is most common on sun-exposed parts of the body. Individuals with dark skin complexion are less likely to develop skin cancer (*STARI*, 2001).

### Signs and Symptoms

Squamous cell carcinoma is a skin lesion that is small, firm, red, flat, and may grow in a cone shape. The surface of the lesion scales and becomes crusted. Squamous cell carcinoma is most common on the face, ears, neck, hands, and arms. The lesions may also occur on the lip, mouth, tongue, or genitals.

## Treatment

Any changes in a preexisting skin growth such as a mole, or the presence of an open sore that fails to heal, should prompt an individual to seek medical attention. Early treatment of precancerous lesions may prevent them from developing into squamous cell carcinoma. The treatment varies with the tumor's size, depth, location and how much it has spread. Treatment may include surgical removal, radiation therapy, and chemotherapy.

## Testing

Squamous cell carcinoma is diagnosed based on the appearance of the skin lesion. A biopsy and examination of the lesion confirms diagnosis.

## STARI

### Description

STARI (Southern Tick-Associated Rash Illness) is caused by *Borrelia lonestari*, which is spread by the bite of the lone star tick *Amblyomma americanum*. Lone star ticks can be found from central Texas and Oklahoma eastward across the southern Unites States and along the Atlantic coast as far north as Maine.

### Signs and Symptoms

STARI is characterized by a red, expanding rash with a central clearing following the bite of the lone star tick. The rash is similar in appearance to erythema migrans, which is associated with Lyme disease.

### Treatment

Oral antibiotic treatment is generally effective in treating cases of STARI.

### Testing

Even though spirochetes have been seen in *A. americanum* ticks by microscopy, attempts to culture them have consistently failed. Modified BSK (Barbour-Stoenner-Kelly) is the best medium for cultivating the Lyme disease spirochete, *B. burgdorferi*, but is apparently not suitable for cultivating the spirochete found in *A. americanum*. A spirochete has been detected in *A. americanum* by DNA analysis and was given the name *Borrelia lonestari*.

## STREP THROAT

### Description

Strep throat is caused by *Streptococcus pyogenes*, which is capable of producing injurious enzymes and toxins. Hyaluronidase, which is also known as spreading factor, is an enzyme produced by *S. pyogenes* that dissolves human connective tissues, allowing the organism to spread deep into the tissues. Strep throat is common among children between 5 and 15. The disease is spread by droplets and close contact.

## Signs and Symptoms

The symptoms appear within one to four days after exposure, including an acute onset of sore throat, malaise, fever, headache, nausea, vomiting, and abdominal pain. Color Plate 60 is a photograph of a person with strep throat.

## Treatment

Strep throat is treated with antibiotics to prevent more serious complications of this infection, including rheumatic fever. Resistance to penicillin is increasing, and cephalosporins may be more effective in some situations. Most sore throats are caused by viruses, not strep. The CDC recommends against treating sore throats with antibiotics unless the strep test is positive (Greene, 2004c).

## Testing

Strep cannot be diagnosed by symptoms or a physical exam alone. A throat swab can be tested for culture, although a rapid antigen test is quicker but less reliable.

## STROKE

### Description

Strokes, which are also known as cerebrovascular accidents (CVAs), occur in the blood vessels of the brain. A blood vessel ruptures within the brain causing death of the brain tissue. Figure 2-79 illustrates an ischemic stroke, in which a cerebral blood vessel becomes occluded. Figure 2-80 illustrates a hemorrhagic stroke, in which a cerebral blood vessel ruptures, causing internal bleeding. A transient ischemic attack (TIA) is a stroke that lasts only a few minutes. It occurs when the blood supply to the brain is briefly interrupted. The symptoms of a TIA are similar to a more severe stroke, but they do not last as long. Most symptoms of a TIA last only about an hour, but they may persist for as much as a day (Internet Stroke Center, 2003).

### Signs and Symptoms

Sudden loss of motor control, loss of sensory perception, and loss of speech are common effects of stroke. Because each hemisphere of the brain controls the opposite side of the body, if the symptoms are present on the right side of the body, the left side of the brain was the site of injury, and vice versa. Other symptoms may include numbness, vision changes, slurred speech, difficulty swallowing, drooling, loss of memory, dizziness, personality changes, loss of consciousness, and uncontrollable eye movements.

### Treatment

Physicians have begun calling strokes a brain attack to stress the importance of immediate treatment. The goal is to get the person to the emergency room immediately, determine the type of stroke, and start therapy—all within three hours of the onset of the stroke. Thrombolytic medicine, like tPA, breaks up blood clots and restores blood flow. Blood thinners

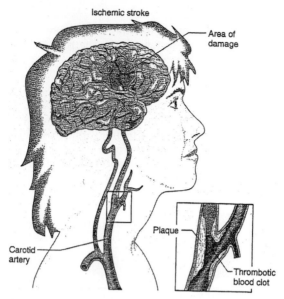

**Figure 2-79** Stroke due to a blockage in the blood vessel in the neck

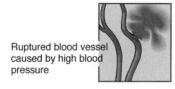

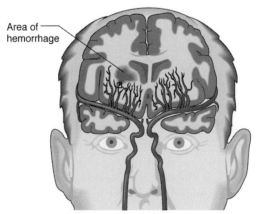

**Figure 2-80** Stroke due to rupture of blood vessel in the brain

such as heparin and coumadin are used to treat strokes. Antiplatelet agents such as aspirin may be used as well. Stroke, many victims have long-term disabilities, but about 10 percent recover completely.

## Testing

Tests used to diagnose strokes may include head CT scan or MRI scan, electrocardiogram to identify heart disorders, echocardiogram, carotid duplex ultrasounds, cerebral angiography, and blood work.

## STRONGYLOIDIASIS

### Description

Strongyloidiasis is an intestinal infection caused by the roundworms *Strongyloides stercoralis* and *S. fülleborni,* which infect humans, chimpanzees, and baboons (Levy, 2004z; *Stongyloidiasis,* 2004). The roundworm may remain in an asymptomatic host for years before causing a fatal infection. According to Polenakovik and Polenakovik (2004), strongyloidiasis is most common in tropical and subtropical regions of the world where the rate of disease may reach 40 percent, although the rate of disease in the United States is only about 4 percent. Strongyloidiasis is transmitted through contaminated soil through the fecal-oral route. The two most severe forms of strongyloidiasis are hyperinfection syndrome and disseminated strongyloidiasis. Hyperinfection syndrome involves an acceleration of the normal life cycle of *S. stercoralis,* leading to excessive worm burden. Disseminated strongyloidiasis involves widespread dissemination of larvae to extraintestinal organs that are not ordinarily part of the parasite life cycle (e.g., CNS, heart, urinary tract, endocrine organs).

### Signs and Symptoms

Common symptoms include itching and rash at the site of larvae penetration (usually the feet), cough, difficulty breathing, fever, wheezing, indigestion, diarrhea, nausea, and vomiting.

### Treatment

Severe cases of strongyloidiasis have a fatality rate of approximately 80 percent, but full recovery is expected with treatment in more mild cases. Strongyloidiasis is treated with anthelmintic medications (e.g., ivermectin and thiabendazole) and antibiotics if bacterial infection is also present. If the peritoneum is compromised, surgical intervention may be required.

### Testing

Tests used in the diagnosis of strongyloidiasis include CBC, stool exam, antigen tests, duodenal aspiration and fluid examination, and sputum examination.

## SUBDURAL HEMATOMA

### Description

An acute subdural hematoma is a rapidly clotting blood collection below the inner layer of the dura, but external to the brain and arachnoid

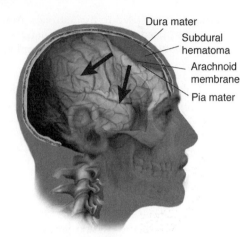

**Figure 2-81** Subdural hematoma

membrane. Acute subdural hematomas are almost always directly the result of blunt force traumas to the head, such as whiplash or violently shaking an infant. Chronic subdural hematomas are less frequently the result of blunt force trauma, and are more likely to be the result of brain atrophy in association with nervous disorders like Alzheimer's disease. Notice in Figure 2-81 that the brain and other cranial tissues are displaced and compressed by intracranial bleeding.

### Signs and Symptoms
Subdural hematoma is characterized by headache, muscle weakness, slurred speech, nausea, vomiting, lethargy, and seizures.

### Treatment
A subdural hematoma is an emergency condition. Treatment includes life-saving measures to support breathing and circulation. Diuretics may be used to reduce swelling. Anticonvulsant medications such as phenytoin are used to control seizures. Drilling a small hole in the skull relieves pressure and allows drainage of the hematoma (Jasmin, 2004).

### Testing
Brain imaging studies, including CT scan and MRI scan, are used to diagnose subdural hematoma.

## SYPHILIS

### Description
Syphilis is a sexually transmitted disease caused by *Treponema pallidum* (Levy, 2003j). *T. pallidum* is a bacterial spirochete with three flagella inserted into each end of the cell, providing it a graceful motility in fluids. Because of its outer layer of lipids, *T. pallidum* causes little response from the immune system and has, therefore, become known as a Teflon

pathogen. Syphilis has often been called the great imitator because so many of the signs and symptoms are indistinguishable from those of other diseases.

## Signs and Symptoms

**Primary Stage:** The primary stage of syphilis is noted by the appearance of a chancre, which is a small, hard ulcer (Figure 2-82) at the site of infection (e.g., penis, anus, vagina, cervix, or mouth) approximately 10 to 90 days after contact. Fluid forms in the center of this painless lesion. Syphilitic chancres abound with treponemes, and they are extremely infectious. The chancre is frequently not visible in females because it appears on the cervix or the vaginal wall.

**Secondary Stage:** About 2 to 12 weeks after the chancre disappears, the secondary stage of the disease may begin in some individuals. The individual suffers from hair loss, swollen lymph nodes, sore throat, malaise, and low-grade fever. Infected individuals may also present with a rash that is unusual in that it can occur on the palms of the hands and the soles of the feet (see Color Plate 61). All secondary syphilitic lesions of the skin and mucous membranes are highly infectious. The secondary stage may either relapse for several weeks, or it may go entirely unnoticed by the infected individual. A person can easily pass the disease to sex partners when primary or secondary stage signs or symptoms are present.

**Tertiary Stage:** In about 25 percent of the cases of syphilis, the disease does not progress beyond the secondary stage, and another 25 percent of the cases become latent and no further symptoms are experienced by the infected individual, whether treated not. The other 50 percent of cases of

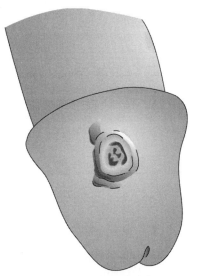

**Figure 2-82** Syphilis chancre

syphilis develop into a tertiary stage 2 to 20 years later. During the latent period, the individual may experience no symptoms of the disease.

During the tertiary stage of syphilis, a rubberlike lesion known as a gumma appears on the bone, viscera, and skin (see Color Plate 62). In the tertiary stage, syphilis may begin to damage the internal organs, including the brain, nerves, eyes, heart, blood vessels, liver, bones, and joints. The aorta may be affected causing it to weaken. A loss of motor control may occur in cases of syphilis in which the central nervous system becomes infected. Syphilis can lead to seizures, blindness, and death. In the United States, the tertiary stage of syphilis is rarely seen due to medical intervention.

## Treatment

Syphilis is treated with antibiotics. Persons who receive syphilis treatment must abstain from sexual contact with new partners until the syphilis sores are completely healed. Persons with syphilis must notify their sex partners so that they also can be tested and receive treatment. Having had syphilis does not protect a person from getting it again.

## Testing

The proper diagnostic tests for syphilis depend on the stage of the disease and may include dark field examination of the primary lesion (in primary syphilis), and blood tests such as Venereal Disease Research Laboratory (VDRL), Rapid Plasmin Reagin (RPR), and Fluorescent Treponemal Antibody Absorption Test (FTA-ABS). In the case of neurosyphilis, a spinal tap is required to make the diagnosis and may be sent for VDRL and/or FTA-ABS (Levy, 2003j).

## TAKAYASU'S ARTERITIS

### Description

Takayasu's arteritis is an inflammatory disease of the aorta and the arteries that arise from it. It is especially prevalent among young, Asian women, and women in general are eight times more likely than men to develop Takayasu's arteritis. The typical age of onset of the disease is between 15 and 30 (Takayasu's Arteritis Foundation, n/d).

### Signs and Symptoms

Takayasu's arteritis is characterized by anemia, fever, night sweats, loss of appetite, arthritis, fatigue, impaired speech and chewing, vision loss, and atrophy of the extremities. Heart failure is likely, stemming from severe hypertension. Takayasu's arteritis can also cause weakness of the arterial walls resulting in aneurysms.

### Treatment

In some cases, Takayasu's arteritis is fatal; some others experience long-term survival. There is no cure or prevention of Takayasu's arteritis. Treatment may include corticosteroids or cyclophosphamide. Other treatment may include surgery to reestablish blood flow and medication to thin the blood. Angiotensin converting enzyme inhibitors (e.g., captopril, enalapril, lisinopril) may be effective in treating hypertension.

## Testing

Tests used in the diagnosis of Takayasu's arteritis include angiography of the aorta, CAT scans, CT scans, ultrasound, magnetic resonance angiography, and MRI. In addition, a physical examination typically reveals absent or weakened blood pressure in the affected arteries, with a contrasting brisk pulse in the legs.

## TAY-SACHS DISEASE

### Description

Tay-Sachs disease is a familial disorder found predominantly in Ashkenazi Jewish families that results in early death (Hart, 2003m). Tay-Sachs disease is caused by a deficiency of hexosaminidase. This enzyme aids in the metabolism of gangliosides, which are found in nerve tissue. Gangliosides, particularly ganglioside GM2, then accumulate in the brain. One in 25 Ashkenazi Jews carries the gene that causes Tay-Sachs. The three forms of Tay-Sachs are infantile, juvenile, and adult.

Symptoms generally appear by six months old. The disease progresses rapidly, and death usually occurs by the age of five.

### Signs and Symptoms

Tay-Sachs is characterized by slowed growth, loss of motor skills, increased startle reaction, blindness, deafness, dementia, listlessness, irritability, seizures, paralysis, and decreased muscle strength.

### Treatment

There is no specific treatment for Tay-Sachs disease, except to treat the symptoms.

### Testing

Enzyme analysis of blood or body tissue for hexosaminidase levels is used to diagnose Tay-Sachs disease. Eye exams reveal a cherry-red spot in the macula.

## TEMPORAL ARTERITIS

### Description

Temporal arteritis is the most common form of arterial inflammation and is also known as giant cell arteritis. It is usually diagnosed in the temporal artery in the side of the head in association with complaints of headaches. The cause of the disease is unknown, but the affected vessels are infiltrated by immune cells due to necrosis of the artery. Loss of some vision is present in about half the cases of temporal arteritis (Egland, 2001; NINDS Temporal Arteritis, 2001).

### Signs and Symptoms

Temporal arteritis is characterized by fever, throbbing headache on one side of the head or the back of the head, scalp tenderness, jaw pain, blurred vision, blindness, fatigue, loss of appetite, weight loss, muscle aches, and excessive sweating.

## Treatment
Temporal arteritis is treated with corticosteroids and medications that suppress the immune system (e.g., cyclophosphamide or methotrexate). If blindness is to be prevented, it is crucial to recognize and treat temporal arteritis early in its progression because it spreads from the temporal arteries to other arteries, such as the ophthalmic arteries of the eye, the carotid arteries, and the aorta. Most people make a full recovery.

## Testing
Blood tests for temporal arteritis are nonspecific. Tests used in the diagnosis of temporal arteritis include liver function tests and a biopsy of the affected artery (Clowse, 2003f).

## TESTICULAR CANCER

## Description
There are two broad categories of testicular cancer (Barker, 2002). The first type is seminoma, and the others are categorized as nonseminomas. The nonseminomas include choriocarcinoma, embryonal carcinoma, teratoma, and yolk sac tumors. Although the causes of testicular cancer are unknown, some of the risk factors include undescended testicles (cryptorchidism), abnormal testicular development, and Klinefelter's syndrome, which is a sex chromosome disorder characterized by low levels of male hormones, sterility, breast enlargement, and small testes.

## Signs and Symptoms
Most testicular cancers are found by men themselves, and any of the following should alert men to see their health-care professional:

- a painless lump or swelling in either testicle
- any enlargement of a testicle or change in the way it feels
- a feeling of heaviness in the scrotum
- a dull ache in the lower abdomen or the groin
- a sudden collection of fluid in the scrotum
- pain or discomfort in a testicle or in the scrotum

## Treatment
The survival rate for testicular cancer ranges between 70 and 95 percent, depending on the type of tumor, the stage of the tumor, and the extent of the disease. Testicular cancer is treated with radiation therapy, chemotherapy, and surgery. Testicular cancer is one of the most treatable cancers (Grund, 2004f).

## Testing
Tests used in the diagnosis of testicular cancer include scrotal ultrasound, chest X-rays, and an abdominal CT scan for potential metastasis. Blood

tests for tumor markers include alpha-fetoprotein (AFP), human chorionic gonadotrophin (beta HCG), and lactic dehydrogenase (LDH). Tissue biopsy is usually part of surgical removal of the testicle.

## TETANUS

### Description

*Clostridium tetani* is the causative agent of the bacterial infection that leads to tetanus, which is also known as lockjaw (Mylonakis, 2003; Tetanus, n/d). *C. tetani* is an obligate anaerobic, endospore-forming, grampositive rod. It is found in soil contaminated with animal feces. The symptoms of tetanus are caused by its neurotoxin, which is released upon the destruction of the bacteria by the immune system. In certain parts of the world, tetanus is a common cause of death among infants who have had their umbilical cords treated with soil, clay, and manure as part of cultural practices. Worldwide, there are assumed to be several hundred thousand cases of tetanus each year. As a result of the widespread use of the DTaP vaccine, tetanus is no longer common in the United States. Tetanus may also occur in newborns from the use of contaminated instruments during delivery, and tetanus may occur in cases of septic abortions.

### Signs and Symptoms

The bacteria themselves cause no inflammation at the site of infection, and they do not generally move from the local site of infection. The tetanus neurotoxin tetanospasmin prevents muscle relaxation causing opposing muscles to contract at the same time. The muscles of the jaw are affected first, spreading to the respiratory muscles where death occurs via asphyxia. Deep puncture wounds with little bleeding, similar to those caused by stepping on a nail, provide an excellent reservoir for *C. tetani*.

### Treatment

Tetanus is treated with tetanus immune globulin, penicillin, wound debridement, and diazepam for muscle spasms. Respiratory support with oxygen, endotracheal tube, and mechanical ventilation may be necessary. Wounds on the head or face seem to be more dangerous than those on the body. A serum is available that helps protect against tetanus; however, it requires a booster shot every 10 years, and many Americans fail to receive their boosters.

### Testing

Diagnosis of tetanus is based on the history and physical findings, and diagnostic studies generally are of little value, as cultures of the wound site are negative for *C. tetani* two thirds of the time. Tests for tetanus include culture of the wound site and a tetanus antibody test.

## TETRALOGY OF FALLOT

### Description

Tetralogy of Fallot is a congenital defect of the newborn's heart. The classic form of tetralogy includes four defects within the heart; however, there are numerous defects under the umbrella term of Tetralogy of Fallot. The first defect is a ventricular septal defect, which is a hole between the right and left ventricles. The second type of defect is a narrowing of the pulmonic outflow tract, which is a tube that connects the heart with the lungs. The third type is an aorta that arises from both ventricles, rather than exclusively from the left ventricle. The fourth type of defect is a thickened muscular wall of the right ventricle. At birth, infants may not show the signs of the cyanosis, but later may develop sudden frightening episodes of bluish skin called tet spells. Tetralogy of Fallot occurs in approximately 5 out of 10,000 infants (Bruckheimer, 2004).

### Signs and Symptoms
Tetralogy is characterized by difficulty feeding infants, failure to gain weight, poor development, cyanosis with pronouncement during periods of agitation, fainting, squatting during episodes of cyanosis, and clubbing of the fingers.

### Treatment
Surgery to repair the defects in the heart yields a positive prognosis, but without surgery, death usually occurs around 20 years old.

### Testing
Tests used for diagnosis include an EKG, CBC, chest X-rays, cardiac catheterization, and an echocardiogram.

## THALASSEMIA

### Description
Thalassemias are hereditary disorders characterized by defective production of hemoglobin. This leads to low production and overdestruction of red blood cells. Hemoglobin contains two chains, alpha and beta globin. Beta thalassemias are caused by a mutation in the beta globin chain. In the major form, children are normal at birth, but develop anemia during the first year of life. The mild form of beta thalassemia produces small red blood cells, with no symptoms. Beta thalassemias occur in people of Mediterranean origin, and to a lesser extent, Chinese, other Asians, and blacks. Alpha thalassemias occur most commonly in people from southeast Asia and China, and are caused by deletion of genes from the globin chain. The most severe form of alpha thalassemia causes a stillborn fetus (Cohen, 2003d; Yaish, 2001).

### Signs and Symptoms
Thalassemia is characterized by fatigue, difficulty breathing, jaundice, bone deformities, and enlarged spleen. Growth failure, bone deformities, and enlarged liver and spleen may occur.

### Treatment
With severe thalassemia, regular blood transfusions and folate supplementation are given. Patients who receive significant numbers of blood

transfusions require therapy to remove iron from the body, called chelation therapy, to reduce damage to the heart, liver, and endocrine systems. Bone marrow transplant is being investigated as a treatment and is most successful in children. In severe thalassemia, death from heart failure can occur between the ages or 20 and 30. Less severe forms of thalassemia usually do not impact life span.

## Testing

Tests used in the diagnosis of thalassemias include peripheral blood smear, CBC, hemoglobin electrophoresis, and osmotic fragility tests.

# THROMBOCYTOPENIA

## Description

Thrombocytopenia refers to a severely reduced platelet (thrombocytes) count. It typically occurs when the bone marrow fails to produce platelets as quickly as they are used, or when platelets are removed too quickly from the blood (Grund, 2004g). One cause of thrombocytopenia is the presence of immune system antibodies in the blood that bind to their platelets. These antibodies may bind to the chemicals in the test tube used to count the platelets, giving a false indication of thrombocytopenia. Thrombocytopenia may be inherited, or it may be caused by impairment of the bone marrow. Thrombocytopenia can result from infections like meningitis, complications of pregnancy, cancers like leukemia or prostate cancer, or blood diseases related to food poisoning.

## Signs and Symptoms

Thrombocytopenia can cause several bleeding disorders. In particular, thrombocytopenia can cause bleeding from the nose and gums, and it may be fatal if spontaneous bleeding inside the head or digestive tract occurs. Bruising and petechial rash are also common symptoms.

## Treatment

The treatment of thrombocytopenia is entirely dependent upon the cause but is aimed at controlling spontaneous bleeding and restoring proper thrombocyte levels in the blood.

## Testing

Tests used in the diagnosis of thrombocytopenia include CBC, bone marrow aspiration or biopsy, PTT coagulation studies, PT coagulation studies, and tests for platelet associated antibodies.

# TONSILLITIS

## Description

Tonsillitis is an inflammation of the tonsils caused by an infection (Newman, 2003c). Tonsillitis is contagious and can spread through contact with the throat or nasal fluids of infected persons. At one time, removing tonsils from the throat was a common practice, called a tonsillectomy. Health-care professionals have since discovered the importance of the tonsils in the immune system, and tonsillitis is now treated with antibiotics.

## Signs and Symptoms

Tonsillitis is characterized by tonsils that are enlarged, red, and often spotted or coated by microorganisms, which appear yellow, gray, or white. Fever, chills, and voice loss are common symptoms. Tonsillitis may begin as sudden sore throat and painful swallowing; however, it may progress into severe respiratory difficulties.

## Treatment

If the cause of the tonsillitis is bacterial, antibiotics are given to cure the infection. Tonsillitis symptoms usually lessen in a few days after treatment starts. The infection usually is cured by then, but may require more than one course of antibiotics. Complications of untreated strep tonsillitis may be severe. A tonsillectomy may be recommended if tonsillitis is severe, comes back, or does not respond to antibiotics.

## Testing

A culture for the streptococcus bacteria may be taken because it is the most common and most dangerous form of tonsillitis. A rapid strep test may also be performed by taking a throat swab for a quick diagnosis.

## TOURETTE'S SYNDROME

### Description

Georges Gille de la Tourette's syndrome, also called Tourette's syndrome, is a disorder characterized by multiple motor and vocal tics that begins before age 18 (Kiriakopoulos, 2003b). Tics can include eye blinking, repeated throat clearing or sniffing, arm thrusting, kicking movements, shoulder shrugging, or jumping. Approximately 2 percent of the general population has Tourette's, although many tics may be subclinical. Tourette's syndrome is four times as likely among males. Tourette's syndrome is believed to be inherited (Soliman, 2004).

### Signs and Symptoms

The most common initial symptom of Tourette's syndrome is a facial tic. Contrary to popular belief, uncontrolled cursing is a rare manifestation of this disease. Tics may occur many times a day, and their severity is timed to certain times of day. Many patients explain their tics as partially voluntary, but necessary. Tourette's syndrome differs from obsessive-compulsive disorder because patients are compelled to do the behaviors out of fear in obsessive-compulsive disorder.

### Treatment

Many patients with Tourette's syndrome have minor symptoms and are not treated, due to the side effects of the medication. Antipsychotic medications such as haloperidol (Haldol) and pimozide are used to treat Tourette's syndrome, as well as risperidone, clonidine, and tetrabenazine.

## Testing

There are no specific lab tests to confirm a diagnosis of Tourette's syndrome.

## TOXIC SHOCK SYNDROME

### Description

Toxic shock syndrome (TSS) is caused by *Staphylococcus aureus* bacteria (Levy, 2004aa). Prior to the mid-1970s, TSS was not prevalent because tampons were made of natural materials. These materials are less absorbent than tampons that contain synthetic materials, which swell with menstrual fluids and blood. These saturated tampons adhere to the vagina and can cause tears in the vaginal wall when removed, allowing bacteria to enter the tissues. Half of the cases of TSS are associated with tampon use; the other half are nosocomial infections. Nosocomial spread of TSS may result from surgical incisions, absorbent packing used after nasal surgery, and among women who have just given birth. TSS has also been found in males and premenstrual females. Any wound caused by a strain of *S. aureus* that produces the TSS-1 toxin may cause TSS.

### Signs and Symptoms

The condition begins with a high fever, rash, and signs of dehydration due to watery diarrhea and vomiting for several days. Color Plate 63 is a photograph of the leg of a person exhibiting a rash due to TSS. Patients may also develop severe low blood pressure, causing shock. The rash is usually isolated to the trunk of the body, although it may spread. Color Plate 46 is a photograph of a person with an eye infection due to TSS caused by *Staphylococcus aureus*.

### Treatment

TSS is best prevented by avoiding the use of tampons, using low absorbency tampons, and changing tampons frequently. Most persons with TSS recover, although approximately 5 percent of the cases of TSS are fatal. Subsequent infection is also likely, with 60 percent of menstruating women experiencing recurrence of TSS. Antibiotic therapy is also used and in some cases, intravenous immunoglobulin may be required.

### Testing

The diagnosis of TSS is based on physical exam, appearance of disease characteristics, and case history. In some cases, blood cultures may be positive for growth of *S. aureus*.

## TOXOCARIASIS

### Description

Toxocariasis is an intestinal infection caused by parasitic roundworms found in the intestine of dogs (*Toxocara canis*) and cats (*T. cati*). In the United States, an estimated 10,000 cases of *Toxocara* infections occur yearly in humans. Ocular larva migrans and visceral larva migrans are the two major forms of toxocariasis (Levy, 2004ae). In most cases, toxocariasis is asymptomatic, but it can be serious in children. Severe cases of toxocariasis are rare, and they usually occur in children who play in or eat dirt contaminated with infected dog or cat feces.

## Signs and Symptoms
Ocular larva migrans occurs when a microscopic worm enters the eye, causes inflammation and the formation of a scar on the retina, and may eventually cause blindness. More severe *Toxocara* infections, although rare, can cause visceral larva migrans, which results in swelling of the organs or central nervous system. Symptoms of visceral larva migrans include fever, coughing, asthma, or pneumonia.

## Treatment
Toxocariasis is treated with antiparasitic drugs in combination with anti-inflammatory medications. Treatment of ocular larva migrans, however, is more difficult and usually consists of measures to prevent progressive damage to the eye. This infection is usually self-limiting and may not require therapy. Certain antiparasitic drugs may also be used such as diethylcarbamazine, albendazole, or mebendazole.

## Testing
Toxocariasis is diagnosed by detection of larvae in the affected tissue. A blood test for antibodies can also be used to detect infection.

## TOXOPLASMOSIS

### Description
Toxoplasmosis is an infection caused by a single-celled protozoan named *Toxoplasma gondii.* It is found throughout the world. According to Wener (2004j), more than 60 million people in the United States probably are infected with *T. gondii,* but the disease is usually asymptomatic. The lifecycle of *T. gondii* is presented in Figure 2-83. Humans can contract toxoplasmosis by ingesting contaminated water or foods such as undercooked meats, although the most common form of transmission is through handling contaminated cat feces. Cats can only spread the protozoan for a few weeks after they become infected (Toxoplasmosis, 2003).

### Signs and Symptoms
The mild flulike symptoms of toxoplasmosis are accompanied by swollen lymph glands or muscle aches and pains that last for a few days to several weeks. *T. gondii* forms tissue cysts throughout the body, but especially in the skeletal muscle, myocardium, and brain. Severe toxoplasmosis can result in damage to the eye or the brain and is ultimately fatal. The effects on a fetus range from convulsions to mental retardation, blindness, and death.

### Treatment
Medications to treat toxoplasmosis include pyrimethamine, sulfonamide drugs, folinic acid, clindamycin, and trimethoprim-sulfamethoxazole.

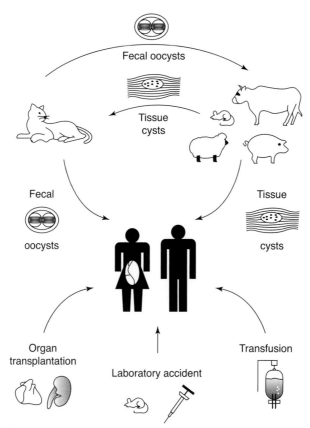

**Figure 2-83** Life cycle of *Toxoplasma gondii*

## Testing

Toxoplasmosis is diagnosed with tests for serologic titers, MRI scans of the head, cranial CT scans, brain biopsy, and slit lamp examination revealing characteristic retinal lesions.

## TRACHEITIS

### Description

Tracheitis is any inflammation of the trachea; however, the term normally refers to a bacterial infection of the trachea resulting in blockage of the windpipe (Newman, 2003e). It is most often caused by *Staphylococcus aureus,* and tracheitis frequently follows viral upper respiratory infections. Typically, young children are affected, possibly because their trachea is easily blocked by swelling.

### Signs and Symptoms

Some of the signs of tracheitis include a deep, barking cough, crowing sounds upon inhalation, high fever, difficulty breathing, and intercostal retractions. Intercostal retractions occur when the muscles between the ribs pull in as the person attempts to breathe.

## Treatment

Due to the blockage of the airway, tracheitis almost always requires hospitalization and the insertion of a breathing tube known as an endotracheal tube. Tracheitis is treated with antibiotics (e.g., penicillin and cephalosporins). Full recovery is expected if the patient can be brought to a medical facility in time.

## Testing

Tests used in the diagnosis of tracheitis include nasopharyngeal culture, tracheal culture, X-rays of the trachea, and examination of purulent tracheal secretions obtained while intubating the patient.

## TREACHER-COLLIN'S SYNDROME

### Description

Treacher-Collins syndrome, which is also known as mandibulofacial cranlosynostosis, is a rare hereditary condition that causes facial defects. A defective treacle gene causes this disease (Jackson, 2004; Stewart, 2003o).

### Signs and Symptoms

Treacher-Collins syndrome is characterized by hearing loss, small jaw, large mouth, a defect in the lower eyelid, ear defects or absence, cleft palate, and scalp hair that extends onto the cheeks. Other signs include a downward-beaked nose, absent zygomatic bones, thin facial skin, and a fishlike appearance to the face.

### Treatment

There is no cure for Treacher-Collins syndrome. Treatment consists of treating any hearing loss and plastic surgery. Children with Treacher-Collins should grow to become normally functioning adults of normal intelligence.

### Testing

There is no specific laboratory test to diagnose Treacher-Collins syndrome.

## TRENCH MOUTH

### Description

Trench mouth is a painful bacterial infection and ulceration of the gums. The term comes from its prevalence among soldiers during World War I. Trench mouth is caused by an excess of bacteria in the mouth, resulting in infection of the gums and painful ulcers. Viruses may allow the normal bacteria of the mouth to overgrow. Risks for trench mouth include poor oral hygiene, poor nutrition, and throat or mouth infection. Trench mouth is a rare disorder of persons 15 to 35 years old. Other names of the disease include Vincent's stomatitis and acute necrotizing ulcerative gingivitis (Owens, 2004; Trench mouth, 2004).

## Signs and Symptoms

Symptoms of trench mouth may appear suddenly, and they include painful gums, bleeding of the gums in response to pressure, red and swollen gums, grayish film on the gums, foul taste in the mouth, and ulcers between the teeth. If the infection spreads, it can cause fever and swollen lymph nodes in the head and neck.

## Treatment

Saltwater rinses, antiseptic solutions, and hydrogen peroxide may be soothing to sore gums. Over-the-counter analgesics, coating agents, and viscous lidocaine may be used for pain. Antibiotics may be prescribed. The dentist is likely to perform a scaling and root planing tooth cleaning. In this procedure, ultrasound is used to clean the teeth and gums. Surgical bone grafting may be necessary in severe cases for trench mouth.

## Testing

Dental X-rays or facial X-rays may be performed to determine the extent of infection and tissue destruction. This disease may also alter the results of a throat swab culture.

## TRICHINOSIS

### Description

Trichinosis, which is also known as trichinellosis, is caused by a species of worm called *Trichinella*, which is spread by eating infected raw or undercooked pork and wild game products. After ingesting the infective *Trichinella* cyst, stomach acid dissolves the outer covering of the cyst and releases the worms, which pass into the small intestine, where they mature within approximately two days. Trichinosis does not spread through contact with infected persons. Although trichinosis was once common in the United States, infection is now rare due to improved standards of care for hogs.

### Signs and Symptoms

The first symptoms of trichinosis typically appear within two days after infection, and further symptoms appear two to eight weeks after ingesting contaminated meat. The first symptoms of trichinosis are nausea, diarrhea, vomiting, fatigue, fever, and abdominal discomfort. Headaches, fevers, chills, cough, eye swelling, arthritis, muscle pain, pruritis, and constipation or diarrhea follow the first symptoms. In severe cases, infected persons may experience difficulty coordinating movements and have heart and breathing problems.

### Treatment

There is no specific treatment for trichinosis once the larvae have invaded the muscles. Albendazole can work on the intestinal forms, but not on the muscle forms. Most people with trichinosis have no symptoms, and their infection is self-limited. More severe infections may be more difficult to treat, especially if the lungs, the heart, or the brain is involved. Trichinosis can be fatal.

## Testing

Tests used in the diagnosis of trichinosis include CBC, muscle biopsy to identify trichinella cysts, serology studies, and CPK showing elevated levels of muscle enzymes.

# TRICHOMONIASIS

## Description

Trichomoniasis is a sexually transmitted disease caused by the single-celled protozoan parasite, *Trichomonas vaginalis*. The vagina is the most common site of infection in women, and the urethra is the most common site of infection in men (Levy, 2004ab).

## Signs and Symptoms

Most men with trichomoniasis are asymptomatic; however, temporary irritation inside the penis, mild discharge, or slight burning after urination or ejaculation may occur. In women, trichomoniasis may present as a frothy, yellow-green vaginal discharge with a strong odor; discomfort during intercourse and urination; irritation and itching of the genitals; and, in rare cases, lower abdominal pain. Symptoms of trichomoniasis usually appear in women within 5 to 28 days after exposure.

## Treatment

Trichomoniasis can usually be cured with metronidazole. Use of alcohol with metronidazole can cause severe nausea and vomiting.

## Testing

Tests used in the diagnosis of trichomoniasis include a wet prep microscopic examination of discharge and a Pap smear. In men, cultures of urethral discharge are used to diagnose the disease.

# TRICHURIASIS

## Description

Trichuriasis is a roundworm infection caused by *Trichuris trichiura*, which is also known as the human whipworm. Infection is most frequent in tropical areas and areas with poor sanitation practices. According to the CDC, 800 million people are infected worldwide, and children are the most likely group of people to become infected. Trichuriasis is known to occur in the southern United States and is spread through the fecal-oral route or through soil contaminated with feces of an infected person or animal (*Trichuriasis*, 2004).

## Signs and Symptoms

Most cases of trichuriasis are asymptomatic. However, severe cases may result in gastrointestinal disorders, rectal prolapse, and the retardation of children's normal growth.

## Treatment

The drug of choice for treatment is mebendazole with albendazole as an alternative.

## Testing

Microscopic inspection of feces is used to test for the presence of *Trichuris trichiura*.

## TRUNCUS ARTERIOSUS

### Description

Truncus arteriosus is a rare heart defect in which one blood vessel arises from both the left and right ventricles of the heart. In the healthy heart pictured in Figure 2-84, the aorta and the pulmonary artery arise from the left and right ventricles, respectively. A large defect is typically present in the septum of the heart between the ventricles as well. The septum divides the heart's left and right side. This defect basically connects the two ventricles into one large ventricle. This decreases the heart's ability to effectively pump blood, and it allows oxygenated blood to mix with deoxygentated blood. Untreated, truncus arteriosus causes increased blood

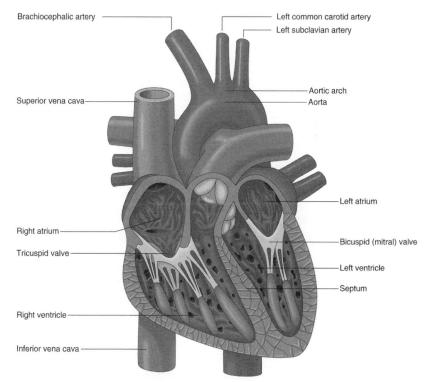

**Figure 2-84** Structures of the heart

pressure in the lungs, and it can cause fluids to fill the lungs (Campbell, 2004; McElhinny & Wernovsky, 2004).

## Signs and Symptoms
Truncus arteriosis is characterized by weakness, poor feeding, difficulty breathing, cyanosis, excessive perspiration, heart failure, and clubbing of the fingertips.

## Treatment
Truncus arteriosis is treated surgically to repair the defect in the heart.

## Testing
Truncus arteriosis is diagnosed with an ECG, chest X-rays, echocardiogram, and, rarely, a heart catheterization.

## TUBERCULOSIS

### Description
There are over 1 billion cases of tuberculosis (TB) infection worldwide, with 8 million to 10 million new cases each year. TB causes the death of over 2 million people each year. The incidence of TB in the United States was declining before 1985. The number of cases has risen since then, due to

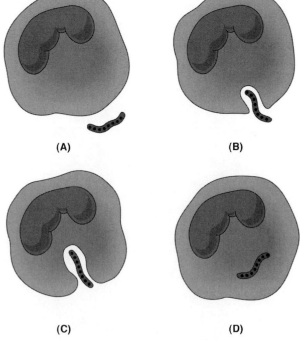

(A)

(B)

(C)

(D)

**Figure 2-85** Phagocytosis of bacteria by a white blood cell

the prevalence of AIDS, increased IV drug use, and increased transmission within closed environments such as prisons and nursing homes. WHO has declared tuberculosis a global emergency (Tuberculosis, 2003, 2002, n/d).

TB is caused by *Mycobacterium tuberculosis*, which is a highly resistant, rod-shaped bacterium with a high lipid content in its cell wall. Up to 60 percent of the dried mass of *M. tuberculosis* is comprised of fats, which is much higher than that of other bacteria. This high lipid content allows this bacterium to be resistant to desiccation and staining. *M. tuberculosis* can survive for weeks in dried sputum and is resistant to antiseptics and many disinfectants.

### Signs and Symptoms

After interacting with the immune system, the bacteria forms a tubercule in the lungs (Figure 2-85 and Figure 2-86). After a few weeks, a caseous, or cheeselike, center forms in the tubercle. The caseous center enlarges in the process of liquefaction, allowing an air-filled tuberculosis cavity to form. Liquefaction continues until the tubercle ruptures, spreading bacteria throughout the respiratory system. TB is often accompanied by hemorrhaging resulting in coughing up blood. Persons with TB are often emaciated and dehydrated due to the chronic nature of the disease process. Other symptoms include fatigue, cough producing phlegm, fever, night sweats, wheezing, excessive sweating, chest pain, and difficulty breathing.

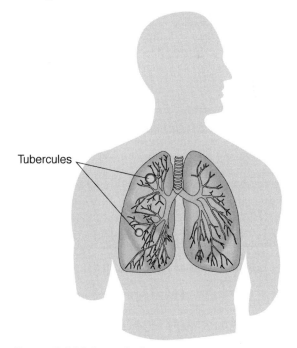

Tubercules

**Figure 2-86** Tuberculosis

## Treatment

One of the primary concerns about TB is that it has become multidrug-resistant, meaning that there are strains of TB that are resistant to all major anti-TB drugs. The goal of treatment is to cure the infection with antitubercular drugs, which includes combinations of rifampin, isoniazid, pyrazinamide, and ethambutol. Treatment is typically continued for six months, but longer courses and different drugs may be required, especially for drug-resistant strains. Prognosis is excellent if pulmonary TB is diagnosed early and treatment is begun, but it can be fatal.

## Testing

Tests used to diagnose TB include chest X-rays, sputum cultures, tuberculin skin test, bronchoscopy, thoracentesis, chest CT scan, and tissue biopsy of lymph nodes or lungs. Biopsies are rarely used to diagnose TB.

## TULAREMIA

### Description

Tularemia was discovered in Tulare County, California, and in 90 percent of the cases in the United States it is acquired by handling rabbits and then rubbing the eyes, hence its alternate name rabbit fever. Tularemia is caused by the bacterium *Francisella tularensis* (Levy, 2004ac). This highly infectious, strictly aerobic, nonmotile, small, gram-negative bacillus is a facultatively intracellular parasite. *F. tularensis* can enter the body through inhalation, ingestion, or minor skin breaks. Ingestion of infected meat leads to infection in the mouth and throat. The bite of arthropods, such as deer flies, ticks, or rabbit lice may also be a mechanism of transmission of the disease (Tularemia, 2002).

### Signs and Symptoms

The first sign of tularemia is a local inflammation and a small ulcer, as indicated in Color Plate 65. About a week after infection, the regional lymph nodes enlarge and fill with pus. Septicemia, pneumonia, and abscesses throughout the body ensue. Other symptoms include headache, muscle pain, conjunctivitis, difficulty breathing, fever, chills, sweating, weight loss, and joint stiffness.

### Treatment

Tularemia is treated with antibiotic therapy. Streptomycin and tetracycline are commonly used in this infection. Tularemia is fatal in about 5 percent of untreated cases and in less than 1 percent with treatment.

### Testing

Tests used in the diagnosis of tularemia include serology, blood culture, and chest X-rays. Tularemia may also alter the results of febrile/cold agglutinins.

## TURNER SYNDROME

### Description

Turner syndrome is a birth defect caused by the absence of an X chromosome in cells of a female, which inhibits sexual development and usually causes infertility (Postellon, 2003; Stewart, 2003p). Turner syndrome is also known as Bonnevie-Ullrich syndrome, gonadal dysgenesis, and monosomy X. Sex is determined by two chromosomes, the X and the Y. Men have an X and a Y, women have two X chromosomes. Turner syndrome occurs in about 1 out of 3,000 live births. Turner syndrome occurs during fetal development. The condition is either diagnosed at birth because of the associated anomalies, or at puberty when there is absent or delayed menses and delayed development of normal secondary sexual characteristics.

### Signs and Symptoms

Girls with Turner syndrome usually have short stature, webbing of the skin of the neck, absent or retarded secondary sexual characteristics, narrowing of the aorta, bicuspid aortic valve, and abnormalities of the eyes and bones. IQ is normal, although some children have learning difficulties. The mutation occurs in some but not all the cells in the body in about 50 percent of the cases.

### Treatment

Treatment may include growth hormone replacement, estrogen therapy, and heart surgery. Women with Turner syndrome can have children through in vitro fertilization.

### Testing

Turner syndrome is diagnosed through karyotyping showing 45 chromosomes with a pattern 45 X,0, ultrasound revealing underdeveloped female reproductive organs, kidney ultrasound, serum luteinizing hormone levels, and echocardiogram. Other tests may indicate estriol in the urine, serum, and an estradiol test.

## TYPHOID

### Description

Typhoid is an acute, contagious, bacterial infection of the digestive system (Levy, 2003k). Typhoid fever is characterized by the presence of necrotic lesions in Peyer's patches, mesenteric glands, and the spleen. The incubation period for typhoid fever is about two weeks, and typhoid is caused by the *Salmonella typhi* bacterium. It is transmitted from one human to another through human feces. Although the incidence of typhoid has diminished in the United States in the last century, typhoid is still a frequent cause of death in countries with developing sanitation standards. Most cases of typhoid in the United States are acquired through foreign travel (Typhoid fever, 2001).

### Signs and Symptoms

Typhoid fever causes rose spots on the chest or abdomen, as pictured in Color Plate 66. Other complications of typhoid include fever, headache, abdominal pain, nosebleed, discoloration of the tongue, and the presence of a whitish furlike material on the tongue.

### Treatment

Typhoid fever is treated with antibiotics to kill the bacteria. With treatment, typhoid usually resolves within four weeks. The prognosis is good with early treatment, but poor if complications develop.

### Testing

Tests used in the diagnosis of typhoid fever include CBC and stool culture, ELISA tests may show Vi antigen for *S. typhi,* and fluorescent antibody studies demonstrate Vi antigen for *S. typhi.* A blood culture during the first week of the fever can show *S. typhi.*

## TYPHUS

### Description

Epidemic typhus, which is also known as louse-borne typhus, is caused by *Rickettsia prowazekii* (Levy, 2004ad). This microbe grows in the intestinal tract of human body lice and is also found in flying squirrels located in the eastern United States. The disease is transmitted when fecal material is rubbed into the bite left by the human body louse, when the human scratches the wound. The louse typically becomes infected with the disease, and leaves when the human becomes febrile. Epidemic typhus is found primarily in crowded areas with poor sanitation, and it is still common in Africa, Central American, and South America. At one time, epidemic typhus was prevalent among sailors aboard ships and soldiers in military camps (Epidemic louse-borne typhus, 1998).

Endemic typhus, which is also known as either murine typhus or flea-borne typhus, is caused by *Rickettsia typhi.* This microbe is harbored in rats and is transmitted by the rat flea to humans, although the flea infests many domestic animals—which may explain the persistence of the disease in urban areas. Endemic typhus is usually self-resolving, and complications are rare. Rat control decreases the occurrence of endemic typhus. The majority of cases contracted in the United States, which is usually less than 100 annually, are reported in the geographic regions of southern Texas and southern California.

### Signs and Symptoms

In cases of epidemic typhus, the tongue may be covered with a white fur or be black and rolled up in the back of the mouth. A measleslike rash is present on the body, which includes the palms of the hands and soles of the feet. The rash begins on the trunk of the body and spreads centrifugally away from the trunk. The neck and face are seldom involved. The mortality rate of epidemic typhus is high (40 percent) when not treated.

Epidemic typhus may also involve fatigue, headache, stupor, neurological impairment, and picking at the bedclothes.

Endemic typhus' symptoms are similar to but less severe than those of epidemic typhus. The rash is different in cases of endemic typhus than it is in either Rocky Mountain spotted fever or epidemic typhus. There is rarely a rash in cases of endemic typhus, and the rash is usually confined to the trunk and extremities if it is present. The rash is rarely found on the palms and soles.

## Treatment

Both epidemic typhus and endemic typhus are treated with antibiotics (e.g., tetracycline, doxycycline, chloramphenicol). Without treatment, death may occur in 10 to 60 percent of patients with epidemic typhus. With timely antibiotic therapy, complete recovery is expected. Less than 2 percent of untreated patients with endemic typhus die (Cooper, 2002).

## Testing

Tests used in the diagnosis of both epidemic typhus and endemic typhus include CBC, serum sodium levels, albumin levels in the blood, liver enzyme tests, renal function tests, and antibody tests for typhus.

## ULCERATIVE COLITIS

### Description

Ulcerative colitis is a disease that causes ulcers in the lining of the rectum and lower part of the colon, but it may affect the entire large intestine (J. Lehrer, 2003b). Figure 2-87 illustrates the appearance of ulcers in conjunction with colitis. The immune system reacts to a virus or a bacterium by causing ongoing inflammation in the intestinal wall. The inflammation causes diarrhea, and the ulcers bleed and produce pus in the lining of the colon. Ulcerative colitis may be misdiagnosed because its symptoms are similar to other intestinal disorders such as Crohn's disease. Crohn's disease causes inflammation deeper within the intestinal wall than ulcerative colitis, and Crohn's disease usually occurs in the small intestine, although it can also occur in the mouth, esophagus, stomach, duodenum, large intestine, appendix, and anus (Ulcerative colitis, 2003).

### Signs and Symptoms

Ulcerative colitis may cause arthritis, inflammation of the eye, liver disease, osteoporosis, skin rashes, and anemia. Ulcerative colitis is characterized by weight loss, loss of appetite, rectal bleeding, loss of body fluids and nutrients, fever, jaundice, bloody diarrhea, nausea, and severe abdominal cramping.

### Treatment

Corticosteroids may be prescribed to reduce inflammation in cases of ulcerative colitis. Medications that may be used to decrease the frequency

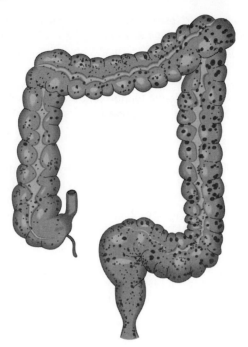

**Figure 2-87** Ulcerative colitis

of attacks include 5-aminosalicylates (e.g., mesalamine) and immunomodulators (e.g., azathioprine) and 6-mercaptopurine. Surgery to remove the colon will cure ulcerative colitis and removes the threat of colon cancer. Patients may need an ostomy or an ileal pouch-anal anastomosis, a procedure that connects the small intestine to the anus to help the patient gain more normal bowel function. Ulcerative colitis may progress rapidly, and a permanent cure is unusual.

### Testing
Tests used in the diagnosis of ulcerative colitis include colonoscopy with biopsy, barium enema, CBC, ESR, and a C-reactive protein (CRP) test.

## UREMIA

### Description
Uremia, which is also known as azotemia, is a disorder of the urinary system characterized by renal insufficiency (Agha, 2003f). Prerenal azotemia is common in hospitalized patients. Decreased volume or pressure of blood flow through the kidney causes blood filtration to drop drastically. Nitrogenous waste products remain in the blood when urine output decreases dramatically. Uremia is characterized by its strong odor and

yellow discoloration of the tissues. Because of the high nitrogenous waste levels in the body, there is a great increase in dehydration and swelling, as observed in Color Plate 67.

## Signs and Symptoms
Uremia is characterized by nausea, vomiting, headache, dizziness, reduced vision, coma, convulsions, stupor, lack of pupil reaction, dry skin, hypertension, and a hard, rapid pulse. Other symptoms include a urinous odor of the breath and perspiration, fatigue, skin pallor, confusion, dry mouth, thirst, and swelling.

## Treatment
Treatment may include hemodialysis or peritoneal dialysis. Intravenous fluids, including blood or blood products, may be used to increase blood volume. Medications (e.g., dopamine and dobutamine) may be used to increase blood pressure and cardiac output. Uremia is reversible if caught within 24 hours, but acute tubular necrosis may occur if not treated.

## Testing
In cases of uremia, urinalysis indicates decreased renal function, low sodium levels with fractional excretion at less than 1 percent, a high urine creatinine to serum creatinine ration, a high urine urea to serum urea (BUN) ratio, and low fractional excretion of urea.

## URINARY TRACT INFECTIONS

### Description
There are a variety of microorganisms that can cause urinary tract infections. These infections are typically categorized by the portion of the urinary tract that is affected, as illustrated in Figure 2-88. Some of the most common microorganisms that cause urinary tract infections include *Neisseria gonorrhea, Chlamydia trachomatis, Escherichia coli, Proteus species*, and *Pseudomonas species*.

### Signs and Symptoms
Urinary tract infections are characterized by pressure in the pelvis, painful burning upon urination, frequent and urgent need to urinate, increased urination at night, cloudy urine, bloody urine, and foul smelling urine. Young children may be asymptomatic or only have a fever. Additional symptoms may include painful sexual intercourse, penis pain, flank pain, and mental changes or confusion (Hart, 2003m).

### Treatment
Urinary tract infection may self-resolve, but due antibiotics are recommended. Commonly used antibiotics include nitrofurantoin, cephalosporins,

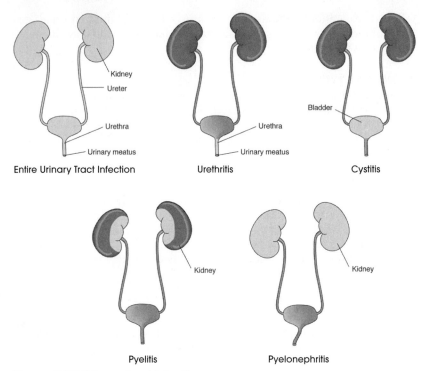

**Figure 2-88** Urinary tract infections

sulfonamides, amoxicillin, trimethoprim-sulfamethoxazole, doxycycline, and quinolones. Phenazopyridine hydrochloride may also be used. In addition, acidifying medications (e.g., ascorbic acid) may decrease the concentration of bacteria in the urine.

### Testing
Tests used in the diagnosis of urinary tract infections include CBC, clean catch urine culture, and catheterized urine specimen. To determine anatomical abnormalities in children, kidney ultrasounds and X-rays taken by a voiding cystourethrogram (VCUG) are recommended.

## URTICARIA

### Description
Urticaria, which are commonly referred to as hives, are raised, itchy, red welts on the surface of the skin. Angiodema is swelling or welts occurring around the face, lips, eyes, hand, feet, or throat. Hives are caused by an allergic reaction to a substance, when histamine and other chemicals are released into the bloodstream. Many substances can trigger hives including medications, foods, pollen, animal dander, and insect bites (Hart, 2003e).

## Signs and Symptoms

In cases of hives, welts may enlarge, spread, and join together to form larger areas of flat, raised skin. They can also change shape. Welts start suddenly and resolve quickly.

## Treatment

Hives may be self-resolving. In severe reactions, especially in the throat, epinephrine or steroids are administered.

## Testing

Hives are diagnosed by their physcial appearance. Tests are performed sometimes to confirm that hives are an allergic reaction. In most cases, the exact cause of hives cannot be identified (Hart, 2003f).

## VARICOSE VEINS

### Description

The name varicose veins comes from the Latin word *varix* meaning twisted (Varicose viens, 2003; Webner, 2003). Varicose veins are enlarged veins that are close to the skin's surface, most commonly found in the legs and feet. Varicose veins, however, may also occur in other areas of the body such as the veins of the esophagus. Varicose veins are caused by excessive venous blood pressure that deforms the veins. Certain cancers may also cause varicose veins. In most cases, varicose veins are only of cosmetic concern, although others experience aching pain. The most positive indicator of varicose veins is the presence of dilated, elongated, and scarred veins that appear through the skin. Predisposing factors for varicose veins include age, pregnancy, obesity, being female, and sitting or standing for long periods. The venous system is illustrated in Figure 2-89.

### Signs and Symptoms

The characteristics of varicose veins of the legs are a sensation of pressure in the legs and feet, swelling, a brownish-gray discoloration of the ankles, itching around a particular vein, and ulcers of the legs or feet. Varicose veins also cause throbbing, burning, muscle cramps.

### Treatment

Treatment for varicose veins begins by avoiding excess standing, elevating the legs when resting or sleeping, and wearing elastic support hose. Surgery such as vein stripping and ligation, or sclerotherapy of veins, in which the veins are injected with a solution that causes scarring to close the vein, may be recommended. Varicose veins tend to worsen over time.

### Testing

Diagnosis of varicose veins is based on appearance of the legs, a duplex ultrasound exam of the extremities, and, rarely, an angiography of the legs may be performed.

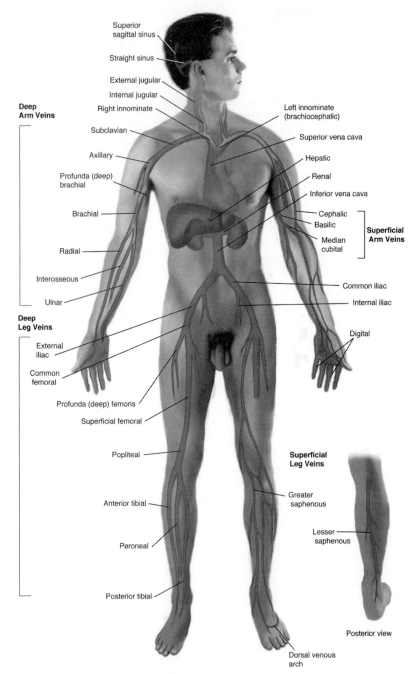

Superior sagittal sinus

Straight sinus

External jugular

Internal jugular

Right innominate

**Deep Arm Veins**

Subclavian

Axillary

Profunda (deep) brachial

Brachial

Radial

Interosseous

Ulnar

**Deep Leg Veins**

External iliac

Common femoral

Profunda (deep) femoris

Superficial femoral

Popliteal

Anterior tibial

Peroneal

Posterior tibial

Left innominate (brachiocephalic)

Superior vena cava

Hepatic

Renal

Inferior vena cava

Cephalic

Basilic

Median cubital

**Superficial Arm Veins**

Common iliac

Internal iliac

Digital

**Superficial Leg Veins**

Greater saphenous

Lesser saphenous

Dorsal venous arch

Posterior view

**Figure 2-89** Veins of the body

## *VIBRIO PARAHAEMOLYTICUS* INFECTION

### Description

*Vibrio parahaemolyticus* is a bacterium that causes gastrointestinal illness in humans. *V. parahaemolyticus* belongs to the same family of bacteria as that which causes cholera. It is found naturally occurring in coastal waters in the United States and Canada and is present in higher concentrations during summer. Most people become infected by eating raw shellfish, particularly oysters, which are natural reservoirs for *V. parahaemolyticus*. Open wounds exposed to seawater may become contaminated with *V. parahaemolyticus*. In Asia, *V. parahaemolyticus* is a common cause of foodborne disease; however, only about 30 to 40 cases of *V. parahaemolyticus* infections are reported each year in the United States (*Vibrio parahaemolyticus*, 2004).

### Signs and Symptoms

Within 24 hours of ingestion, *V. parahaemolyticus* begins to cause watery diarrhea, abdominal cramping, nausea, vomiting, fever, and chills.

### Treatment

Severe disease is rare, and *V. parahaemolyticus* infection is normally self-limiting and lasts about three days. Treatment is not necessary in most cases of *V. parahaemolyticus* infection, and there is no evidence that antibiotic treatment decreases the severity or the length of the illness. In severe or prolonged illnesses, antibiotics such as tetracycline, ampicillin, or ciprofloxacin can be used.

### Testing

Vibrio infection is diagnosed through testing for the presence of organisms in feces, wound, or blood cultures.

## *VIBRIO VULNIFICUS* INFECTIONS

### Description

*Vibrio vulnificus* is a bacterium that lives in brackish saltwater and causes gastrointestinal illness in humans. *V. vulnificus* belongs to the same family of bacteria as that which causes cholera. It is found naturally occurring in coastal waters in the United States and Canada and is present in higher concentrations during summer. Most people become infected by eating raw or undercooked shellfish, particularly oysters (*Vibrio vulnificus*, 2004).

### Signs and Symptoms

Open wounds exposed to seawater may become contaminated with *V. parahaemolyticus*, resulting in a local infection leading to skin breakdown and ulceration. Among otherwise healthy people, ingestion of *V. vulnificus* can cause vomiting, diarrhea, and abdominal pain. In the immunocompromised, particularly those with chronic liver disease, *V. vulnificus* can infect the bloodstream causing a severe and life-threatening illness that is fatal about 50 percent of the time. This systemic illness is characterized by fever and chills, septic shock, and blistering skin lesions. *V. vulnificus* is a rare cause of disease, and there is no evidence for person-to-person transmission of *V. vulnificus*.

## Treatment

*V. vulnificus* infection is treated with antibiotics like doxycycline or a third-generation cephalosporin (e.g., ceftazidime) as appropriate.

## Testing

Infection is diagnosed by routine stool, wound, or blood cultures.

## VIRAL GASTROENTERITIS

## Description

Gastroenteritis is an inflammation of the stomach and small and large intestines (Figure 2-90). Viral gastroenteritis is caused by a variety of viruses (e.g., rotaviruses, adenoviruses, caliciviruses, astroviruses, Norwalk

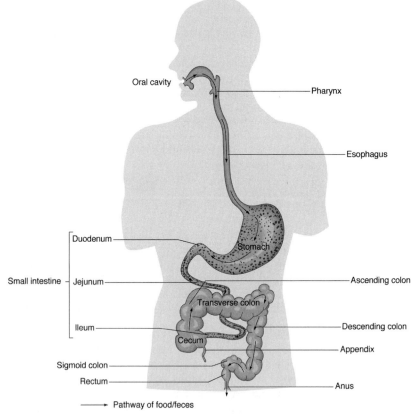

**Figure 2-90** Gastroenteritis

virus, Noroviruses), and it is often refered to as stomach flu, although it is not caused by the influenza viruses. Viral gastroenteritis is contagious, and it is spread through direct contact with infected persons. Each virus is seasonal, with rotavirus and astrovirus infections occurring between October and April, and with adenovirus infections occurring throughout the year.

## Signs and Symptoms
Viral gastroenteritis is characterized by watery diarrhea, vomiting, headache, fever, and abdominal cramps. In general, symptoms begin two days following infection and last up to 10 days, depending on the causal virus.

## Treatment
The CDC recommends that oral rehydration solution be used when diarrhea first occurs to prevent dehydration. Oral rehydration solution is available at pharmacies without a prescription. Medications, including antibiotics, should be avoided unless specifically recommended by a physician.

## Testing
Rotavirus infection can be diagnosed by laboratory testing of a stool specimen. Tests to detect other viruses that cause gastroenteritis are not in routine use.

## VISA AND VRSA

### Description
VISA (Vancomycin-Intermediate *Stapylococcus aureus*) and VRSA (Vancomycin-Resistant *Stapylococcus aureus*) are antibiotic-resistant bacteria that spread among people having close physical contact with infected patients or contaminated material like bandages. VISA and VRSA infections are rare, with only eight cases of infection caused by VISA and two cases of infection caused by VRSA having been reported in the United States (VISA/VRSA, 2003). Persons who have been treated with vancomycin and other antimicrobial agents, persons with diseases like diabetes and kidney disease, persons with previous infections of methicillin-resistant *Staphylococcus aureus,* persons who have been recently hospitalized, and persons who have had intravenous catheters are at an increased risk of developing VISA and VRSA. Otherwise healthy individuals, however, are not likely to develop VISA or VRSA infections.

### Signs and Symptoms
Staph bacteria can cause serious and fatal infections (such as bloodstream infections, surgical wound infections, and pneumonia). In the past, most serious staph bacterial infections were treated with a type of antimicrobial agent related to penicillin. Over the past 50 years, treatment of these infections has become more difficult because staph bacteria have become resistant to various antimicrobial agents, including the commonly used penicillin-related antibiotics.

## Treatment

VISA and VRSA cannot be successfully treated with vancomycin because these organisms have mutated, and they are no longer susceptible to vancomycin. To date, all VISA and VRSA isolates have been treated successfully with several Food and Drug Administration (FDA) approved drugs.

## Testing

Not all susceptibility testing methods detect VISA and VRSA isolates. Two out of three confirmed VRSA isolates were not reliably detected by automated testing systems. In addition, VISA isolates are not detected by disk diffusion. Methods that do detect VISA and VRSA are the vancomycin screen agar plate (BHIA with 6 μg/ml of vancomycin) and nonautomated MIC methods [reference broth microdilution, agar dilution, and Etest® using a 0.5 McFarland standard to prepare inoculum (AB Biodisk, Piscatway, NJ)]. Laboratories that use automated methods or disk diffusion should also include a vancomycin screen plate for enhanced detection of VISA and VRSA. If possible, laboratories should incorporate the vancomycin screen agar plate for testing all *S. aureus*. Alternatively, the screening may be limited to MRSA isolates, because nearly all VISA and all VRSA were also MRSA. *S. aureus* isolates that grow on the vancomycin screen agar plate should be checked for purity and the organism identity confirmed. Vancomycin susceptibility should be retested by a nonautomated MIC method incubated for a full 24 hours.

## VITILIGO

### Description

Vitiligo is an idiopathic disorder in which the melanocytes stop producing pigment and are destroyed (Kantor, 2004f). The loss of pigment results in white, patchy spots on the affected part, which can occur anywhere on the body. Vitiligo affects about 1 percent of the U.S. population. The cause of vitiligo is unknown, but autoimmunity may be a factor. People with certain autoimmune diseases such as hyperthyroidism or pernicious anemia appear to develop vitiligo.

### Signs and Symptoms

Lesions appear as flat depigmented areas with a darker boarder. The edges are sharply defined but irregular. Frequently affected areas are the face, elbows and knees, hands and feet, and genitalia.

### Treatment

Vitiligo is difficult to treat, but treatment may include narrowband ultraviolet light therapy, trimethylpsoralen, methoxsalen, pimecrolimus, tacrolimus, and corticosteroids. Skin grafts may be used in treating vitiligo. Depigmentation may be progressive.

### Testing

Physical examination is sufficient for diagnosis, but a skin biopsy may be needed to rule out other causes of pigment loss.

## VON GIERKE DISEASE

### Description

Von Gierke disease is a group of inherited metabolic disorders that involve increased glycogen storage (Stewart, 2003o). When both parents have the mutated gene, children have a 25 percent chance of inheriting the disease. Patients with von Gierke disease lack proteins responsible for transporting or breaking down the components of glycogen. This causes glycogen to accumulate in the tissues, which causes various symptoms.

### Signs and Symptoms

Von Gierke disease is characterized by severe hypoglycemia, frequent need to eat, stunted growth, hepatamegaly, gout, and bleeding disorders. Patients also exhibit doll-like features, including puffy cheeks and a protruding abdomen. There is also an increased risk of infection and ulcers of the mouth or bowels in one type of von Gierke disease.

### Treatment

Treatment for this disease includes avoiding low blood sugar, fruit and milk sugar, and overnight fasting. Night time feedings occur through a tube through the nose into the stomach. Allopurinol can lower blood uric acid and decrease the risk for gout. Quality of life has improved dramatically due to early treatment. The rate of severe problems such as liver tumors, kidney failure, gout, and life-threatening low blood sugar have been greatly reduced.

### Testing

Tests used to diagnose von Gierke disease indicate enlarged liver with accumulation of glycogen and fat on the liver, tumors of the liver, hypoglycemia, high blood uric acid levels, high blood lactic acid levels, and high triglyceride levels. Liver biopsies may be taken, and genetic tests are performed.

## VON WILLEBRAND DISEASE

### Description

Von Willebrand disease is the most common bleeding disorder in the United States, affecting approximately 2 percent of the population (Cohen, 2004b). Von Willebrand disease is a hereditary disorder that results from a deficiency in the ability to make von Willebrand factor, which is a protein that helps blood clot. Although von Willebrand disease occurs in men and women equally, women are more likely to notice the symptoms due to heavy or abnormal bleeding during their menstrual periods and after childbirth. Most cases of von Willebrand disease are mild. Von Willebrand disease is exacerbated by the use of aspirin and other nonsteroidal antiinfammatory drugs. Bleeding may also occur after surgery.

### Signs and Symptoms

Von Willebrand disease is characterized by nosebleed, bleeding of the gums, bruising, skin rash, and abnormal menstrual bleeding.

## Treatment

Although most bleeding associated with von Willebrand disease is mild and not necessary to treat, cryoprecipitate or 1-deamino-8-D-arginine vasopressin (DDAVP) can be given to raise the levels of von Willebrand factor in the event of trauma or scheduled surgery.

## Testing

Diagnostic tests for von Willebrand disease measure platelet count, bleeding time, levels of von Willebrand factor, platelet aggregation, and ristocetin co-factor levels.

## WAARDENBURG SYNDROME

### Description

Waardenburg syndrome is a rare inherited disease causing deafness and albinism. There are four types of Waardenburg syndrome, resulting from mutations occurring on different genes. Type 3 is known as Klein-Waardenburg syndrome, and Type 4 is called Waardenburg-Shah syndrome. Waardenburg syndrome affects about 1 in every 30,000 people (Stewart, 2003r).

### Signs and Symptoms

All forms of Waardenburg syndrome cause hearing loss and partial albinism. The albinism is incomplete and may appear as a white forelock in an otherwise dark head of hair, extremely pale light-blue eyes, or two different colored eyes. Affected individuals may also have wide separation of the inner corners of the eyes, a broad nasal bridge, and other color changes of the skin. Waardenburg syndrome may also cause a decrease in intellectual functioning, cleft lip, partial contracture of the joints, and constipation.

### Treatment

No cure or specific treatment is available for Waardenburg syndrome.

### Testing

Waardenburg syndrome is diagnosed by genetic testing of the PAX3 gene on chromosome *2q35* and genetic testing of the MITF gene on chromosome *3p13*. Type 4 Waardenburg syndrome may also require genetic testing of the endothelin-3, endothelin receptor B, or SOX10 gene. Audiometry hearing evaluation and biopsy of the colon for the presence of neural ganglia are also conducted.

## WATERHOUSE-FRIDERICHSEN SYNDROME

### Description

Waterhouse-Friderichsen syndrome is a failure of the adrenal glands to secrete appropriate levels of corticosteroids due to bleeding within the adrenal cortex. The disease usually affects children, and it is characterized by a septic bacterial infection with a rapidly deteriorating progression leading to cardiovascular collapse and death. If a bacterial infection known as meningococcemia occurs during anticoagulant therapy, after surgery, or during pregnancy, it may lead to an acute adrenal crisis resulting in sudden death (Karakousis et al., 2001).

## Signs and Symptoms

Waterhouse-Friderichsen syndrome manifests with congestion of the blood vessels and insufficient levels of platelets disrupting proper blood clotting. Massive hemorrhaging ensues, which results in a pinpoint red rash of the skin along with bruising over the body. Because the adrenal gland is highly vascular, it may be the site of massive hemorrhaging and necrosis.

## Treatment

Waterhouse-Friderichsen syndrome is treated with antibiotic therapy.

## Testing

Tests used in the diagnosis of Waterhouse-Friderichsen syndrome include blood tests, cerebrospinal fluid tests, aspirate tests, and imaging exams.

## WEGENER'S GRANULOMATOSIS

### Description

Wegener's granulomatosis is a rare disorder that causes vasculitis in the upper respiratory tract, lungs, and kidneys (Blaivas, 2003c; Sharma & Thompson, 2004). Other areas of the body may be affected, and arthritis is common. Wegener's granulomatosis is an autoimmune disorder of unknown cause. Destructive lesions develop in the upper and lower respiratory tract and the kidney. In the kidney, these lesions cause glomerulonephritis that may result in bloody urine and kidney failure.

### Signs and Symptoms

Although Wegener's granulomatosis may be asymptomatic, early symptoms may include fatigue, fever, nosebleed, pain, and sores around the opening of the nose. Sinusitis, ear infections, and deep central facial pain are common. Night sweats, eye inflammation, loss of appetite, and bloody urine may also occur. Skin lesions are common, especially rashes on the legs. Kidney disease is necessary to diagnose Wegener's granulomatosis. Other symptoms may include coughing up blood, cough, difficulty breathing, eye inflamation, hearing loss, and chest pain.

### Treatment

Treatment with corticosteroids, cyclophosphamide, methotrexate, or azathioprine produces long-term remission in over 90 percent of Wegener's granulomatosis cases. The kidney disease can progress rapidly. If untreated, kidney failure and death are almost certain.

### Testing

Tests used in the diagnosis of Wegener's granulomatosis include open lung biopsy, upper airway biopsy, nasal mucosal biopsy, bronchoscopy with transtracheal biopsy, and kidney biopsy. In addition, urinalysis, chest X-rays, bone marrow aspiration, and blood tests for autoantibodies may also be performed.

## WERNICKE-KORSAKOFF SYNDROME

### Description

Wernicke-Korsakoff syndrome is a brain disorder involving loss of specific brain functions caused by a thiamine (vitamin $B_1$) deficiency. Wernicke-Korsakoff syndrome includes two separate sets of symptoms, one of which starts when the other subsides. The cause of Wernicke syndrome is malnutrition, especially lack of thiamine. Heavy alcohol use interferes with the metabolism of thiamine, so even in cases where alcoholics eat a balanced diet, the metabolic problem persists because thiamine is not absorbed. Korsakoff syndrome, or Korsakoff psychosis, tends to develop as Wernicke's symptoms diminish. It involves impairment of memory. Patients create detailed, believable stories about experiences or situations to cover gaps in memory. This is not usually a deliberate attempt to deceive, because the patient often believes it to be true (Campellone, 2004n).

### Signs and Symptoms

Wernicke-Korsakoff syndrome is characterized by double vision, eye movement abnormalities, eyelid drooping, loss of muscle coordination, and profound loss of memory. Hallucinations and the inability to form new memories may also occur. As the disease progresses, confabulation, which is creating stories to explain behavior with little relation to reality, occurs. Symptoms of alcohol withdrawal may also be present.

### Treatment

Wernicke-Korsakoff is treated with thiamine, which may improve symptoms of confusion or delirium, difficulties with vision and eye movement, and incoordination. Thiamine does not improve loss of memory. Without treatment, Wernicke-Korsakoff syndrome progresses steadily to death. With treatment, progression of the disorder may be slowed or stopped.

### Testing

Diagnosis of Wernicke-Korsakoff syndrome includes examination of the nervous and muscular systems, reflexes, tests of gait, test of the eyes, and a nutritional assessment. Serum B1 levels may be low, pyruvate is elevated, and transketolase activity is decreased. Serum or urine alcohol levels may be elevated. Liver enzymes may be elevated.

## WEST NILE

### Description

West Nile virus is a flavivirus commonly found in Africa, West Asia, and the Middle East (Levy, 2004af). It is not known from where the United States virus originated, but it is most closely related genetically to strains found in the Middle East. It is not known how long it has been in the

United States, but CDC scientists believe the virus has been in the United States since 1999. The virus can infect humans, birds, mosquitoes, horses, and other mammals. More severe diseases due to this virus are West Nile encephalitis, West Nile meningitis, and West Nile meningoencephalitis (West Nile virus, 2003).

## Signs and Symptoms

Signs of West Nile virus infection are similar to those of other viral infections. There is nothing that can be found on physical examination to diagnose West Nile virus infection. West Nile virus usually causes mild disease in people, characterized by flulike symptoms lasting only a few days with no long-term health effects. A rash is present in 20 to 50 percent of patients. True muscle weakness in the presence of other related symptoms is suggestive of West Nile virus infection.

## Treatment

There is no human vaccine available for West Nile virus at present, and it is likely there will not be one for several years. Research trials are under way to determine whether ribavirin, an antiviral drug used to treat hepatitis C, may be useful in treating West Nile infection. In general, the likely outcome of a mild West Nile virus infection is excellent, but approximately 10 percent of patients with brain inflammation do not survive. The spread of disease is being limited through mosquito control.

## Testing

Diagnostic tests that may be used if West Nile virus is suspected include CBC, lumbar puncture and cerebrospinal fluid testing, head CT scans are normal, and head MRI scan indicates inflammation in about a third of cases. The most accurate way to diagnose West Nile infection is serology testing to detect the presence of antibodies against West Nile virus in cerebrospinal fluid or blood serum. Rarely, a sample of blood or CSF may be sent to a lab to be cultured, and the virus can be identified in body fluids using a polymerase chain reaction (PCR) test, but these methods can provide false negative results.

## WHIPPLE'S DISEASE

### Description

Whipple's disease is a rare condition that causes inadequate absorption of nutrients from the intestinal tract due to infection of the intestine (Bobustuc & Gilbert, 2002). Whipple's disease is caused by *Tropheryma whippelii*. The disorder primarily affects middle-aged white men. Without treatment, it is uniformly fatal. This slowly progressive disease has the hallmarks of arthritis, chronic diarrhea, and a fever of unknown origin. Less than 1000 cases have been reported since 1907.

### Signs and Symptoms

Whipple's disease is characterized by abdominal pain, fatty stools, fever, diarrhea, weight loss, gastrointestinal bleeding, chest pain, inflammation of the tongue, arthritis, leg swelling, gray to brown skin discoloration, and memory loss.

## Treatment
Whipple's disease is treated with prolonged antibiotic therapy and dietary supplements.

## Testing
Tests used in the diagnosis of Whipple's disease include small bowel biopsy, CBC, fecal fat levels, D-xylose absorption tests, and albumin levels (Mylonakis, 2002).

## WHITMORE'S DISEASE

### Description
Whitmore's disease, which is also known as melioidosis, is caused by *Burkholderia pseudomallei*. Whitmore's disease is predominantly a disease of tropical climates, especially in Southeast Asia, where it is endemic. *B. pseudomallei* is found in contaminated water and soil and is spread to humans and animals through direct contact. *B. pseudomallei* is an organism that has been considered as a potential agent for biological warfare and biological terrorism (*Burkholderia cepacia infection,* 2004).

### Signs and Symptoms
Acute infection is localized as a nodule and results from a break in the skin. The acute form produces fever and general muscle aches, and may progress rapidly to infect the bloodstream. Pulmonary infection ranges from mild bronchitis to severe pneumonia. The onset of pulmonary melioidosis is typically accompanied by a high fever, headache, loss of appetite, and general muscle soreness. Chest pain is common, but a nonproductive or productive cough with normal sputum is the hallmark of this form of Whitmore's disease. The symptoms of the bloodstream infection vary, but typically include respiratory distress, severe headache, fever, diarrhea, development of pus-filled lesions on the skin, muscle tenderness, and disorientation. Acute bloodstream infection is typically of short duration, and abscesses are present throughout the body. Chronic melioidosis involves the joints, organs, lymph nodes, skin, brain, liver, lung, bones, and spleen.

### Treatment
There is no vaccine for Whitmore's disease. Most cases are treated with antibiotics. *Burkholderia psuedomallei* is treated with imipenem, penicillin, doxycycline, amoxicillin-clavulanic acid, azlocillin, ceftazidime, ticarcillin-vulanic acid, ceftriaxone, and aztreonam. Treatment should be initiated early, and, although bloodstream infection can be fatal, the other types of Whitmore's disease are not.

### Testing
Whitmore's disease is diagnosed by isolating *Burkholderia pseudomallei* from the blood, urine, sputum, or skin lesions. Detecting and measuring antibodies to the bacteria in the blood is another means of diagnosis.

## WILMS' TUMOR

### Description

Wilms' tumor is one of the most common tumors of the abdomen in children and the most common type of kidney tumor (Blackman, 2004j; Paulino & Coppes, 2003). The cause is unknown, but it is associated with certain birth defects including urinary tract abnormalities, absence of the iris, and enlargement of one side of the body. It occurs among some siblings and twins, suggesting a genetic link. The involved genes are those affecting genitourinary development. It is estimated to occur in about 1 out of 250,000 children, especially at three years of age. Wilms' tumor is rare after the age of eight.

### Signs and Symptoms

Wilms' tumor is characterized by an abdominal mass, abdominal pain, swelling of the abdomen, bloody urine, fever, nausea, vomiting, hypertension, constipation, and increased growth of one side of the body. A missing iris of the eye may also be associated with Wilms' tumor.

### Treatment

Wilms' tumor is treated by radiation therapy, chemotherapy, and surgical exploration and removal of the tumor. Regional lymph nodes, abdominal organs, and other tissues are examined and removed if the tumor has metastasized. Children with a localized tumor have a 90 percent cure rate when treated.

### Testing

Tests used to diagnose Wilms' tumor include CBC, BUN, creatinine levels, creatinine clearance, urinalysis for bloody urine or protein, abdominal ultrasound, chest X-rays, intravenous pyelogram (IVP), and CT scans of the abdomen.

## XANTHOMAS

### Description

Xanthomas is a skin condition with fat deposits consisting of immune system cells beneath the surface of the skin (Drayer, 2003c; Horenstein & McNeil, 2004). Xanthomas may be a symptom of underlying metabolic disorders associated with an increase in fats in the blood (e.g., diabetes, biliary cirrhosis, cancer, familial hypercholesterolemia). Xanthomas are most frequently seen on the elbows, joints, tendons, knees, hands, feet, or buttocks. Xanthelasma palpebra is a type of xanthoma of the eyelids.

### Signs and Symptoms

Xanthomas are characterized by painless skin lesions under the skin. The nodules have a flat surface, are soft to the touch, are yellow, and have sharply defined margins.

### Treatment

The goal is to control underlying disorders. The growths can be surgically removed, but they may reappear. They may also be removed with acid. If xanthomas are present in the blood vessels, they can cause a fatality by contributing to atherosclerosis.

## Testing

Diagnosis is primarily on how the skin growth looks, especially if there is a history of an underlying disorder. A biopsy of the growth will show a fatty deposit. Lab studies of the fat levels in the body are also conducted.

## YAWS

### Description

Yaws is a contagious, nonvenereal, treponemal infection in humans that presents mainly in children younger than 15 years (Klein, 2001). Infection with *Treponema pertenue*, a subspecies of *Treponema pallidum*, causes the disease. The disease occurs primarily in warm, humid, tropical areas of Africa, Asia, South America, and Oceania, among poor rural populations where conditions of overcrowding and poor sanitation prevail. Yaws does not occur in the United States. The primary route of infection is through direct person-to-person contact.

### Signs and Symptoms

Yaws is characterized by ulcerative skin lesions that are teaming with spirochetes, which can be transmitted through direct contact with the skin and through trauma such as bites (see Color Plate 68). Yaws is classified into four stages. During the primary stage, lesions develop at the original site of infection. The secondary stage involves widespread dissemination of treponemes resulting in multiple skin lesions similar to those present during the primary stage of yaws. During the latent stage of yaws, there are no observable signs or symptoms of disease. The tertiary stage is characterized by bone, joint, and soft tissue deformities.

### Treatment

Yaws is treated with antibiotics, especially benzathine penicillin.

### Testing

Although yaws is usually diagnosed based on clinical findings, serodiagnostic tests for venereal syphilis are used as well. Dark-field examination of early lesions will be positive, and biopsy of late lesions may be needed to show characteristic histopathology.

## YELLOW FEVER

### Description

Yellow fever is a viral infection transmitted by mosquitoes and characterized by fever, jaundice, kidney failure, and bleeding (Kotton, 2002a; *Yellow Fever*, 2003). Yellow fever is caused by an arbovirus transmitted by the bite of mosquitoes. This disease is common in South America and in sub-Saharan Africa and occurs almost exclusively among forestry and agricultural workers. Humans and monkeys are both hosts in the transmission cycle of this infection.

## Signs and Symptoms

Yellow fever can be divided into an early stage, a period of remission, and a period of intoxication. The early stage is characterized by headache, muscle aches, fever, loss of appetite, vomiting, and jaundice. Most people recover during a period of remission in which symptoms subside. About 15 percent of patients move on to a third stage characterized by multiorgan dysfunction. The period of intoxication is characterized by liver failure, kidney failure, hemorrhaging, brain dysfunction. Thirty percent of cases that advance to the period of intoxication die.

## Treatment

There is no specific treatment for yellow fever, which is a rare cause of illness in travelers. Most countries have regulations and requirements for yellow fever vaccination. Yellow fever vaccine is a live virus vaccine that has been used for several decades. A single dose confers immunity lasting 10 years or more. Yellow fever is a severe infection that can cause death in up to 40 percent of affected individuals.

## Testing

Yellow fever is diagnosed based on case history, physical exam, and a history of travel to endemic countries. The diagnosis is confirmed by blood tests that reveal the virus, viral antigens, or antibodies.

## YERSINIOSIS

### Description

Yersiniosis is an infectious disease caused by a bacterium of the genus *Yersinia*. In the United States, most human illness is caused by one species, *Y. enterocolitica*. Infection with *Y. enterocolitica* can cause a variety of symptoms depending on the age of the person infected. Infection with *Y. enterocolitica* occurs most often in young children. Infection is most often acquired by eating contaminated food, especially raw or undercooked pork products. The preparation of raw pork intestines (chitterlings) may be particularly risky. Infants can be infected if their caretakers handle raw chitterlings and then do not adequately clean their hands before handling the infant or the infant's toys, bottles, or pacifiers. Drinking contaminated unpasteurized milk or untreated water can also transmit the infection (Butler, 1983; *Yersinia enterocolitica*, 2004).

### Signs and Symptoms

Common symptoms in children are fever, abdominal pain, and diarrhea, which is often bloody. Symptoms typically develop a week after exposure and may last three weeks or longer. In older children and adults, right-sided abdominal pain and fever may be the predominant symptoms, and may be confused with appendicitis. In a small proportion of cases, complications such as skin rash, joint pains, or spread of bacteria to the bloodstream can occur. Occasionally, some persons develop joint pain, most commonly in the knees, ankles, or wrists. These joint pains usually develop about one month after the initial episode of diarrhea and generally resolve after six months. A skin rash, called erythema nodosum, may also appear on the legs and trunk. In most cases, erythema nodosum resolves spontaneously within a month.

## Treatment

Uncomplicated cases of diarrhea due to *Y. enterocolitica* usually resolve on their own without antibiotic treatment. In more severe or complicated infections, antibiotics such as aminoglycosides, doxycycline, trimethoprim-sulfamethoxazole, or fluoroquinolones may be useful.

## Testing

*Y. enterocolitica* infections are generally diagnosed by detecting the organism in the stools. Many laboratories do not routinely test for *Y. enterocolitica*, so it is important to notify laboratory personnel when infection with this bacterium is suspected so that special tests can be done. The organism can also be recovered from other sites, including the throat, lymph nodes, joint fluid, urine, bile, and blood.

## ZOLLINGER-ELLISON SYNDROME

### Description

Zollinger-Ellison syndrome is caused by tumors, called gastrinomas, usually found in the head of the pancreas and the upper small bowel that produce the hormone gastrin (Radebold, 2003; Stone, 2004h). High levels of gastrin cause overproduction of stomach acid, which leads to ulcers in the stomach and small bowel. Patients with Zollinger-Ellison syndrome may experience abdominal pain and diarrhea. About two-thirds of gastrinomas are malignant and may spread to the liver and nearby lymph nodes. Patients with multiple gastrinomas may result in a condition called Multiple Endocrine Neoplasia type I (MEN I). MEN I patients often have tumors of the pituitary gland and parathyroid glands. To date, there have been approximately 60 reported cases of this disease.

### Signs and Symptoms

Zollinger-Ellison syndrome is characterized by abdominal pain, hematemeisis, and diarrhea. Ulcers of the intestine are common.

### Treatment

Zollinger-Ellison syndrome is treated with acid-suppressing medications called proton pump inhibitors (e.g., omeprazole and lansoprazole). Early diagnosis and surgical resection are associated with a cure rate of only 20 to 25 percent. Zollinger-Ellison syndrome progresses slowly, and patients may live for many years after tumors are discovered.

### Testing

Diagnosis of Zollinger-Ellison syndrome includes increased gastrin levels, a positive secretin stimulation test, a positive calcium infusion test, abdominal CT scans, exploratory surgery, and octreotide scans demonstrating tumors in the pancreas and small bowel.

# Appendix

Internet Websites for Further Information

American College of Allergy, Asthma, and Immunology,

    htttp://allergy.mcg.edu.

American Heart Association, www.americanheart.org.

American Osteopathic College of Dermatology, www.aocd.org.

British Association of Cancer United Patients, www.cancerbacup.org.

Center for Disease Control and Prevention, www.cdc.gov.

eMedicine, www.emedicine.com

Internet Stroke Center, www.strokecenter.org.

Kirksville College of Osteopathic Medicine,

    www.kcom.edu/faculty/chamberlain/Website/intmic.htm.

March of Dimes, www.marchofdimes.com.

Mayo Clinic, www.mayoclinic.com.

*Medical Microbiology, 4th Edition,*

    http://gsbs.utmb.edu/microbook.htm.

MedlinePlus, www.nlm.nih.gov.

National Cancer Institute, www.nci.nih.gov.

National Center for Infectious Diseases, Division of Parasitic Diseases,

www.dpd.cdc.gov.

National Center for Infectious Diseases, www.cdc.gov/ncid.

National Digestive Diseases Information Clearinghouse,

www.niddk.nih.gov.

National Human Genome Research Institute, www.genome.gov.

National Institute of Allergy and Infectious Diseases,

www.niaid.nih.gov.

National Institute of Neurological Disorders and Stroke,

www.ninds.nih.gov.

National Institutes of Health, www.nih.gov.

National Library of Medicine, www.nlm.gov.

*Todar's Online Textbook of Bacteriology,*

www.bact.wisc.edu/microtextbook/disease/overview.html.

U.S. Food and Drug Administration, www.fda.gov.

University of Iowa Virtual Hospital, www.vh.org.

World Health Organization, www.who.int

# References

Abbuhl, S. 2004. Chancroid. *eMedicine*, Retrieved November 11, 2004, from: http://www.emedicine.com/EMERG/topic95.htm.

*Acanthamoeba infection*. 2004. *DPD*, Retrieved November 12, 2004, from the National Center for Infectious Diseases, Division of Parasitic Diseases. Centers for Disease Control and Prevention: http://www.cdc.gov/ncid.

Accetta, D. 2004. Anaphylaxis. *MedlinePlus*, Retrieved March 8, 2005, from the U.S. National Library of Medicine and the National Institutes of Health: http://www.nlm.nih.gov/medlineplus/ency/article/000844.htm.

Agha, I. 2003a. Analgesic nephropathy. *MedlinePlus*, Retrieved March 8, 2005, from the U.S. National Library of Medicine and the National Institutes of Health: http://www.nlm.nih.gov/medlineplus/ency/article/000482.htm.

Agha, I. 2003b. Glomerulonephritis. *MedlinePlus*, Retrieved November 11, 2004, from the U.S. National Library of Medicine and the National Institutes of Health: http://www.nlm.nih.gov/medlineplus/ency/article/000484.htm.

Agha, I. 2003c. Interstitial nephritis. *MedlinePlus*, Retrieved November 10, 2004, from the U.S. National Library of Medicine and the National Institutes of Health: http://www.nlm.nih.gov/medlineplus/ency/article/000464.htm.

Agha, I. 2003d. Nephrolithiasis. *MedlinePlus*, Retrieved November 10, 2004, from the U.S. National Library of Medicine and the National Institutes of Health: http://www.nlm.nih.gov/medlineplus/ency/article/000458.htm.

Agha, I. 2003e. Polycystic kidney disease. *MedlinePlus*, Retrieved November 10, 2004, from the U.S. National Library of Medicine and the National Institutes of Health: http://www.nlm.nih.gov/medlineplus/ency/article/000502.htm.

Agha, I. 2003f. Prerenal azotemia. *MedlinePlus*, Retrieved November 10, 2004, from the U.S. National Library of Medicine and the National Institutes of Health: http://www.nlm.nih.gov/medlineplus/ency/article/000508.htm.

Aicardi Syndrome Foundation. 2004. Aicardi syndrome. Retrieved March 8, 2005, from http://www.aicardisyndrome.org/index.php?pname=whatis.

Akroush, A. 1997. Fatal familial insomnia. Retrieved November 11, 2004, from: http://www.personal.umd.umich.edu/~jcthomas/JCTHOMAS/1997%20Case%20Studies/AAkroush.htm.l.

Albuisson, J. 2003. Aase Syndrome. Retrieved February 27, 2005, from http://www.orpha.net/consor/cgi-bin/OC_Exp.php?Lng=GB&Expert=917.

All about hantavirus. 2003. Retrieved July 26, 2003, from the National Center for Infectious Diseases, Division of Viral and Rickettsial Diseases, Special Pathogens Branch. Centers for Disease Control and Prevention: http://www.cdc.gov/ncidod/diseases/hanta/hps/index.htm.

Alström Syndrome International. 2005. Retrieved March 8, 2005, from http://www.jax.org/alstrom/.

Alter, B., & Lipton, J. 2004. Anemia, Falconi's. *eMedicine*. Retrieved March 12, 2005, from http://www.emedicine.com/ped/topic3022.htm.

Amaldo, F. 2004a. Arterial embolism. *MedlinePlus*, Retrieved November 11, 2004, from the U.S. National Library of Medicine and the National Institutes of Health: http://www.nlm.nih.gov/medlineplus/ency/article/001102.htm.

Amaldo, F. 2004b. Coronary heart disease. *MedlinePlus*, Retrieved November 11, 2004, from the U.S. National Library of Medicine and the National Institutes of Health: http://www.nlm.nih.gov/medlineplus/ency/article/007115.htm.

American Diabetes Association. 2005. All about diabetes. Retrieved March 12, 2005, from http://www.diabetes.org/about-diabetes.jsp.

Anadiotis, G. 2003. Galactose-1-Phosphate Uridyltransferase deficiency. *eMedicine*, Retrieved November 11, 2004, from: http://www.emedicine.com/ped/topic818.htm.

Anemia. 2003. *MEDLINEplus*. Retrieved July 24, 2003, from the U.S. National Library of Medicine and the National Institutes of Health: http://www.nlm.nih.gov/medlineplus/anemia.html.

Angelo, S. 2002. Age-related hearing loss. *MedlinePlus*, Retrieved November 10, 2004, from the U.S. National Library of Medicine and the National Institutes of Health: http://www.nlm.nih.gov/medlineplus/ency/article/001045.htm.

Ania, B. 2002. Mycetoma. *eMedicine*, Retrieved November 11, 2004, from: http://www.emedicine.com/med/topic30.htm.

*Angiostrongylus cantonensis infection.* 2004. *DPD*, Retrieved November 12, 2004, from the National Center for Infectious Diseases, Division of Parasitic Diseases. Centers for Disease Control and Prevention: http://www.cdc.gov/ncidod/dpd/parasites/angiostrongylus/factsht_angiostrongylus.htm.

*Anisakiasis.* 2004. *DPDx*, Retrieved November 12, 2004, from the National Center for Infectious Diseases, Division of Parasitic Diseases. Centers for Disease Control and Prevention: http://www.dpd.cdc.gov/dpdx/HTM.L/Anisakiasis.htm.

Anthrax. 2003. Retrieved July 26, 2003, from the National Center for Infectious Diseases, Division of Bacterial and Mycotic Diseases. Centers for Disease Control and Prevention: http://www.cdc.gov/ncidod/dbmd/diseaseinfo/anthrax_g.htm.

Anthrax. 2002. Retrieved July 19, 2003, from the U.S. Food and Drug Administration: http://www.fda.gov/cber/vaccine/anthrax.htm.

Arnold, G. 2003. Phenylketonuria. *eMedicine*, Retrieved November 11, 2004, from: http://www.emedicine.com/ped/topic1787.htm.

*Ascaris infection.* 2004. *DPD*, Retrieved November 12, 2004, from the National Center for Infectious Diseases, Division of Parasitic Diseases. Centers for Disease Control and Prevention: http://www.cdc.gov/ncidod/dpd/parasites/ascaris/factsht_ascaris.htm.

Aspergillosis. 2002. Retrieved July 26, 2003, from the National Center for Infectious Diseases, Division of Bacterial and Mycotic Diseases. Centers for Disease Control and Prevention: http://www.cdc.gov/ncidod/dbmd/diseaseinfo/aspergillosis_t.htm.

Atherosclerosis. (n/d). Retrieved June 4, 2003, from the American Heart Association: http://www.americanheart.org/presenter.jhtml?identifier=4440.

Autism Society of America. 2005. What is autism? Retrieved March 8, 2005, from http://www.autism-society.org/site/PageServer?pagename=whatisautism.

Aventura, M. 2002. Retinoblastoma. *eMedicine*, Retrieved November 11, 2004, from: http://www.emedicine.com/oph/topic346.htm.

*Babesiosis.* 2004. *DPDx*, Retrieved November 12, 2004, from the National Center for Infectious Diseases, Division of Parasitic Diseases. Centers for Disease Control and Prevention: http://www.dpd.cdc.gov/dpdx/HTM.L/Babesiosis.htm.

*Bacterial vaginosis.* 2004. *STD Prevention,* Retrieved November 12, 2004, from the National Center for HIV, STD and TB Prevention, Division of Sexually Transmitted Diseases. Centers for Disease Control and Prevention: http://www.cdc.gov/std/ BV/STDFact-Bacterial-Vaginosis. htm.

*Bacterial vaginosis.* 2002. *MMWR,* Retrieved November 12, 2004, from the National Center for HIV, STD and TB Prevention, Division of Sexually Transmitted Diseases. Centers for Disease Control and Prevention: http://www.cdc.gov/STD/ treatment/5-2002TG.htm.#BacterialVaginosis.

Balevicience, G., & Schwartz, R. 2005. Osler-Weber-Rendu syndrome. *eMedicine.* Retrieved March 14, 2005, from http://www.emedicine.com/derm/ topic782.htm.

Baloghova, J. 2003. Mucopolysaccharidoses Type I-VII. *eMedicine,* Retrieved November 11, 2004, from: http://www.emedicine.com/derm/topic710.htm.

Banerjee, A. 2004a. Fifth disease. *MedlinePlus,* Retrieved November 11, 2004, from the U.S. National Library of Medicine and the National Institutes of Health: http://www.nlm.nih.gov/medlineplus/ency/article/000977.htm.

Banerjee, A. 2004b. Measles. *MedlinePlus,* Retrieved November 10, 2004, from the U.S. National Library of Medicine and the National Institutes of Health: http://www.nlm.nih.gov/medlineplus/ency/article/001569.htm.

Banerjee, A. 2004c. Mumps. *MedlinePlus,* Retrieved November 10, 2004, from the U.S. National Library of Medicine and the National Institutes of Health: http://www.nlm.nih.gov/medlineplus/ency/article/001557.htm.

Bardorf, C. 2001. Nystagmus, acquired. *eMedicine,* Retrieved November 11, 2004, from: http://www.emedicine.com/oph/topic339.htm.

Barker, J. 2002. Seminoma. *eMedicine,* Retrieved November 11, 2004, from: http://www.emedicine.com/ped/topic2078.htm.

Barret, A. 2004. Pick's disease. *eMedicine.* Retrieved March 14, 2005, from http://www.emedicine.com/neuro/topic311.htm.

Batres, L. 2003. Beriberi. *eMedicine.* Retrieved March 8, 2005, from http:// www.emedicine.com/ped/topic229.htm.

*Baylisascaris infection.* 2004. *DPD,* Retrieved November 12, 2004, from the National Center for Infectious Diseases, Division of Parasitic Diseases. Centers for Disease Control and Prevention: http://www.cdc.gov/ncidod/dpd/parasites/baylisacaris/ default.htm.

Beryllium Network. 2004. Beryllium poses danger for workers and their families. Retrieved November 11, 2004, from: http://www.chronicberylliumdisease.com/.

Besa, E. 2004. Hairy cell leukemia. *eMedicine,* Retrieved November 11, 2004, from: http://www.emedicine.com/med/topic937.htm.

Besa, E., & Woermann, U. 2002. Paroxysmal nocturnal hemoglobinuria. *eMedicine,* Retrieved November 11, 2004, from: http://www.emedicine.com/med/ topic2696.htm.

Best, R. 2002. Anencephaly. *eMedicine,* Retrieved November 11, 2004, from: http:// www.emedicine.com/neuro/topic639.htm.

Bjerke, H. 2002. Flail chest. *eMedicine*: Retrieved June 9, 2003, from http://www .emedicine.com/med/topic2813.htm.

Blackman, S. 2004a. Asperger's syndrome. *MedlinePlus,* Retrieved November 10, 2004, from the U.S. National Library of Medicine and the National Institutes of Health: http://www.nlm.nih.gov/medlineplus/ency/article/001549.htm.

Blackman, S. 2004b. Caput succedaneum. *MedlinePlus,* Retrieved March 10, 2005, from the U.S. National Library of Medicine and the National Institutes of Health: http://www.nlm.nih.gov/medlineplus/ency/article/001587.htm.

Blackman, S. 2004c. Ewing's sarcoma. *MedlinePlus,* Retrieved November 11, 2004, from the U.S. National Library of Medicine and the National Institutes of Health: http://www.nlm.nih.gov/medlineplus/ency/article/001302.htm.

Blackman, S. 2004d. Kwashiorkor. *MedlinePlus*, Retrieved March 13, 2005, from the U.S. National Library of Medicine and the National Institutes of Health: http://www.nlm.nih.gov/medlineplus/ency/article/001604.htm.

Blackman, S. 2004e. Lesch-Nyhan syndrome. *MedlinePlus*, Retrieved March 13, 2005, from the U.S. National Library of Medicine and the National Institutes of Health: http://www.nlm.nih.gov/medlineplus/ency/article/001655.htm.

Blackman, S. 2004f. Neuroblastoma. *MedlinePlus*, Retrieved November 10, 2004, from the U.S. National Library of Medicine and the National Institutes of Health: http://www.nlm.nih.gov/medlineplus/ency/article/001408.htm.

Blackman, S. 2004g. Osteosarcoma. *MedlinePlus*, Retrieved November 10, 2004, from the U.S. National Library of Medicine and the National Institutes of Health: http://www.nlm.nih.gov/medlineplus/ency/article/001650.htm.

Blackman, S. 2004h. Retinoblastoma. *MedlinePlus*, Retrieved November 10, 2004, from the U.S. National Library of Medicine and the National Institutes of Health: http://www.nlm.nih.gov/medlineplus/ency/article/001030.htm.

Blackman, S. 2004i. Rhabdomyosarcoma. *MedlinePlus*, Retrieved November 10, 2004, from the U.S. National Library of Medicine and the National Institutes of Health: http://www.nlm.nih.gov/medlineplus/ency/article/001429.htm.

Blackman, S. 2004j. Wilms' tumor. *MedlinePlus*, Retrieved November 10, 2004, from the U.S. National Library of Medicine and the National Institutes of Health: http://www.nlm.nih.gov/medlineplus/ency/article/001575.htm.

*Blastomycosis.* 2004. *DBMD*, Retrieved November 12, 2004, from the National Center for Infectious Diseases, Division of Bacterial and Mycotic Diseases. Centers for Disease Control and Prevention: http://www.cdc.gov/ncidod/dbmd/diseaseinfo/blastomycosis_t.htm.

Blaivas, A. 2004a. Chronic bronchitis. *MedlinePlus*, Retrieved November 11, 2004, from the U.S. National Library of Medicine and the National Institutes of Health: http://www.nlm.nih.gov/medlineplus/ency/article/000119.htm.

Blaivas, A. 2004b. Chronic obstructive pulmonary disease. *MedlinePlus*, Retrieved November 11, 2004, from the U.S. National Library of Medicine and the National Institutes of Health: http://www.nlm.nih.gov/medlineplus/ency/article/000091.htm.

Blaivas, A. 2004c. Pleurisy. *MedlinePlus*, Retrieved November 10, 2004, from the U.S. National Library of Medicine and the National Institutes of Health: http://www.nlm.nih.gov/medlineplus/ency/article/001371.htm.

Blaivas, A. 2003a. Obesity hypoventilation syndrome. *MedlinePlus*, Retrieved November 10, 2004, from the U.S. National Library of Medicine and the National Institutes of Health: http://www.nlm.nih.gov/medlineplus/ency/article/000085.htm.

Blaivas, A. 2003b. Silicosis. *MedlinePlus*, Retrieved November 10, 2004, from the U.S. National Library of Medicine and the National Institutes of Health: http://www.nlm.nih.gov/medlineplus/ency/article/000134.htm.

Blaivas, A. 2003c. Wegener's granulomatosis. *MedlinePlus*, Retrieved November 10, 2004, from the U.S. National Library of Medicine and the National Institutes of Health: http://www.nlm.nih.gov/medlineplus/ency/article/000135.htm.

Bobustuc, G., & Gilbert, M. 2002. Whipple Disease. *eMedicine*, Retrieved November 11, 2004, from: http://www.emedicine.com/neuro/topic397.htm.

Body lice. 2000. Retrieved July 26, 2003, from the National Center for Infectious Diseases, Division of Parasitic Infections. Centers for Disease Control and Prevention: http://www.cdc.gov/ncidod/dpd/parasites/lice/factsht_body_lice.htm.

Bordetella pertussis. 2001. Retrieved July 26, 2003, from the Office of Laboratory Safety, Health Canada: http://www.hc-sc.gc.ca/pphb-dgspsp/msds-ftss/msds20e.html.

Botulism. 2001. Retrieved July 26, 2003, from the National Center for Infectious Diseases, Division of Bacterial and Mycotic Diseases. Centers for Disease Control and Prevention: http://www.cdc.gov/ncidod/dbmd/diseaseinfo/botulism_g.htm.

Bourgon, D., & Outwater, E. 2004. Ectopic pregnancy. *eMedicine*. Retrieved March 12, 2005, from http://www.emedicine.com/radio/topic231.htm.

*Brainerd Diarrhea*. 2003. CDC, Retrieved November 12, 2004, from the National Center for Infectious Diseases, Division of Bacterial and Mycotic Diseases. Centers for Disease Control and Prevention: http://www.cdc.gov/ncidod/dbmd/diseaseinfo/brainerddiarrhea_g.htm.

Brooks, D. 2004. Retinitis pigmentosa. *MedlinePlus*, Retrieved November 10, 2004, from the U.S. National Library of Medicine and the National Institutes of Health: http://www.nlm.nih.gov/medlineplus/ency/article/001029.htm.

Brooks, M. 2001. Pregnancy, eclampsia. *eMedicine*. Retrieved July 25, 2003, from http://www.emedicine.com/emerg/topic796.htm.

Brose, M. 2004a. Multiple myeloma. *MedlinePlus*, Retrieved November 10, 2004, from the U.S. National Library of Medicine and the National Institutes of Health: http://www.nlm.nih.gov/medlineplus/ency/article/000583.htm.

Brose, M. 2004b. Non-Hodgkin's lymphoma. *MedlinePlus*, Retrieved November 10, 2004, from the U.S. National Library of Medicine and the National Institutes of Health: http://www.nlm.nih.gov/medlineplus/ency/article/000581.htm.

Brose, M. 2004c. Pheochromocytoma. *MedlinePlus*, Retrieved November 10, 2004, from the U.S. National Library of Medicine and the National Institutes of Health: http://www.nlm.nih.gov/medlineplus/ency/article/000340.htm.

Brose, M. 2004d. Prostate cancer. *MedlinePlus*, Retrieved November 10, 2004, from the U.S. National Library of Medicine and the National Institutes of Health: http://www.nlm.nih.gov/medlineplus/ency/article/000380.htm.

Brose, M. 2004e. Renal cell carcinoma. *MedlinePlus*, Retrieved November 10, 2004, from the U.S. National Library of Medicine and the National Institutes of Health: http://www.nlm.nih.gov/medlineplus/ency/article/000516.htm.

Brown, T. 2003a. Diabetes. *MedlinePlus*, Retrieved November 11, 2004, from the U.S. National Library of Medicine and the National Institutes of Health: http://www.nlm.nih.gov/medlineplus/ency/article/001214.htm.

Brown, T. 2003b. Diabetes insipidus. *MedlinePlus*, Retrieved November 11, 2004, from the U.S. National Library of Medicine and the National Institutes of Health: http://www.nlm.nih.gov/medlineplus/ency/article/000377.htm.

*Brucellosis*. 2004. DBMD, Retrieved November 12, 2004, from the National Center for Infectious Diseases, Division of Bacterial and Mycotic Diseases. Centers for Disease Control and Prevention: http://www.cdc.gov/ncidod/dbmd/diseaseinfo/brucellosis_g.htm.

Bruckheimer, E. 2004. Tetralogy of Fallot. *MedlinePlus*, Retrieved November 10, 2004, from the U.S. National Library of Medicine and the National Institutes of Health: http://www.nlm.nih.gov/medlineplus/ency/article/001567.htm.

Bucurescu, G., & Suleman, A. 2005. Neurosarcoidosis. *eMedicine*. Retrieved March 14, 2005, from http://www.emedicine.com/neuro/topic649.htm.

Burke, B. 2004. Thrombophlebitis. *MedlinePlus*, Retrieved November 10, 2004, from the U.S. National Library of Medicine and the National Institutes of Health: http://www.nlm.nih.gov/medlineplus/ency/article/001108.htm.

Burke, D., & Hauser, R. 2001. Essential tremor. *eMedicine*. Retrieved March 12, 2005, from http://www.emedicine.com/neuro/topic129.htm.

*Burkholderia cepacia infection*. 2004. CDC, Retrieved November 12, 2004, from the National Center for Infectious Diseases, Division of HealthCare Quality Promotion. Centers for Disease Control and Prevention: http://www.cdc.gov/ncidod/hip/B_cepacia.htm.

Butler T. 1983. *Plague and other Yersinia infections*. New York: Plenum Press.

Cha-Kim, A. 2004. Guillain-Barre syndrome. *eMedicine*, Retrieved November 11, 2004, from: http://www.emedicine.com/pmr/topic48.htm.

Campbell, B. 2004. Truncus arteriosus. *MedlinePlus*, Retrieved November 10, 2004, from the U.S. National Library of Medicine and the National Institutes of Health: http://www.nlm.nih.gov/medlineplus/ency/article/001111.htm.

Campellone, J. 2004a. Bell's palsy. *MedlinePlus*. Retrieved March 8, 2005, from the U.S. National Library of Medicine and the National Institutes of Health: http://www.nlm.nih.gov/medlineplus/ency/article/000773.htm.

Campellone, J. 2004b. Encephalitis. *MedlinePlus*, Retrieved November 11, 2004, from the U.S. National Library of Medicine and the National Institutes of Health: http://www.nlm.nih.gov/medlineplus/ency/article/001415.htm.

Campellone, J. 2004c. Epilepsy. *MedlinePlus*, Retrieved November 11, 2004, from the U.S. National Library of Medicine and the National Institutes of Health: http://www.nlm.nih.gov/medlineplus/ency/article/000694.htm.

Campellone, J. 2004d. Essential tremor. *MedlinePlus*, Retrieved November 11, 2004, from the U.S. National Library of Medicine and the National Institutes of Health: http://www.nlm.nih.gov/medlineplus/ency/article/000762.htm.

Campellone, J. 2004f. Guillain-Barre syndrome. *MedlinePlus*, Retrieved November 11, 2004, from the U.S. National Library of Medicine and the National Institutes of Health: http://www.nlm.nih.gov/medlineplus/ency/article/000684.htm.

Campellone, J. 2004g. Meniere's disease. *MedlinePlus*, Retrieved November 10, 2004, from the U.S. National Library of Medicine and the National Institutes of Health: http://www.nlm.nih.gov/medlineplus/ency/article/000702.htm.

Campellone, J. 2004h. Multiple sclerosis. *MedlinePlus*, Retrieved November 10, 2004, from the U.S. National Library of Medicine and the National Institutes of Health: http://www.nlm.nih.gov/medlineplus/ency/article/000737.htm.

Campellone, J. 2004i. Myasthenia gravis. *MedlinePlus*, Retrieved November 10, 2004, from the U.S. National Library of Medicine and the National Institutes of Health: http://www.nlm.nih.gov/medlineplus/ency/article/000712.htm.

Campellone, J. 2004j. Neuralgia. *MedlinePlus*, Retrieved November 10, 2004, from the U.S. National Library of Medicine and the National Institutes of Health: http://www.nlm.nih.gov/medlineplus/ency/article/001407.htm.

Campellone, J. 2004k. Neurosarcoidosis. *MedlinePlus*, Retrieved November 10, 2004, from the U.S. National Library of Medicine and the National Institutes of Health: http://www.nlm.nih.gov/medlineplus/ency/article/000720.htm.

Campellone, J. 2004l. Parkinson's disease. *MedlinePlus*, Retrieved November 10, 2004, from the U.S. National Library of Medicine and the National Institutes of Health: http://www.nlm.nih.gov/medlineplus/ency/article/000755.htm.

Campellone, J. 2004m. Peripheral neuropathy. *MedlinePlus*, Retrieved November 10, 2004, from the U.S. National Library of Medicine and the National Institutes of Health: http://www.nlm.nih.gov/medlineplus/ency/article/000593.htm.

Campellone, J. 2004n. Wernicke-Korsakoff syndrome. *MedlinePlus*, Retrieved November 10, 2004, from the U.S. National Library of Medicine and the National Institutes of Health: http://www.nlm.nih.gov/medlineplus/ency/article/000771.htm.

*Cancer of the Pancreas*. 2002. Retrieved November 11, 2004, from the National Cancer Institute. U.S. National Institutes of Health: http://www.nci.nih.gov/cancertopics/wyntk/pancreas/page6.

*Capillariasis*. 2004. *DPDx*, Retrieved November 12, 2004, from the National Center for Infectious Diseases, Division of Parasitic Diseases. Centers for Disease Control and Prevention: http://www.dpd.cdc.gov/dpdx/HTM.L/Capillariasis.htm.

Castro, L. 2003. Chromoblastomycosis. *eMedicine*, Retrieved November 11, 2004, from: http://www.emedicine.com/DERM/topic855.htm.

CDC. 2002. *B Virus (Cercopithecine herpesvirus 1) Infection.* Retrieved November 12, 2004, from the National Center for Infectious Diseases. Centers for Disease Control and Prevention: http://www.cdc.gov/ncidod/diseases/bvirus.htm.

*Cellulitis.* 2004. *The MayoClinic,* Retrieved November 12, 2004, from the Mayo Foundation for Medical Education and Research: http://www.mayoclinic.com/ invoke.cfm?objectid=2875823B-229A-4555-9C0FC8019E4254BC&dsection=3.

*Chagas disease.* 2004. *DPD,* Retrieved November 12, 2004, from the National Center for Infectious Diseases, Division of Parasitic Diseases. Centers for Disease Control and prevention: http://www.cdc.gov/ncidod/dpd/parasites/chagasdisease/ factsht_chagas_disease.htm.

Chan, L. 2003. Bullous pemphigoid. *eMedicine,* Retrieved November 11, 2004, from: http://www.emedicine.com/derm/topic64.htm.

Cheema, J., & Harcke, H. 2003. Blount's disease. *eMedicine.* Retrieved March 8, 2005, from http://www.emedicine.com/radio/topic83.htm.

Chen, A. 2004a. Muscular dystrophy. *MedlinePlus,* Retrieved November 10, 2004, from the U.S. National Library of Medicine and the National Institutes of Health: http://www.nlm.nih.gov/medlineplus/ency/article/001190.htm.

Chen, A. 2004b. Osteoarthritis. *MedlinePlus,* Retrieved November 10, 2004, from the U.S. National Library of Medicine and the National Institutes of Health: http://www.nlm.nih.gov/medlineplus/ency/article/000423.htm.

Chen, A. 2004c. Plantar fasciitis. *MedlinePlus,* Retrieved November 10, 2004, from the U.S. National Library of Medicine and the National Institutes of Health: http://www.nlm.nih.gov/medlineplus/ency/article/007021.htm.

Chen, A. 2004d. Scoliosis. *MedlinePlus,* Retrieved November 10, 2004, from the U.S. National Library of Medicine and the National Institutes of Health: http:// www.nlm.nih.gov/medlineplus/ency/article/001241.htm.

Chen, A. 2003a. Blount's disease. *MedlinePlus.* Retrieved March 10, 2005, from the U.S. National Library of Medicine and the National Institutes of Health: http://www.nlm.nih.gov/medlineplus/ency/article/001584.htm.

Chen, A. 2003b. Legg-Calve-Perthes disease. *MedlinePlus,* Retrieved November 10, 2004, from the U.S. National Library of Medicine and the National Institutes of Health: http://www.nlm.nih.gov/medlineplus/ency/article/001264.htm.

Chen, A. 2003c. Osgood-Schlatter disease. *MedlinePlus,* Retrieved November 10, 2004, from the U.S. National Library of Medicine and the National Institutes of Health: http://www.nlm.nih.gov/medlineplus/ency/article/001258.htm.

Chen, H. 2005. Cri du chat syndrome. *eMedicine.* Retrieved March 11, 2005, from http://www.emedicine.com/ped/topic504.htm.

Chen, H. 2003a. Klinefelter syndrome. *eMedicine,* Retrieved November 11, 2004, from: http://www.emedicine.com/ped/topic1252.htm.

Chen, H. 2003b. Marfan syndrome. *eMedicine,* Retrieved November 11, 2004, from http://www.emedicine.com/PED/topic1372.htm.

Chen, P. 2004a. Asherman's syndrome. *MedlinePlus.* Retrieved March 8, 2005, from the U.S. National Library of Medicine and the National Institutes of Health: http://www.nlm.nih.gov/medlineplus/ency/article/001483.htm.

Chen, P. 2004b. Endometriosis. *MedlinePlus,* Retrieved November 11, 2004, from the U.S. National Library of Medicine and the National Institutes of Health: http://www.nlm.nih.gov/medlineplus/ency/article/000915.htm.

Chen, P. 2004c. Ovarian cysts. *MedlinePlus,* Retrieved November 10, 2004, from the U.S. National Library of Medicine and the National Institutes of Health: http://www.nlm.nih.gov/medlineplus/ency/article/001504.htm.

Chen, P. 2004d. Sheehan's syndrome. *MedlinePlus,* Retrieved March 14, 2005, from the U.S. National Library of Medicine and the National Institutes of Health: http://www.nlm.nih.gov/medlineplus/ency/article/001175.htm.

Chijide, V. 2002. Balantidiasis. *eMedicine,* Retrieved November 12, 2004, from: http://www.emedicine.com/med/topic203.htm.

Chlamydia in the United States. 2001. Retrieved July 20, 2003, from the Division of Sexually Transmitted Diseases Prevention, National Center for HIV, STD, and TB Prevention. Centers for Disease Control and Prevention: http://www.cdc.gov/nchstp/dstd/Fact_Sheets/chlamydia_facts.htm

*Chronic fatigue syndrome.* 2003. CDC, Retrieved November 12, 2004, from the National Center for Infectious Diseases. Centers for Disease Control and Prevention: http://www.cdc.gov/ncidod/diseases/cfs/info.htm.

Chuang, T. 2003a. Keratoacanthoma. *eMedicine,* Retrieved November 11, 2004, from: http://www.emedicine.com/derm/topic206.htm.

Chuang, T., & Stitle, L. 2003. Lichen planus. *eMedicine,* Retrieved November 11, 2004, from: http://www.emedicine.com/derm/topic233.htm.

Cirrhosis of the liver. 2002. Retrieved June 7, 2003, from the National Digestive Diseases Information Clearinghouse, National Institutes of Health: http://www.niddk.nih.gov/health/digest/pubs/cirrhosi/cirrhosi.htm.

Cleft Palate Association. (n/d). About cleft lip and palate. Retrieved May 30, 2003, from http://www.cleftline.org/aboutclp.

Cleft Palate Foundation. 2003. About cleft lip and palate. Retrieved May 30, 2005, from http://www.cleftline.org/aboutclp/.

Clowse, M. 2003a. Henoch-Schonlein purpura. *MedlinePlus,* Retrieved November 10, 2004, from the U.S. National Library of Medicine and the National Institutes of Health: http://www.nlm.nih.gov/medlineplus/ency/article/000425.htm.

Clowse, M. 2003b. Raynaud's phenomenon. *MedlinePlus,* Retrieved November 10, 2004, from the U.S. National Library of Medicine and the National Institutes of Health: http://www.nlm.nih.gov/medlineplus/ency/article/000412.htm.

Clowse, M. 2003c. Reiter's syndrome. *MedlinePlus,* Retrieved November 10, 2004, from the U.S. National Library of Medicine and the National Institutes of Health: http://www.nlm.nih.gov/medlineplus/ency/article/000440.htm.

Clowse, M. 2003d. Sjogren syndrome. *MedlinePlus,* Retrieved November 10, 2004, from the U.S. National Library of Medicine and the National Institutes of Health: http://www.nlm.nih.gov/medlineplus/ency/article/000456.htm.

Clowse, M. 2003e. Systemic sclerosis (scleroderma). *MedlinePlus,* Retrieved November 10, 2004, from the U.S. National Library of Medicine and the National Institutes of Health: http://www.nlm.nih.gov/medlineplus/ency/article/000429.htm.

Clowse, M. 2003f. Temporal arteritis. *MedlinePlus,* Retrieved November 10, 2004, from the U.S. National Library of Medicine and the National Institutes of Health: http://www.nlm.nih.gov/medlineplus/ency/article/000448.htm.

Coccidioidomycosis. 2002. Retrieved July 26, 2003, from the National Center for Infectious Diseases, Division of Bacterial and Mycotic Diseases. Centers for Disease Control and Prevention: http://www.cdc.gov/ncidod/dbmd/diseaseinfo/coccidioidomycosis_t.htm.

Cohen, E. 2004a. Hemophilia A. *MedlinePlus,* Retrieved November 10, 2004, from the U.S. National Library of Medicine and the National Institutes of Health: http://www.nlm.nih.gov/medlineplus/ency/article/000538.htm.

Cohen, E. 2004b. Von Willebrand's disease. *MedlinePlus,* Retrieved November 12, 2004, from the U.S. National Library of Medicine and the National Institutes of Health: http://www.nlm.nih.gov/medlineplus/ency/article/000544.htm.

Cohen, E. 2003a. Hemolytic anemia. *MedlinePlus,* Retrieved November 10, 2004, from the U.S. National Library of Medicine and the National Institutes of Health: http://www.nlm.nih.gov/medlineplus/ency/article/000571.htm.

Cohen, E. 2003b. Fanconi's anemia. *MedlinePlus,* Retrieved March 12, 2005, from the U.S. National Library of Medicine and the National Institutes of Health: http://www.nlm.nih.gov/medlineplus/ency/article/000334.htm.

Cohen, E. 2003c. Sickle cell anemia. *MedlinePlus,* Retrieved November 10, 2004, from the U.S. National Library of Medicine and the National Institutes of Health: http://www.nlm.nih.gov/medlineplus/ency/article/000527.htm.

Cohen, E. 2003d. Thalassemia. *MedlinePlus,* Retrieved November 10, 2004, from the U.S. National Library of Medicine and the National Institutes of Health: http://www.nlm.nih.gov/medlineplus/ency/article/000587.htm.

Cohen, E. 2002. Primary brain tumor. *MedlinePlus,* Retrieved November 11, 2004, from the U.S. National Library of Medicine and the National Institutes of Health: http://www.nlm.nih.gov/medlineplus/ency/article/000768.htm.

Cole, C. 2002. Carbon monoxide poisoning. *eMedicine:* Retrieved June 9, 2003, from http://www.emedicine.com/aaem/topic92.htm.

Cooper, D. 2004a. Osteoporosis. *MedlinePlus,* Retrieved November 10, 2004, from the U.S. National Library of Medicine and the National Institutes of Health: http://www.nlm.nih.gov/medlineplus/ency/article/000360.htm.

Cooper, D. 2002b. Typhus. *MedlinePlus.* Retrieved July 26, 2003, from the U.S. National Library of Medicine and the National Institutes of Health: http://www.nlm.nih.gov/medlineplus/ency/article/001363.htm.

COPD International. 2005. Retrieved March 11, 2005, from http://www.copd-international.com/.

Corrigan, E. 1997. Cushing's fact sheet. Retrieved May 29, 2003, from the Cushing's Support and Research Foundation: http://world.std.com/~csrf/factsheet.html#cushing.

Crawford, A. 2002. Neurofibromatosis. *eMedicine,* Retrieved November 11, 2004, from: http://www.emedicine.com/orthoped/topic525.htm.

Crawford, G. 2003. Erythrasma. *MedlinePlus,* Retrieved November 11, 2004, from the U.S. National Library of Medicine and the National Institutes of Health: http://www.nlm.nih.gov/medlineplus/ency/article/001470.htm.

Crowe, M. 2004. Molluscum contagiosum. *eMedicine,* Retrieved November 11, 2004, from: http://www.emedicine.com/ped/topic1759.htm.

Cryptosporidiosis. 2003. Retrieved July 26, 2003, from the National Center for Infectious Diseases, Division of Parasitic Infections. Centers for Disease Control and Prevention: http://www.cdc.gov/ncidod/dpd/parasites/cryptosporidiosis/default.htm.

Cutler, C. 2003. Paroxysmal nocturnal hemoglobinuria. *MedlinePlus,* Retrieved November 10, 2004, from the U.S. National Library of Medicine and the National Institutes of Health: http://www.nlm.nih.gov/medlineplus/ency/article/000534.htm.

Cystic fibrosis research directions. 1997. Retrieved May 30, 2003, from the National Institutes of Health, National Institute of Diabetes and Digestive and Kidney Disorders: http://www.niddk.nih.gov/health/endo/pubs/cystic/cystic.htm.

*Cysticercosis.* 2003. *DPD,* Retrieved November 12, 2004, from the National Center for Infectious Diseases, Division of Parasitic Diseases. Centers for Disease Control and Prevention: http://www.cdc.gov/ncidod/dpd/parasites/cysticercosis/factsht_cysticercosis.htm.

Cytomegalovirus (CMV) infection. 2002. Retrieved July 26, 2003, from the National Center for Infectious Diseases, Centers for Disease Control and Prevention: http://www.cdc.gov/ncidod/diseases/cmv.htm.

Davey, M., & Altman, L. 2003. Suspected cases of monkeypox are rising. *New York Times*. Electronic Version, June 10: Retrieved June 10, 2003, from http://www.nytimes.com/2003/06/10/national/10DOGS.html?th.

Davis, L., & Benbensity, K. 2003. Erysipelas. *eMedicine*. Retrieved March 12, 2005, from http://www.emedicine.com/derm/topic129.htm.

De Beus, A. 2004. Retinitis pigmentosa. *eMedicine*, Retrieved November 11, 2004, from: http://www.emedicine.com/oph/topic704.htm.

Debemardo, R. 2004a. Nabothian cyst. *MedlinePlus*, Retrieved November 10, 2004, from the U.S. National Library of Medicine and the National Institutes of Health: http://www.nlm.nih.gov/medlineplus/ency/article/001514.htm.

*Dengue fever*. 2003. CDC, Retrieved November 12, 2004, from the National Center for Infectious Diseases, Division of Vector-Borne Infectious Diseases. Centers for Disease Control and Prevention: http://www.cdc.gov/ncidod/dvbid/dengue/index.htm.

Devarajan, P. 2004. Alport syndrome. *eMedicine*, Retrieved November 11, 2004, from: http://www.emedicine.com/ped/topic74.htm.

*Dientamoeba fragilis infection*. 2004. DPD, Retrieved November 12, 2004, from the National Center for Infectious Diseases, Division of Parasitic Diseases. Centers for Disease Control and Prevention: http://www.cdc.gov/ncidod/dpd/parasites/dientamoeba/factsht_dientamoeba.htm.

*DiGeorge syndrome*. 2002. Retrieved November 11, 2004, from: http://nvnv.essortment.com/digeorgesyndrom_ruuh.htm.

*DiGeorge syndrome* NCBI. 2004. Retrieved November 11, 2004, from the National Center for Biotechnology Information, National Library of Medicine. National Institute of Health: http://www.ncbi.nlm.nih.gov/books/bv.fcgi?call=bv.View.ShowSection&rid=gnd.section.150.

*DiGeorge syndrome* NPIRC. 2004. *Info4PI*, Retrieved November 11, 2004, from National Primary Immunodeficiency Resource Center. Jeffrey Modell Foundation: http://npi.jmfworld.org/patienttopatient/index.cfm?section=patient-topatient&content=syndromes&area=3&CFID= 5494170&CFTOKEN=75925349.

Dixon, T. 1999. Anthrax. *New England Journal of Medicine*, 341:815–826.

Do, T. 2002. Muscular dystrophy. *eMedicine*. Retrieved March 13, 2005, from http://www.emedicine.com/orthoped/topic418.htm.

Donaldson, J. 2003. Mastoiditis. *eMedicine*, Retrieved November 11, 2004, from: http://www.emedicine.com/ped/topic1379.htm.

Donegan, W., Spratt, J., & Orsini, J. (Eds.). 2002. *Cancer of the Breast*. Philadelphia: W.B. Saunders.

Douglas, R. 2002. Scleritis. *MedlinePlus*, Retrieved November 10, 2004, from the U.S. National Library of Medicine and the National Institutes of Health: http://www.nlm.nih.gov/medlineplus/ency/article/001003.htm.

DPD. 2004. *Acanthamoeba infection*. Retrieved November 12, 2004, from the National Center for Infectious Diseases, Division of Parasitic Diseases. Centers for Disease Control and Prevention: http://www.cdc.gov/ncid.

*Dracunculiasis*. 2004. DPD, Retrieved November 12, 2004, from the National Center for Infectious Diseases, Division of Parasitic Diseases. Centers for Disease Control and Prevention: http://www.cdc.gov/ncidod/dpd/parasites/guineaworm/factsht_guineaworm.htm.

Drayer, J. 2003a. Acrodermatitis. *MedlinePlus*. Retrieved November 24, 2004, from the U.S. National Library of Medicine and the National Institutes of Health: http://www.nlm.nih.gov/medlineplus/ency/article/001446.htm.

Drayer, J. 2003b. Ichthyosis vulgaris. *MedlinePlus*. Retrieved March 13, 2005, from the U.S. National Library of Medicine and the National Institutes of Health: http://www.nlm.nih.gov/medlineplus/ency/article/001451.htm.

Drayer, J. 2003c. Xanthelasma and Xanthoma. *MedlinePlus*, Retrieved November 10, 2004, from the U.S. National Library of Medicine and the National Institutes of Health: http://www.nlm.nih.gov/medlineplus/ency/article/001447.htm.

Ebola hemorrhagic fever. 2002. Retrieved July 26, 2003, from the National Center for Infectious Diseases, Division of Viral and Rickettsial Diseases, Special Pathogens Branch. Centers for Disease Control and Prevention: http://www.cdc.gov/ncidod/dvrd/spb/mnpages/dispages/ebola.htm.

Edwards, B. 2003. Encephalitis. Retrieved March 16, 2004, from the Brain and Nervous Systems Center of the Mayo Clinic: http://www.mayoclinic.com/invoke.cfm?id=DS00226.

Egland, A. 2001. Temporal arteritis. *eMedicine*: Retrieved June 4, 2003, from http://www.emedicine.com/EMERG/topic568.htm.

Enneking, W. 1995. Osteosarcoma. *Musculoskeletal Pathology*. Retrieved May 29, 2003, from http://www.med.ufl.edu/medinfo/ortho/ostsarc.html#A1.

Epidemic louse-borne typhus. 1998. Retrieved July 26, 2003, from the World Health Organization, Geneva: http://www.who.int/inf-fs/en/fact162.html.

Epstein-Barr virus and infectious mononucleosis. 2002. Retrieved July 26, 2003, from the National Center for Infectious Diseases, Centers for Disease Control and Prevention: http://www.cdc.gov/ncidod/diseases/ebv.htm.

*Erythroblastosis fetalis*. 2002. *MedlinePlus*, Retrieved November 10, 2004, from the U.S. National Library of Medicine and the National Institutes of Health: http://www.nlm.nih.gov/medlineplus/ency/article/001298.htm.

Facts about Down syndrome. 2003. Retrieved May 30, 2003, from the National Institutes of Health, National Institute for Child Health and Human Development: http://www.nichd.nih.gov/publications/pubs/downsyndrome/down.htm#DownSyndrome.

Farrar, R. 1989. Erysipelothrix rhusiopathiae: an occupational pathogen. *Pubmed*, Retrieved November 11, 2004, from National Library of Medicine, Department of Health and Human Services. National Center of Biotechnology Information: http://www.ncbi.nlm.nih.gov/entrez/query.fcgi?cmd=Retrieve&db=PubMed&dopt=Abstract&list_uids= 90030167.

*Fascioliasis*. 2004. *DPDx*, Retrieved November 12, 2004, from the National Center for Infectious Diseases, Division of Parasitic Diseases. Centers for Disease Control and Prevention: http://www.dpd.cdc.gov/dpdx/HTM.L/Fascioliasis.htm.

Feinberg, E. 2004a. Episcleritis. R *MedlinePlus*, Retrieved November 11, 2004, from the U.S. National Library of Medicine and the National Institutes of Health: http://www.nlm.nih.gov/medlineplus/ency/article/001019.htm.

Feinberg, E. 2004b. Glaucoma. *MedlinePlus*, Retrieved November 11, 2004, from the U.S. National Library of Medicine and the National Institutes of Health: http://www.nlm.nih.gov/medlineplus/ency/article/001620.htm.

Feinberg, E. 2004c. Macular degeneration. *MedlinePlus*, Retrieved November 10, 2004, from the U.S. National Library of Medicine and the National Institutes of Health: http://www.nlm.nih.gov/medlineplus/ency/article/001000.htm.

Felter, R. 2001. Pediatrics, Epiglottis. *eMedicine*, Retrieved November 11, 2004, from: http://www.emedicine.com/emerg/topic375.htm.

*Filariasis*. 2004. *DPDx*, Retrieved November 12, 2004, from the National Center for Infectious Diseases, Division of Parasitic Diseases. Centers for Disease Control and Prevention: http://www.dpd.cdc.gov/dpdx/HTM.L/Filariasis.htm.

Fine, S. 2002. Treponematosis (endemic syphilis). *eMedicine*, Retrieved November 11, 2004, from: http://www.emedicine.com/med/topic2305.htm.

Fishman, A. 2002. Kaposi sarcoma. *eMedicine*, Retrieved November 11, 2004, from: http://www.emedicine.com/med/topic1218.htm.

Foye, P. 2004. De Quervain tenosynovitis. *eMedicine*, Retrieved November 11, 2004, from: http://www.emedicine.com/pmr/topic36.htm.

Frank, C. 2004. Hallux valgus. *eMedicine*, Retrieved November 11, 2004, from: http://www.emedicine.com/orthoped/topic126.htm.

Franklin, D. 1984. Pain killer abuse spells renal damage. *Science News*. 125 (10): 151–152.

Frasseto, L. 2004. Bartter's syndrome. *eMedicine*, Retrieved March 8, 2005, from http://www.emedicine.com/med/topic213.htm.

Fratterelli, D. 2002. DiGeorge syndrome. *eMedicine*, Retrieved November 11, 2004, from: http://www.emedicine.com/ped/topic589.htm.

Freedman, K. 2004. Carpal tunnel syndrome. *MedlinePlus*. Retrieved March 10, 2005, from the U.S. National Library of Medicine and the National Institutes of Health: http://www.nlm.nih.gov/medlineplus/ency/article/000433.htm.

Fretz, P., & Hughes, J. 2003. Adenocarcinoma: Lung tumors. Retrieved May 29, 2003, from the Virtual Hospital, University of Iowa Health Care:http://www.vh.org/adult/provider/radiology/LungTumors/PathologicTypes/Text/Adenocarcinoma.html.

Freytes, C. 2002. Lymphoma, Follicular. *eMedicine*, Retrieved November 11, 2004, from: http://www.emedicine.com/med/topic1362.htm.

Frye, R., & Tamer, M. 2005. Bacterial overgrowth syndrome. *eMedicine*, Retrieved March 10, 2005, from http://www.emedicine.com/med/topic198.htm.

Frye, R., & Tamer, M. 2002. Malabsorption syndromes. *eMedicine*, Retrieved November 11, 2004, from: http://www.emedicine.com/ped/topic1356.htm.

Fung, K. 2004. Otosclerosis. *MedlinePlus*, Retrieved November 10, 2004, from the U.S. National Library of Medicine and the National Institutes of Health: http://www.nlm.nih.gov/medlineplus/ency/article/001036.htm.

Gatti, J. 2003. Hypospadias. *eMedicine*, Retrieved November 11, 2004, from: http://www.emedicine.com/ped/topic1136.htm.

Gaudier, F. 2003. Placenta previa. *MedlinePlus*, Retrieved November 10, 2004, from the U.S. National Library of Medicine and the National Institutes of Health: http://www.nlm.nih.gov/medlineplus/ency/article/000900.htm.

Gaufberg, S. 2004. Abruptio placentae. *eMedicine*, Retrieved November 11, 2004, from: http://www.emedicine.com/emerg/topic12.htm.

Genital herpes. 2001. Retrieved July 26, 2003, from the National Center for HIV, STDs, and TB Prevention, Division of HIV/AIDS Prevention. Centers for Disease Control and Prevention: http://www.cdc.gov/nchstp/dstd/Fact_Sheets/facts_Genital_Herpes.htm.

*Gerstmann-Straussler-Scheinker disease.* 2003. Retrieved November 11, 2004, from the National Institute of Neurological Disorders and Stroke. National Institutes of Health: http://www.ninds.nih.gov/health_and_medical/disorders/gss.htm.

Giardiasis. 2001. Retrieved July 26, 2003, from the National Center for Infectious Diseases, Division of Parasitic Infections. Centers for Disease Control and Prevention: http://www.cdc.gov/ncidod/dpd/parasites/giardiasis/factsht_giardia.htm.

Giardino, A., & Giardino, E. 2004. Fibromyalgia. *eMedicine*. Retrieved March 12, 2005, from http://www.emedicine.com/ped/topic777.htm.

Gilbert, S. 2004a. Hypospadias. *MedlinePlus*, Retrieved November 11, 2004, from the U.S. National Library of Medicine and the National Institutes of Health: http://www.nlm.nih.gov/medlineplus/ency/article/001286.htm.

Gilbert, S. 2004b. Orchitis. *MedlinePlus*, Retrieved November 10, 2004, from the U.S. National Library of Medicine and the National Institutes of Health: http://www.nlm.nih.gov/medlineplus/ency/article/001280.htm.

Gilbert, S. 2004c. Prostatitis. *MedlinePlus*, Retrieved November 10, 2004, from the U.S. National Library of Medicine and the National Institutes of Health: http://www.nlm.nih.gov/medlineplus/ency/article/000523.htm.

Gilbert, S. 2004d. Unilateral hydronephrosis. *MedlinePlus*, Retrieved November 10, 2004, from the U.S. National Library of Medicine and the National Institutes of Health: http://www.nlm.nih.gov/medlineplus/ency/article/000506.htm.

Gilbert, S. 2003a. Balanitis. *MedlinePlus*. Retrieved March 8, 2005, from the U.S. National Library of Medicine and the National Institutes of Health: http://www.nlm.nih.gov/medlineplus/ency/article/000862.htm.

Gilbert, S. 2003b. Hydrocele. *MedlinePlus*, Retrieved November 10, 2004, from the U.S. National Library of Medicine and the National Institutes of Health: http://www.nlm.nih.gov/medlineplus/ency/article/000518.htm.

*Gnathostomiasis*. 2004. DPDx, Retrieved November 12, 2004, from the National Center for Infectious Diseases, Division of Parasitic Diseases. Centers for Disease Control and Prevention:http://ww.dpd.cdc.gov/dpdx/HTM.L/gnathostomiasis.htm.

Goldenring, J. 2004a. Aicardi syndrome. *MedlinePlus*. Retrieved March 8, 2005, from the U.S. National Library of Medicine and the National Institutes of Health: http://www.nlm.nih.gov/medlineplus/ency/article/001664.htm.

Goldenring, J. 2004b. Gastroschisis. *MedlinePlus*, Retrieved November 11, 2004, from the U.S. National Library of Medicine and the National Institutes of Health: http://www.nlm.nih.gov/medlineplus/ency/article/000992.htm.

Goldenring, J. 2004c. Hydrocephalus. *MedlinePlus*, Retrieved November 10, 2004, from the U.S. National Library of Medicine and the National Institutes of Health: http://www.nlm.nih.gov/medlineplus/ency/article/001571.htm.

Goldenring, J. 2004d. Neonatal conjunctivitis. *MedlinePlus*, Retrieved November 10, 2004, from the U.S. National Library of Medicine and the National Institutes of Health: http://www.nlm.nih.gov/medlineplus/ency/article/001606.htm.

Goldenring, J. 2004e. Pertussis. *MedlinePlus*, Retrieved November 10, 2004, from the U.S. National Library of Medicine and the National Institutes of Health: http://www.nlm.nih.gov/medlineplus/ency/article/001561.htm.

Goldenring, J. 2004f. Phenylketonuria. *MedlinePlus*, Retrieved November 10, 2004, from the U.S. National Library of Medicine and the National Institutes of Health: http://www.nlm.nih.gov/medlineplus/ency/article/001166.htm.

Goldenring, J. 2004g. Reye's syndrome. *MedlinePlus*, Retrieved November 10, 2004, from the U.S. National Library of Medicine and the National Institutes of Health: http://www.nlm.nih.gov/medlineplus/ency/article/001565.htm.

Goldenring, J. 2004h. Rickets. *MedlinePlus*, Retrieved November 10, 2004, from the U.S. National Library of Medicine and the National Institutes of Health: http://www.nlm.nih.gov/medlineplus/ency/article/000344.htm.

Goldenring, J. 2004i. Sudden infant death syndrome. *MedlinePlus*, Retrieved March 14, 2005, from the U.S. National Library of Medicine and the National Institutes of Health: http://www.nlm.nih.gov/medlineplus/ency/article/001566.htm.

Goldenring, J. 2003a. Hand-foot-mouth disease. *MedlinePlus*, Retrieved November 10, 2004, from the U.S. National Library of Medicine and the National Institutes of Health: http://www.nlm.nih.gov/medlineplus/ency/article/000965.htm.

Goldenring, J. 2003b. Scarlet fever. *MedlinePlus*, Retrieved November 10, 2004, from the U.S. National Library of Medicine and the National Institutes of Health: http://www.nlm.nih.gov/medlineplus/ency/article/000974.htm.

Gonorrhea. 2001. Retrieved July 26, 2003, from the National Center for HIV, STD, and TB Prevention, Division of Sexually Transmitted Diseases. Centers for Disease Control and Prevention: http://www.cdc.gov/nchstp/dstd/Fact_Sheets/FactsGonorrhea.htm.

Gowda, A., & Nzerue, C. 2003. Pyelonephritis, chronic. *eMedicine*: Retrieved June 9, 2003, from http://www.emedicine.com/med/topic2841.htm.

*Gnathostomiasis.* 2004. *DPDx*, Retrieved November 12, 2004, from the National Center for Infectious Diseases, Division of Parasitic Diseases. Centers for Disease Control and Prevention: http://www.dpd.cdc.gov/dpdx/HTM.L/ gnathostomiasis.htm.

Graham, P. 2004. Roseola. *MedlinePlus*, Retrieved November 10, 2004, from the U.S. National Library of Medicine and the National Institutes of Health: http://www.nlm.nih.gov/medlineplus/ency/article/000968.htm.

Graham, P. 2003. Craniotabes. *MedlinePlus*. Retrieved March 8, 2005, from the U.S. National Library of Medicine and the National Institutes of Health: http://www.nlm.nih.gov/medlineplus/ency/article/001591.htm.

Graham, P. 2002. Bartter's syndrome. *MedlinePlus*. Retrieved March 8, 2005, from the U.S. National Library of Medicine and the National Institutes of Health: http://www.nlm.nih.gov/medlineplus/ency/article/000308.htm.

Green, R. 2003. Lung cancer. *MedlinePlus*, Retrieved November 10, 2004, from the U.S. National Library of Medicine and the National Institutes of Health: http://www.nlm.nih.gov/medlineplus/ency/article/007194.htm.

Greene, A. 2004a. Common cold. *MedlinePlus*, Retrieved November 11, 2004, from the U.S. National Library of Medicine and the National Institutes of Health: http://www.nlm.nih.gov/medlineplus/ency/article/000678.htm.

Greene, A. 2004b. Ear infection. *MedlinePlus*, Retrieved November 10, 2004, from the U.S. National Library of Medicine and the National Institutes of Health: http://www.nlm.nih.gov/medlineplus/ency/article/000638.htm.

Greene, A. 2004c. Strep throat. *MedlinePlus*, Retrieved November 10, 2004, from the U.S. National Library of Medicine and the National Institutes of Health: http://www.nlm.nih.gov/medlineplus/ency/article/000639.htm.

Greene, A. 2003. The flu. *MedlinePlus*, Retrieved November 10, 2004, from the U.S. National Library of Medicine and the National Institutes of Health: http://www.nlm.nih.gov/medlineplus/ency/article/000080.htm.

Grethlein, S. 2004. Multiple myeloma. *eMedicine*, Retrieved November 11, 2004, from: http://www.emedicine.com/med/topic1521.htm.

Grigsby, D. 2003. Malnutrition. *eMedicine*. Retrieved March 13, 2005, from http://www.emedicine.com/ped/topic1360.htm.

Grund, S. 2004a. Hepatocellular carcinoma. *MedlinePlus*, Retrieved November 10, 2004, from the U.S. National Library of Medicine and the National Institutes of Health: http://www.nlm.nih.gov/medlineplus/ency/article/ 000280.htm.

Grund, S. 2004b. Hodgkin's lymphoma. *MedlinePlus*, Retrieved November 10, 2004, from the U.S. National Library of Medicine and the National Institutes of Health: http://www.nlm.nih.gov/medlineplus/ency/article/000580.htm.

Grund, S. 2004c. Kaposi's sarcoma. *MedlinePlus*, Retrieved November 10, 2004, from the U.S. National Library of Medicine and the National Institutes of Health: http://www.nlm.nih.gov/medlineplus/ency/article/000661.htm.

Grund, S. 2004d. Leukoplakia. *MedlinePlus*, Retrieved November 10, 2004, from the U.S. National Library of Medicine and the National Institutes of Health: http://www.nlm.nih.gov/medlineplus/ency/article/001046.htm.

Grund, S. 2004e. Squamous cell cancer. *MedlinePlus*, Retrieved November 10, 2004, from the U.S. National Library of Medicine and the National Institutes of Health: http://www.nlm.nih.gov/medlineplus/ency/article/000829.htm.

Grund, S. 2004f. Testicular cancer. *MedlinePlus*, Retrieved November 10, 2004, from the U.S. National Library of Medicine and the National Institutes of Health: http://www.nlm.nih.gov/medlineplus/ency/article/001288.htm.

Grund, S. 2004g. Thrombocytopenia. *MedlinePlus,* Retrieved November 10, 2004, from the U.S. National Library of Medicine and the National Institutes of Health: http://www.nlm.nih.gov/medlineplus/ency/article/000586.htm.

*Haemophilus influenzae* serotype b (Hib) disease. 2003. Retrieved July 19, 2003, from the Division of Bacterial and Mycotic Diseases, Centers for Disease Control and Prevention: http://www.cdc.gov/ncidod/dbmd/diseaseinfo/haeminfluserob_t.htm.

Hait, E. 2002. Cystic fibrosis. *MedlinePlus,* Retrieved November 11, 2004, from the U.S. National Library of Medicine and the National Institutes of Health: http://www.nlm.nih.gov/medlineplus/ency/article/000107.htm.

*Hand, foot, and mouth disease.* 2001. *CDC,* Retrieved November 12, 2004, from the National Center for Infectious Diseases, Respiratory and Enteric Viruses Branch. Centers for Disease Control and Prevention:http://www.cdc.gov/ncidod/dvrd/revb/enterovirus/hfhf.htm.

Hanly, E. 2004. Buerger disease. *eMedicine,* Retrieved November 11, 2004, from: http://www.emedicine.com/med/topic253.htm.

*Hansen's disease.* 2004. *CDC,* Retrieved November 12, 2004, from the National Center for Infectious Diseases, Division of Bacterial and Mycotic Diseases. Centers for Disease Control and Prevention: http://www.cdc.gov/ncidod/dbmd/diseaseinfo/hansens_t.htm.

Harris, G. 2004. Legg-Calve-Perthes disease. *eMedicine,* Retrieved November 11, 2004, from: http://www.emedicine.com/orthoped/topic458.htm.

Hart, J. 2004a. Albinism. *MedlinePlus.* Retrieved March 8, 2005, from the U.S. National Library of Medicine and the National Institutes of Health: http://www.nlm.nih.gov/medlineplus/ency/article/001479.htm.

Hart, J. 2004b. Autism. *MedlinePlus,* Retrieved March 8, 2005, from the U.S. National Library of Medicine and the National Institutes of Health: http://www.nlm.nih.gov/medlineplus/ency/article/001526.htm.

Hart, J. 2004c. Beriberi. *MedlinePlus,* Retrieved March 8, 2005, from the U.S. National Library of Medicine and the National Institutes of Health: http://www.nlm.nih.gov/medlineplus/ency/article/000339.htm.

Hart, J. 2004d. Gangrene. *MedlinePlus,* Retrieved November 11, 2004, from the U.S. National Library of Medicine and the National Institutes of Health: http://www.nlm.nih.gov/medlineplus/ency/article/007218.htm.

Hart, J. 2004e. Genital warts. *MedlinePlus,* Retrieved November 10, 2004, from the U.S. National Library of Medicine and the National Institutes of Health: http://www.nlm.nih.gov/medlineplus/ency/article/000886.htm.

Hart, J. 2004f. Heart failure. *MedlinePlus,* Retrieved November 11, 2004, from the U.S. National Library of Medicine and the National Institutes of Health: http://www.nlm.nih.gov/medlineplus/ency/article/000158.htm.

Hart, J. 2004g. Mesothelioma. *MedlinePlus,* Retrieved November 10, 2004, from the U.S. National Library of Medicine and the National Institutes of Health: http://www.nlm.nih.gov/medlineplus/ency/article/000115.htm.

Hart, J. 2004h. Mononucleosis. *MedlinePlus,* Retrieved November 10, 2004, from the U.S. National Library of Medicine and the National Institutes of Health: http://www.nlm.nih.gov/medlineplus/ency/article/000591.htm.

Hart, J. 2004i. Morning sickness. *MedlinePlus,* Retrieved November 10, 2004, from the U.S. National Library of Medicine and the National Institutes of Health: http://www.nlm.nih.gov/medlineplus/ency/article/003119.htm.

Hart, J. 2004j. Pericarditis. *MedlinePlus,* Retrieved November 10, 2004, from the U.S. National Library of Medicine and the National Institutes of Health: http://www.nlm.nih.gov/medlineplus/ency/article/000182.htm.

Hart, J. 2004k. Pernicious anemia. *MedlinePlus*, Retrieved November 10, 2004, from the U.S. National Library of Medicine and the National Institutes of Health: http://www.nlm.nih.gov/medlineplus/ency/article/000569.htm.

Hart, J. 2004l. Polycythemia vera. *MedlinePlus*, Retrieved November 10, 2004, from the U.S. National Library of Medicine and the National Institutes of Health: http://www.nlm.nih.gov/medlineplus/ency/article/000589.htm.

Hart, J. 2004m. Psittacosis. *MedlinePlus*, Retrieved November 10, 2004, from the U.S. National Library of Medicine and the National Institutes of Health: http://www.nlm.nih.gov/medlineplus/ency/article/000088.htm.

Hart, J. 2004n. Splenomegaly. *MedlinePlus*, Retrieved November 10, 2004, from the U.S. National Library of Medicine and the National Institutes of Health: http://www.nlm.nih.gov/medlineplus/ency/article/003276.htm.

Hart, J. 2003b. Heart Attack. *MedlinePlus*, Retrieved November 10, 2004, from the U.S. National Library of Medicine and the National Institutes of Health: http://www.nlm.nih.gov/medlineplus/ency/article/000195.htm.

Hart, J. 2003b. Hemorrhoids. *MedlinePlus*, Retrieved November 10, 2004, from the U.S. National Library of Medicine and the National Institutes of Health: http://www.nlm.nih.gov/medlineplus/ency/article/000292.htm.

Hart, J. 2003c. Hepatitis. *MedlinePlus*, Retrieved November 10, 2004, from the U.S. National Library of Medicine and the National Institutes of Health: http://www.nlm.nih.gov/medlineplus/ency/article/001154.htm.

Hart, J. 2003d. Hernia. *MedlinePlus*, Retrieved November 10, 2004, from the U.S. National Library of Medicine and the National Institutes of Health: http://www.nlm.nih.gov/medlineplus/ency/article/000960.htm.

Hart, J. 2003e. Hives. *MedlinePlus*, Retrieved November 10, 2004, from the U.S. National Library of Medicine and the National Institutes of Health: http://www.nlm.nih.gov/medlineplus/ency/article/000845.htm.

Hart, J. 2003f. Hypertensive heart disease. *MedlinePlus*, Retrieved November 11, 2004, from the U.S. National Library of Medicine and the National Institutes of Health: http://www.nlm.nih.gov/medlineplus/ency/article/000163.htm.

Hart, J. 2003g. Stroke. *MedlinePlus*, Retrieved November 10, 2004, from the U.S. National Library of Medicine and the National Institutes of Health: http://www.nlm.nih.gov/medlineplus/ency/article/000726.htm.

Hart, J. 2003h. Peptic ulcer. *MedlinePlus*, Retrieved November 10, 2004, from the U.S. National Library of Medicine and the National Institutes of Health: http://www.nlm.nih.gov/medlineplus/ency/article/000206.htm.

Hart, J. 2003i. Pneumonia. *MedlinePlus*, Retrieved November 10, 2004, from the U.S. National Library of Medicine and the National Institutes of Health: http://www.nlm.nih.gov/medlineplus/ency/article/000145.htm.

Hart, J. 2003j. Ringworm. *MedlinePlus*, Retrieved November 10, 2004, from the U.S. National Library of Medicine and the National Institutes of Health: http://www.nlm.nih.gov/medlineplus/ency/article/001439.htm.

Hart, J. 2003k. Sinusitis. *MedlinePlus*, Retrieved November 10, 2004, from the U.S. National Library of Medicine and the National Institutes of Health: http://www.nlm.nih.gov/medlineplus/ency/article/000647.htm.

Hart, J. 2003l. Tay-Sachs disease. *MedlinePlus*, Retrieved November 10, 2004, from the U.S. National Library of Medicine and the National Institutes of Health: http://www.nlm.nih.gov/medlineplus/ency/article/001417.htm.

Hart, J. 2003m. Urinary tract infection. *MedlinePlus*, Retrieved November 10, 2004, from the U.S. National Library of Medicine and the National Institutes of Health: http://www.nlm.nih.gov/medlineplus/ency/article/000521.htm.

Hart, J. 2004. Canavan disease. *MedlinePlus*, Retrieved November 11, 2004, from the U.S. National Library of Medicine and the National Institutes of Health: http://www.nlm.nih.gov/medlineplus/ency/article/001586.htm.

*Health Matters*. 2001. The common cold. Retrieved March 16, 2004, from the National Institute of Allergy and Infectious Diseases, National Institutes of Health, U.S. Department of Health and Human Services: http://www.niaid.nih.gov/factsheets/cold.htm.

Hecht, B. 2004. Pelvic inflammatory disease. *MedlinePlus*, Retrieved November 10, 2004, from the U.S. National Library of Medicine and the National Institutes of Health: http://www.nlm.nih.gov/medlineplus/ency/article/000888.htm.

*Hendra virus disease and nipah virus encephalitis*. 2004. CDC, Retrieved November 12, 2004, from the National Center for Infectious Diseases, Special Pathogens Branch. Centers for Disease Control and Prevention: http://www.cdc.gov/ncidod/dvrd/spb/mnpages/dispages/nipah.htm.

*Hereditary bleeding disorders*. 2004. CDC, Retrieved November 12, 2004, from the National Center on Birth Defects and Developmental Disabilities. Centers for Disease Control and Prevention: http://www.cdc.gov/ncbddd/hbd/hemophilia.htm.

*Heterophyes heterophyes*. 2004. *Graphic Images of Parasites*, Retrieved November 12, 2004, from the College of Biological Sciences. The Ohio State University: http://www.biosci.ohio-state.edu/~parasite/heterophyes.htm.l.

*Heterophyiasis*. 2004. *DPDx*, Retrieved November 12, 2004, from the National Center for Infectious Diseases, Division of Parasitic Diseases. Centers for Disease Control and Prevention: http://www.dpd.cdc.gov/dpdx/HTM.L/heterophyiasis.htm.

*Histoplasmosis*. 2003. Retrieved July 26, 2003, from the National Center for Infectious Diseases, Division of Bacterial and Mycotic Diseases. Centers for Disease Control and Prevention: http://www.cdc.gov/ncidod/dbmd/diseaseinfo/histoplasmosis_g.htm.

Hiong, C., & Cunha, B. 2004. Escherichia coli infections. *eMedicine*. Retrieved March 12, 2005, from http://www.emedicine.com/med/topic734.htm.

*Hookworm infection*. 1999. *DPDx*, Retrieved November 12, 2004, from the National Center for Infectious Diseases, Division of Parasitic Diseases. Centers for Disease Control and Prevention: http://www.cdc.gov/ncidod/dpd/parasites/hookworm/factsht_hookworm.htm.

Horenstein, M., & McNeil, J. 2004. Xanthomas. *eMedicine*, Retrieved November 11, 2004, from: http://www.emedicine.com/derm/topic461.htm.

Howard, S. 2003. Melanoma. *MedlinePlus*, Retrieved November 10, 2004, from the U.S. National Library of Medicine and the National Institutes of Health: http://www.nlm.nih.gov/medlineplus/ency/article/000850.htm.

Huang, H. 2002. Burkitt lymphoma. *eMedicine*, Retrieved November 11, 2004, from: http://www.emedicine.com/med/topic256.htm.

*Human ehrlichiosis in the United States*. 2000. CDC, Retrieved November 12, 2004, from the National Center for Infectious Diseases, Viral and Rickettsial Zoonoses Branch. Centers for Disease Control and Prevention: http://www.cdc.gov/ncidod/dvrd/ehrlichia/Index.htm.

Human papilloma virus. 1997. Retrieved May 29, 2003, from the Department of Gynecology and Obstetrics, University of Iowa: http://obgyn.uihc.uiowa.edu/Patinfo/Adhealth/hpv.htm.

Hurtado, R. 2003. Pharyngitis. *MedlinePlus*. Retrieved March 15, 2004, from http://www.nlm.nih.gov/medlineplus/ency/article/000655.htm.

Hydrocephalus. 2003. *MEDLINEplus*. Retrieved July 25, 2003, from the U.S. National Library of Medicine and the National Institutes of Health: http://www.nlm.nih.gov/medlineplus/hydrocephalus.html.

*Hymenolepiasis*. 2004. *DPDx*, Retrieved November 12, 2004, from the National Center for Infectious Diseases, Division of Parasitic Diseases. Centers for Disease Control and Prevention: http://www.dpd.cdc.gov/dpdx/HTM.L/ Hymenolepiasis.htm.

Incesu, L., & Khosla, A. 2004. Meningitis, bacterial. *eMedicine*. Retrieved March 14, 2005, from http://www.emedicine.com/radio/topic441.htm.

Influenza (the flu). 2003. Retrieved July 26, 2003, from the National Center for Infectious Diseases, Division of Viral and Rickettsial Diseases, Special Pathogens Branch. Centers for Disease Control and Prevention: http://www.cdc.gov/ncidod/ diseases/flu/fluinfo.htm.

Internet Stroke Center. 2003. Retrieved July 25, 2003, from the University of Washington in St. Louis: http://www.strokecenter.org/prof/index.html.

Interstitial cystitis. 2002. Retrieved June 9, 2003, from the National Kidney and Urologic Diseases Information Clearinghouse, National Institutes of Health: http://www.niddk.nih.gov/health/urolog/pubs/cystitis/cystitis.htm.

Jackson, I. 2004. Congenital syndromes. *eMedicine*. Retrieved March 15, 2005, from http://www.emedicine.com/plastic/topic183.htm.

Jain, T. 2004a. Gynecomastia. *MedlinePlus*, Retrieved November 11, 2004, from the U.S. National Library of Medicine and the National Institutes of Health: http://www.nlm.nih.gov/medlineplus/ency/article/003165.htm.

Jain, T. 2004b. Paget's disease. *MedlinePlus*, Retrieved March 14, 2005, from the U.S. National Library of Medicine and the National Institutes of Health: http://www.nlm.nih.gov/medlineplus/ency/article/000414.htm.

Jain, T. 2003c. Goiter. *MedlinePlus*, Retrieved November 11, 2004, from the U.S. National Library of Medicine and the National Institutes of Health: http://www.nlm.nih.gov/medlineplus/ency/article/001178.htm.

Jinnah, H. 2002. Lesch-Nyhan syndrome. *eMedicine*. Retrieved March 13, 2005, from http://www.emedicine.com/neuro/topic630.htm.

Jasmin, L. 2004. Subdural hematoma. *MedlinePlus*, Retrieved November 10, 2004, from the U.S. National Library of Medicine and the National Institutes of Health: http://www.nlm.nih.gov/medlineplus/ency/article/000713.htm.

Johnson, C. 2004. Acute Mountain Sickness. Medlineplus. Retrieved May 29, 2005, from the U.S. National Library of Medicine and the National Institutes of Health: http://www.nlm.nih.gov/medlineplus/ency/article/000133.htm.

Johnson, M. 2003. Indiana University School of Medicine. Retrieved February 27, 2005, from http://web.indstate.edu/thcme/micro/actncard.html.

Jonnalagadda, S. 2004a. Malabsorption. *MedlinePlus*, Retrieved November 10, 2004, from the U.S. National Library of Medicine and the National Institutes of Health: http://www.nlm.nih.gov/medlineplus/ency/article/000299.htm.

Joy, S., & Lyon, D. 2004. Placenta previa. *eMedicine*, Retrieved November 11, 2004, from: http://www.emedicine.com/med/topic3271.htm.

Jung, L. 2004. Sjogren syndrome. *eMedicine*, Retrieved November 11, 2004, from: http://www.emedicine.com/ped/topic2811.htm.

Kang, Y. 2002. Orchitis. *MEDLINEplus*. Retrieved July 25, 2003, from the U.S. National Library of Medicine and the National Institutes of Health: http://www .nlm.nih.gov/medlineplus/ency/article/001280.htm.

Kantor, J. 2004a. Eczema. *MedlinePlus*, Retrieved November 11, 2004, from the U.S. National Library of Medicine and the National Institutes of Health: http://www .nlm.nih.gov/medlineplus/ency/article/000853.htm.

Kantor, J. 2004b. Melasma. *MedlinePlus*, Retrieved November 10, 2004, from the U.S. National Library of Medicine and the National Institutes of Health: http://www.nlm.nih.gov/medlineplus/ency/article/000836.htm.

Kantor, J. 2004c. Pemphigus vulgaris. *MedlinePlus*, Retrieved November 10, 2004, from the U.S. National Library of Medicine and the National Institutes of Health: http://www.nlm.nih.gov/medlineplus/ency/article/000882.htm.

Kantor, J. 2004d. Scabies. *MedlinePlus*, Retrieved March 14, 2005, from the U.S. National Library of Medicine and the National Institutes of Health: http://www.nlm.nih.gov/medlineplus/ency/article/000830.htm.

Kantor, J. 2004e. Seborrheic dermatitis. *MedlinePlus*, Retrieved November 10, 2004, from the U.S. National Library of Medicine and the National Institutes of Health: http://www.nlm.nih.gov/medlineplus/ency/article/000963.htm.

Kantor, J. 2004f. Vitiligo. *MedlinePlus*, Retrieved November 10, 2004, from the U.S. National Library of Medicine and the National Institutes of Health: http://www.nlm.nih.gov/medlineplus/ency/article/000831.htm.

Kaplan, L. 1991. Clinical assessment and multispecialty management of Apert syndrome. *Clinics in Plastic Surgery*. 18(2): 217–225.

Kapner, M. 2003. Gingivitis. *MedlinePlus*, Retrieved November 11, 2004, from the U.S. National Library of Medicine and the National Institutes of Health: http://www.nlm.nih.gov/medlineplus/ency/article/001056.htm.

Kapoor, D., & Davila, W. 2004. Endometriosis. *eMedicine*. Retrieved March 12, 2005, from http://www.emedicine.com/med/topic3419.htm.

Karakousis, P., Page, K., Varello, M., Howlett, P., & Stieritz, D. 2001. Case report: Waterhouse-Friderichsen syndrome after infection with group A Streptococcus. *Mayo Clinic Procedures*, 76:1167–1170.

Kaufman, D. 2003. Sarcoidosis. *MedlinePlus*, Retrieved November 10, 2004, from the U.S. National Library of Medicine and the National Institutes of Health: http://www.nlm.nih.gov/medlineplus/ency/article/000076.htm.

*Kawasaki syndrome*. 2003. *CDC*, Retrieved November 12, 2004, from the National Center for Infectious Diseases. Centers for Disease Control and Prevention: http://www.cdc.gov/ncidod/diseases/kawasaki/index.htm.

Keller, S. 2004. Myocarditis. *MedlinePlus*, Retrieved November 10, 2004, from the U.S. National Library of Medicine and the National Institutes of Health: http://www.nlm.nih.gov/medlineplus/ency/article/000149.htm.

Kelsch, R. 2003. Geographic tongue. *eMedicine*. Retrieved March 12, 2005, from http://www.emedicine.com/derm/topic664.htm.

Khoury, G., & Deeba, S. 2001. Pancreatitis. *eMedicine*: Retrieved June 7, 2003, from http://www.emedicine.com/EMERG/topic354.htm.

Kibbi, A. 2002. Erythrasma. *eMedicine*, Retrieved November 11, 2004, from: http://www.emedicine.com/derm/topic140.htm.

King, R. 2002. Osteomyelitis. *eMedicine*: Retrieved June 1, 2003, from http://www.emedicine.com/emerg/topic349.htm#section~treatment.

Kiriakopoulos, E. 2003a. Eye movements-uncontrollable. *MedlinePlus*, Retrieved November 10, 2004, from the U.S. National Library of Medicine and the National Institutes of Health: http://www.nlm.nih.gov/medlineplus/ency/article/003037.htm.

Kiriakopoulos, E. 2003b. Gilles de la Tourette syndrome. *MedlinePlus*, Retrieved March 15, 2005, from the U.S. National Library of Medicine and the National Institutes of Health: http://www.nlm.nih.gov/medlineplus/ency/article/000733.htm.

Kiriakopoulos, E. 2003c. Huntington's disease. *MedlinePlus*, Retrieved November 10, 2004, from the U.S. National Library of Medicine and the National Institutes of Health: http://www.nlm.nih.gov/medlineplus/ency/article/000770.htm.

Klein, N. 2004. Pinta. *eMedicine*, Retrieved November 11, 2004, from: http://www.emedicine.com/med/topic1836.htm.

Klein, N. 2001. Yaws. *eMedicine*, Retrieved November 11, 2004, from: http://www.emedicine.com/med/topic2431.htm.

Klein, S., & Garcia, C. 1973. Asherman's syndrome: A critique and current review. *Fertility and Sterility*. 24(9):722–735.

Koening, A. 2002. Scleroderma. *eMedicine*, Retrieved November 11, 2004, from: http://www.emedicine.com/med/topic2076.htm.

Konety, B., & Pirtskhalaishvili, G. 2002. Transitional cell carcinoma, renal. *eMedicine*: Retreived May 29, 2003, from http://www.emedicine.com/med/topic2003.htm.

Koren, A. 2003a. Goodpasture's syndrome. *MedlinePlus*, Retrieved November 11, 2004, from the U.S. National Library of Medicine and the National Institutes of Health: http://www.nlm.nih.gov/medlineplus/ency/article/000142.htm.

Koren, A. 2003b. Hypertension. *MedlinePlus*, Retrieved November 11, 2004, from the U.S. National Library of Medicine and the National Institutes of Health: http://www.nlm.nih.gov/medlineplus/ency/article/000468.htm.

Koren, A. 2001a. Chronic renal failure. *MEDLINEplus*. Retrieved June 9, 2003, from the U.S. National Library of Medicine and the National Institutes of Health: http://www.nlm.nih.gov/medlineplus/ency/article/000471.htm.

Koren, A. 2001b. Nephrolithiasis. *MedlinePlus*. Retrieved June 9, 2003, from the U.S. National Library of Medicine and the National Institutes of Health: http://www.nlm.nih.gov/medlineplus/ency/article/000458.htm.

Kotton, C. 2003a. Hantavirus. *MedlinePlus*, Retrieved November 10, 2004, from the U.S. National Library of Medicine and the National Institutes of Health: http://www.nlm.nih.gov/medlineplus/ency/article/001382.htm.

Kotton, C. 2003b. Lyme disease. *MedlinePlus*, Retrieved November 10, 2004, from the U.S. National Library of Medicine and the National Institutes of Health: http://www.nlm.nih.gov/medlineplus/ency/article/001319.htm.

Kotton, C. 2002a. Yellow fever. *MedlinePlus*, Retrieved November 10, 2004, from the U.S. National Library of Medicine and the National Institutes of Health: http://www.nlm.nih.gov/medlineplus/ency/article/001365.htm.

Kotton, C. 2002b. Pulmonary tuberculosis. *MedlinePlus*, Retrieved November 10, 2004, from the U.S. National Library of Medicine and the National Institutes of Health: http://www.nlm.nih.gov/medlineplus/ency/article/000077.htm.

Krafchik, B. 2003. Kasabach-Merritt syndrome. *eMedicine*, Retrieved November 11, 2004, from: http://www.emedicine.com/med/topic1221.htm.

Lambert, M. 2005. Bell palsy. *eMedicine*, Retrieved March 8, 2005, from http://www.emedicine.com/emerg/topic56.htm.

Lamont, D. 2001. Systemic lupus erythematosus. *eMedicine*, Retrieved November 11, 2004, from: http://www.emedicine.com/EMERG/topic564.htm.

*Lassa fever*. 2004. *CDC*, Retrieved November 12, 2004, from the National Center for Infectious Diseases, Special Pathogens Branch. Centers for Disease Control and Prevention: http://www.cdc.gov/ncidod/dvrd/spb/mnpages/dispages/lassaf.htm.

Legionellosis: Legionnaire's disease (LD) and Pontiac fever. 2001. Retrieved July 26, 2003, from the National Center for Infectious Disease, Division of Bacterial and Mycotic Diseases. Centers for Disease Control and Prevention: http://www.cdc.gov/ncidod/dbmd/diseaseinfo/legionellosis_g.htm.

Lehrer, J. 2003a. Plummer-Vinson syndrome/esophageal web. *MedlinePlus*, Retrieved March 14, 2005, from the U.S. National Library of Medicine and the National Institutes of Health: http://www.nlm.nih.gov/medlineplus/ency/article/001158.htm.

Lehrer, J. 2003b. Ulcerative colitis. *MedlinePlus*, Retrieved November 10, 2004, from the U.S. National Library of Medicine and the National Institutes of Health: http://www.nlm.nih.gov/medlineplus/ency/article/000250.htm.

Lehrer, M. 2003a. Impetigo. *MedlinePlus*, Retrieved November 10, 2004, from the U.S. National Library of Medicine and the National Institutes of Health: http://www.nlm.nih.gov/medlineplus/ency/article/000860.htm.

Lehrer, M. 2003b. Lichen planus. *MedlinePlus*, Retrieved November 10, 2004, from the U.S. National Library of Medicine and the National Institutes of Health: http://www.nlm.nih.gov/medlineplus/ency/article/000867.htm.

Lehrer, M. 2003c. Liver spots. *MedlinePlus*, Retrieved November 10, 2004, from the U.S. National Library of Medicine and the National Institutes of Health: http://www.nlm.nih.gov/medlineplus/ency/article/001141.htm.

Lehrer, M. 2003d. Molluscum contagiosum. *MedlinePlus*, Retrieved November 10, 2004, from the U.S. National Library of Medicine and the National Institutes of Health: http://www.nlm.nih.gov/medlineplus/ency/article/000826.htm.

Lehrer, M. 2003e. Paronychia. *MedlinePlus*, Retrieved November 10, 2004, from the U.S. National Library of Medicine and the National Institutes of Health: http://www.nlm.nih.gov/medlineplus/ency/article/001444.htm.

Lehrer, M. 2003f. Pityriasis. *MedlinePlus*, Retrieved November 10, 2004, from the U.S. National Library of Medicine and the National Institutes of Health: http://www.nlm.nih.gov/medlineplus/ency/article/000871.htm.

Lehrer, M. 2003g. Ulcerative colitis. *MedlinePlus*, Retrieved November 10, 2004, from the U.S. National Library of Medicine and the National Institutes of Health: http://www.nlm.nih.gov/medlineplus/ency/article/000250.htm.

*Leishmania infection.* 2004. *DPD*, Retrieved on November 12, 2004, from the National Center for Infectious Diseases, Division of Parasitic Diseases. Centers for Disease Control and Prevention: http://www.cdc.gov/ncidod/dpd/parasites/leishmania/factsht_leishmania.htm.

Leptospirosis. 2001. Retrieved July 26, 2003, from the National Center for Infectious Disease, Division of Bacterial and Mycotic Diseases. Centers for Disease Control and Prevention: http://www.cdc.gov/ncidod/dbmd/diseaseinfo/leptospirosis_g.htm.

Levine, N. 2002. Acanthosis nigricans. *eMedicine*, Retrieved November 11, 2004, from: http://www.emedicine.com/derm/topic1.htm.

Levy, A. 2002. Sickle cell anemia. *MedlinePlus*. Retrieved June 5, 2003, from the U.S. National Library of Medicine and the National Institutes of Health: http://www.nlm.nih.gov/ency/article/000527.htm.

Levy, D. 2004a. Atypical mycobacterial infection. *MedlinePlus*, Retrieved November 10, 2004, from the U.S. National Library of Medicine and the National Institutes of Health: http://www.nlm.nih.gov/medlineplus/ency/article/000640.htm.

Levy, D. 2004b. Blastomycosis. *MedlinePlus*, Retrieved November 12, 2004, from the U.S. National Library of Medicine and the National Institutes of Health: http://www.nlm.nih.gov/medlineplus/ency/article/000102.htm.

Levy, D. 2004c. Diphtheria. *MedlinePlus*, Retrieved November 11, 2004, from the U.S. National Library of Medicine and the National Institutes of Health: http://www.nlm.nih.gov/medlineplus/ency/article/001608.htm.

Levy, D. 2004d. E. coli enteritis. *MedlinePlus*, Retrieved November 11, 2004, from the U.S. National Library of Medicine and the National Institutes of Health: http://www.nlm.nih.gov/medlineplus/ency/article/000296.htm.

Levy, D. 2004e. Erysipelas. *MedlinePlus*, Retrieved November 11, 2004, from the U.S. National Library of Medicine and the National Institutes of Health: http://www.nlm.nih.gov/medlineplus/ency/article/000618.htm.

Levy, D. 2004f. Gonorrhea-female. *MedlinePlus,* Retrieved November 11, 2004, from the U.S. National Library of Medicine and the National Institutes of Health: http://www.nlm.nih.gov/medlineplus/ency/article/000656.htm.

Levy, D. 2004g. Herpes labialis. *MedlinePlus,* Retrieved November 11, 2004, from the U.S. National Library of Medicine and the National Institutes of Health: http://www.nlm.nih.gov/medlineplus/ency/article/000606.htm.

Levy, D. 2004h. Herpes zoster. *MedlinePlus,* Retrieved November 10, 2004, from the U.S. National Library of Medicine and the National Institutes of Health: http://www.nlm.nih.gov/medlineplus/ency/article/000858.htm.

Levy, D. 2004i. Histoplasmosis. *MedlinePlus,* Retrieved November 10, 2004, from the U.S. National Library of Medicine and the National Institutes of Health: http://www.nlm.nih.gov/medlineplus/ency/article/001082.htm.

Levy, D. 2004j. Leptospirosis. *MedlinePlus,* Retrieved November 10, 2004, from the U.S. National Library of Medicine and the National Institutes of Health: http://www.nlm.nih.gov/medlineplus/ency/article/001376.htm.

Levy, D. 2004k. Lymphogranuloma venereum. *MedlinePlus,* Retrieved November 10, 2004, from the U.S. National Library of Medicine and the National Institutes of Health: http://www.nlm.nih.gov/medlineplus/ency/article/000634.htm.

Levy, D. 2004l. Meningitis. *MedlinePlus,* Retrieved November 10, 2004, from the U.S. National Library of Medicine and the National Institutes of Health: http://www.nlm.nih.gov/medlineplus/ency/article/000607.htm.

Levy, D. 2004m. Meningitis-cryptococcal. *MedlinePlus,* Retrieved November 11, 2004, from the U.S. National Library of Medicine and the National Institutes of Health: http://www.nlm.nih.gov/medlineplus/ency/article/000642.htm.

Levy, D. 2004n. Meningococcemia. *MedlinePlus,* Retrieved November 10, 2004, from the U.S. National Library of Medicine and the National Institutes of Health: http://www.nlm.nih.gov/medlineplus/ency/article/001349.htm.

Levy, D. 2004o. Mucormycosis. *MedlinePlus,* Retrieved November 10, 2004, from the U.S. National Library of Medicine and the National Institutes of Health: http://www.nlm.nih.gov/medlineplus/ency/article/000649.htm.

Levy, D. 2004p. Nocardia infection. *MedlinePlus,* Retrieved November 10, 2004, from the U.S. National Library of Medicine and the National Institutes of Health: http://www.nlm.nih.gov/medlineplus/ency/article/000679.htm.

Levy, D. 2004q. Osteomyelitis. *MedlinePlus,* Retrieved November 10, 2004, from the U.S. National Library of Medicine and the National Institutes of Health: http://www.nlm.nih.gov/medlineplus/ency/article/000437.htm.

Levy, D. 2004r. Parinaud's syndrome. *MedlinePlus,* Retrieved November 10, 2004, from the U.S. National Library of Medicine and the National Institutes of Health: http://www.nlm.nih.gov/medlineplus/ency/article/000736.htm.

Levy, D. 2004s. Q fever. *MedlinePlus,* Retrieved November 10, 2004, from the U.S. National Library of Medicine and the National Institutes of Health: http://www.nlm.nih.gov/medlineplus/ency/article/001337.htm.

Levy, D. 2004t Rabies. *MedlinePlus,* Retrieved November 10, 2004, from the U.S. National Library of Medicine and the National Institutes of Health: http://www.nlm.nih.gov/medlineplus/ency/article/001334.htm.

Levy, D. 2004u. Recurrent cystitis. *MedlinePlus,* Retrieved November 11, 2004, from the U.S. National Library of Medicine and the National Institutes of Health: http://www.nlm.nih.gov/medlineplus/ency/article/000515.htm.

Levy, D. 2004v. Schistosomiasis. *MedlinePlus,* Retrieved November 10, 2004, from the U.S. National Library of Medicine and the National Institutes of Health: http://www.nlm.nih.gov/medlineplus/ency/article/001321.htm.

Levy, D. 2004x. Scrofula. *MedlinePlus,* Retrieved March 14, 2005, from the U.S. National Library of Medicine and the National Institutes of Health: http://www.nlm.nih.gov/medlineplus/ency/article/001354.htm.

Levy, D. 2004y. Sporotrichosis. *MedlinePlus,* Retrieved November 10, 2004, from the U.S. National Library of Medicine and the National Institutes of Health: http://www.nlm.nih.gov/medlineplus/ency/article/001338.htm.

Levy, D. 2004z. Strongyloidiasis. *MedlinePlus,* Retrieved November 10, 2004, from the U.S. National Library of Medicine and the National Institutes of Health: http://www.nlm.nih.gov/medlineplus/ency/article/000630.htm.

Levy, D. 2004aa. Toxic shock syndrome. *MedlinePlus,* Retrieved November 10, 2004, from the U.S. National Library of Medicine and the National Institutes of Health: http://www.nlm.nih.gov/medlineplus/ency/article/000653.htm.

Levy, D. 2004ab. Trichomoniasis. *MedlinePlus,* Retrieved November 10, 2004, from the U.S. National Library of Medicine and the National Institutes of Health: http://www.nlm.nih.gov/medlineplus/ency/article/001331.htm.

Levy, D. 2004ac. Tularemia. *MedlinePlus,* Retrieved November 10, 2004, from the U.S. National Library of Medicine and the National Institutes of Health: http://www.nlm.nih.gov/medlineplus/ency/article/000856.htm.

Levy, D. 2004ad. Typhus. *MedlinePlus,* Retrieved November 10, 2004, from the U.S. National Library of Medicine and the National Institutes of Health: http://www.nlm.nih.gov/medlineplus/ency/article/001363.htm.

Levy, D. 2004ae. Visceral larva migrans. *MedlinePlus,* Retrieved November 10, 2004, from the U.S. National Library of Medicine and the National Institutes of Health: http://www.nlm.nih.gov/medlineplus/ency/article/000633.htm.

Levy, D. 2004af. West Nile virus. *MedlinePlus,* Retrieved November 10, 2004, from the U.S. National Library of Medicine and the National Institutes of Health: http://www.nlm.nih.gov/medlineplus/ency/article/007186.htm.

Levy, D. 2004ag. Whipworm infection. *MedlinePlus,* Retrieved November 10, 2004, from the U.S. National Library of Medicine and the National Institutes of Health: http://www.nlm.nih.gov/medlineplus/ency/article/001364.htm.

Levy, D. 2003a. Dengue fever. *MedlinePlus,* Retrieved November 11, 2004, from the U.S. National Library of Medicine and the National Institutes of Health: http://www.nlm.nih.gov/medlineplus/ency/article/001374.htm.

Levy, D. 2003b. Hookworm. *MedlinePlus,* Retrieved November 10, 2004, from the U.S. National Library of Medicine and the National Institutes of Health: http://www.nlm.nih.gov/medlineplus/ency/article/000629.htm.

Levy, D. 2003c. Inhalation anthrax. *MedlinePlus,* Retrieved November 10, 2004, from the U.S. National Library of Medicine and the National Institutes of Health: http://www.nlm.nih.gov/medlineplus/ency/article/000641.htm.

Levy, D. 2003d. Legionnaire's disease. *MedlinePlus,* Retrieved November 10, 2004, from the U.S. National Library of Medicine and the National Institutes of Health: http://www.nlm.nih.gov/medlineplus/ency/article/000616.htm.

Levy, D. 2003e. Lymphadenitis and lymphangitis. *MedlinePlus,* Retrieved November 10, 2004, from the U.S. National Library of Medicine and the National Institutes of Health: http://www.nlm.nih.gov/medlineplus/ency/article/001301.htm.

Levy, D. 2003f. Malaria. *MedlinePlus,* Retrieved November 10, 2004, from the U.S. National Library of Medicine and the National Institutes of Health: http://www.nlm.nih.gov/medlineplus/ency/article/000621.htm.

Levy, D. 2003g. Plague. *MedlinePlus,* Retrieved November 10, 2004, from the U.S. National Library of Medicine and the National Institutes of Health: http://www.nlm.nih.gov/medlineplus/ency/article/000596.htm.

Levy, D. 2003h. Rocky Mountain spotted fever. *MedlinePlus,* Retrieved November 10, 2004, from the U.S. National Library of Medicine and the National Institutes of Health: http://www.nlm.nih.gov/medlineplus/ency/article/000654.htm.

Levy, D. 2003i. Smallpox. *MedlinePlus,* Retrieved November 10, 2004, from the U.S. National Library of Medicine and the National Institutes of Health: http://www.nlm.nih.gov/medlineplus/ency/article/001356.htm.

Levy, D. 2003j. Syphilis. *MedlinePlus*, Retrieved November 10, 2004, from the U.S. National Library of Medicine and the National Institutes of Health: http://www.nlm.nih.gov/medlineplus/ency/article/001327.htm.

Levy, D. 2003k. Typhoid fever. *MedlinePlus*, Retrieved November 10, 2004, from the U.S. National Library of Medicine and the National Institutes of Health: http://www.nlm.nih.gov/medlineplus/ency/article/001332.htm.

Lewis, M., & McClay, J. 2004. Scrofula. *eMedicine*. Retrieved March 14, 2005, from http://www.emedicine.com/ent/topic524.htm.

Listeriosis. 2003. Retrieved July 19, 2003, from the National Center for Infectious Disease, Division of Bacterial and Mycotic Diseases, Center for Disease Control and Prevention: http://www.cdc.gov/ncidod/dbmd/diseaseinfo/listeriosis_g .htm#symptom.

Lorenzo, N. 2004. Meniere disease. *eMedicine*, Retrieved November 11, 2004, from: http://www.emedicine.com/emerg/topic308.htm.

Lowery, R. 2004. Blepharitis, adult. eMedicine, Retrieved November 11, 2004, from: http://www.emedicine.com/oph/topic81.htm.

Lyme disease. 2001. Retrieved July 26, 2003, from the National Center for Infectious Diseases, Division of Vector-Borne Infectious Disease. Centers for Disease Control and Prevention: http://www.cdc.gov/ncidod/dvbid/lyme/ index.htm.

*Lymphocytic choriomeningitis.* 2004. *CDC*, Retrieved November 12, 2004, from the National Center for Infectious Diseases, Special Pathogens Branch. Centers for Disease Control and Prevention: http://www.cdc.gov/ncidod/dvrd/spb/mnpages/ dispages/lcmv.htm.

Mack, D. 2003. Dientamoeba fragilis infection. *eMedicine*, Retrieved November 12, 2004, from: http://www.emedicine.com/ped/topic563.htm.

Mahon, C., & Manuselis, G. 2000. *Textbook of Diagnostic Microbiology. 2ⁿᵈ Edition.* Philadelphia: Saunders.

Malaria. 2002. Retrieved July 26, 2003, from the National Center for Infectious Diseases, Division of Parasitic Infections. Centers for Disease Control and Prevention: http://www.cdc.gov/ncidod/dpd/parasites/malaria/default.htm.

Manian, P. and Resnick, M. 2004. Hydroneprhosis and hydroureter. *eMedicine*. Retrieved March 13, 2005, from http://www.emedicine.com/med/topic1055.htm.

*Marburg hemorrhagic fever.* 2004. *CDC*, Retrieved November 12, 2004, from the National Center for Infectious Diseases, Special Pathogens Branch. Centers for Disease Control and Prevention: http://www.cdc.gov/ncidod/dvrd/spb/*mnpages*/ dispages/marburg.htm.

Marchiano, D. 2004. Ectopic pregnancy. *MedlinePlus*, Retrieved November 11, 2004, from the U.S. National Library of Medicine and the National Institutes of Health: http://www.nlm.nih.gov/medlineplus/ency/article/000895.htm.

Marcincuk, M. 2004. Inner ear, presbycusis. *eMedicine*, Retrieved November 11, 2004, from: http://www.emedicine.com/ent/topic224.htm.

Marill, K. 2001. Endocarditis. *eMedicine*: Retrieved June 4, 2003, from http://www .emedicine.com/EMERG/topic164.htm.

Maxton, D. 2004. Haemochromatosis. Netdoctor, Retrieved November 11, 2004, from: http://www.netdoctor.co.uk/diseases/facts/haemochromatosis.htm.

McElhinny, D., & Wernovsky, G. 2004. Truncus arteriosus. *eMedicine*, Retrieved November 11, 2004, from: http://www.emedicine.com/ped/topic2316.htm.

McGovern, M. 2003. Gaucher disease. *eMedicine*, Retrieved November 11, 2004, from: http://www.emedicine.com/ped/topic837.htm.

McGovern, M. 2002. Niemann-Pick disease. *eMedicine*, Retrieved November 11, 2004, from: http://www.emedicine.com/ped/topic2889.htm.

McKinley Health Center. 2002. Herpes simplex (cold sores). Retrieved March 11, 2005, from the University of Illinois at Urbana-Champagne: http://www.mckinley.uiuc.edu/Handouts/herpsimp/herpsimp.html.

McNeil, D. June 16, 2003. Tenth of HIV cases in a study in Europe are resistant to drugs. *New York Times*.

Measles. (n/d). Retrieved July 26, 2003, from the National Immunization Program, Centers for Disease Control and Prevention: http://www.cdc.gov/nip/publications/pink/meas.pdf.

Meningococcal diseases. 2003. Retrieved March 16, 2004, from the Division of Bacterial and Mycotic Diseases, Centers for Disease Control and Prevention, http://www.cdc.gov/ncidod/dbmd/diseaseinfo/meningococcal_g.htm.

Michelini, G. 2004. Hyperemesis gravidarum. *eMedicine*, Retrieved November 11, 2004, from: http://www.emedicine.com/med/topic1075.htm.

Miethke, M., & Raugi, G. 2003. Leiomyoma. *eMedicine*: Retrieved May 29, 2003, from http://www.emedicine.com/DERM/topic217.htm.

Minnaganti, V. 2002. Isosporiasis. *eMedicine*, Retrieved November 12, 2004, from http://www.emedicine.com/med/topic1194.htm.

Mishky, P. 2004. Eczema. *eMedicine*. Retrieved March 12, 2005, from http://www.emedicinehealth.com/articles/8545-1.asp.

Mixed Gliomas: The Cancer BACUP Factsheet. 2001. Retrieved May 29, 2003, from the British Association of Cancer United Patients: http://www.cancerbacup.org.uk/info/mixedglioma.htm.

Molmenti, H. 2004. Peritonitis. *MedlinePlus*, Retrieved November 10, 2004, from the U.S. National Library of Medicine and the National Institutes of Health: http://www.nlm.nih.gov/medlineplus/ency/article/001335.htm.

Molmenti, H. 2002. Meckel's diverticulum. *MedlinePlus*, Retrieved November 10, 2004, from the U.S. National Library of Medicine and the National Institutes of Health: http://www.nlm.nih.gov/medlineplus/ency/article/000234.htm.

*Monkey B Virus*. 1998. *Biological Safety*, Retrieved November 12, 2004, from Environmental Health and Safety. University of Florida: http://www.ehs.ufl.edu/Bio/monkeyb.htm.

Monkeypox fact sheet. 1998. Retrieved June 10, 2003, from the World Health Organization, Geneva: http://www.who.int/inf-fs/en/fact161.html.

Montemarano, A. 2003. Melasma. *eMedicine*. Retrieved March 13, 2005, from http://www.emedicine.com/derm/topic260.htm.

Muir, A. 2003a. Gastritis. *MedlinePlus*, Retrieved November 11, 2004, from the U.S. National Library of Medicine and the National Institutes of Health: http://www.nlm.nih.gov/medlineplus/ency/article/001150.htm.

Muir, A. 2003b. Hirschsprung's disease. *MedlinePlus*, Retrieved November 10, 2004, from the U.S. National Library of Medicine and the National Institutes of Health: http://www.nlm.nih.gov/medlineplus/ency/article/001140.htm.

Mukherjee, S. 2001. Gilbert syndrome. *eMedicine*, Retrieved November 11, 2004, from: http://www.emedicine.com/med/topic870.htm.

Mulinda, J. 2004. Goiter. *eMedicine*. Retrieved March 12, 2005, from http://www.emedicine.com/med/topic916.htm.

Multiple Congenital Anomaly/Mental Retardation (MCA/MR) Syndromes. 1999. U.S. National Library of Medicine. Retrieved February 27, 2005, from http://www.nlm.nih.gov/mesh/jablonski/syndromes/syndrome001.html.

Mumps. (n/d). Retrieved July 26, 2003, from the National Immunization Program, Centers for Disease Control and Prevention: http://www.cdc.gov/nip/publications/pink/mumps.pdf.

Muniz, A. 2004. Croup. *eMedicine*, Retrieved November 11, 2004, from: http://www.emedicine.com/ped/topic510.htm.

*Mycobacterium avium* complex. 2003. Retrieved from the National Center for Infectious Diseases, Division of Bacterial and Mycotic Diseases. Centers for Disease Control and Prevention: http://www.cdc.gov/ncidod/dbmd/diseaseinfo/mycobacteriumavium_t.htm.

*Mycoplasma pneumoniae*. 2002. Retrieved from the National Center for Infectious Diseases, Division of Bacterial and Mycotic Diseases. Centers for Disease Control and Prevention: http://www.cdc.gov/ncidod/dbmd/diseaseinfo/mycoplasmapneum_t.htm.

Mylonakis, E. 2003. Tetanus. *MedlinePlus*, Retrieved November 10, 2004, from the U.S. National Library of Medicine and the National Institutes of Health: http://www.nlm.nih.gov/medlineplus/ency/article/000615.htm.

Mylonakis, E. 2002. Whipple's disease. *MedlinePlus*, Retrieved November 10, 2004, from the U.S. National Library of Medicine and the National Institutes of Health: http://www.nlm.nih.gov/medlineplus/ency/article/000209.htm.

Nachimuthu, S., & Piccione, P. 2004. Crohn's disease. *eMedicine*. Retrieved March 10, 2005, from http://www.emedicine.com/med/topic477.htm.

*Naegleria infection*. 2004. *DPD*, Retrieved November 12, 2004, from National Center for Infectious Diseases, Division of Parasitic Diseases. Centers for Disease Control and Prevention: http://www.cdc.gov/ncidod/dpd/parasites/naegleria/factsht_naegleria.htm.

National Human Genome Research Institute. 2003. Learning about cystic fibrosis. Retrieved May 30, 2003, from the National Institutes of Health: http://www.genome.gov/page.cfm?pageID=10001213.

National Institute for Child Health and Human Development. 2003. Facts about Down syndrome. Retrieved May 30, 2003, from the National Institutes of Health: http://www.nichd.nih.gov/publications/pubs/downsyndrome/down.htm #DownSyndrome.

Nazziola, E., & Lafleur, J. 2004. Mountain sickness. *eMedicine*. Retrieved March 13, 2005, from http://www.emedicinehealth.com/articles/6323-1.asp.

Neiberger, R. 2004. Nephritis. *eMedicine*. Retrieved March 14, 2005, from http://www.emedicine.com/ped/topic1561.htm.

Neville, H. 2003. Hirschsprung disease. *eMedicine*, Retrieved November 11, 2004, from: http://www.emedicine.com/ped/topic1010.htm.

New variant CJD: Fact sheet. 2003. *Bovine Spongiform Encephalopathy and Creutzfeldt-Jacob Disease*. Atlanta: National Center for Infectious Diseases (NCID).

Newicki, R., & Szarmach, H. 2003. Chediak-Higashi syndrome. *eMedicine*. Retrieved March 10, 2005, from http://www.emedicine.com/derm/topic704.htm.

Newman, J. 2003a. Geographic tongue. *MedlinePlus*, Retrieved March 12, 2005, from the U.S. National Library of Medicine and the National Institutes of Health: http://www.nlm.nih.gov/medlineplus/ency/article/001049.htm.

Newman, J. 2003b. Gingivostomatitis. *MedlinePlus*, Retrieved November 11, 2004, from the U.S. National Library of Medicine and the National Institutes of Health: http://www.nlm.nih.gov/medlineplus/ency/article/001052.htm.

Newman, J. 2003c. Mastoiditis. *MedlinePlus*, Retrieved November 10, 2004, from the U.S. National Library of Medicine and the National Institutes of Health: http://www.nlm.nih.gov/medlineplus/ency/article/001034.htm.

Newman, J. 2003d. Tonsillitis. *MedlinePlus*, Retrieved November 10, 2004, from the U.S. National Library of Medicine and the National Institutes of Health: http://www.nlm.nih.gov/medlineplus/ency/article/001043.htm.

Newman, J. 2003e. Tracheitis. *MedlinePlus*, Retrieved November 10, 2004, from the U.S. National Library of Medicine and the National Institutes of Health: http://www.nlm.nih.gov/medlineplus/ency/article/000988.htm.

Newmark, C. 2003a. Alström syndrome. Retrieved March 8, 2005, from the U.S. National Library of Medicine and the National Institutes of Health: http://www.nlm.nih.gov/medlineplus/ency/article/001665.htm.

Newmark, C. 2003b. Myelomeningocele. *MedlinePlus*, Retrieved November 10, 2004, from the U.S. National Library of Medicine and the National Institutes of Health: http://www.nlm.nih.gov/medlineplus/ency/article/001558.htm.

NFID. 2003. Facts about diphtheria for adults. Retrieved March 12, 2005, from the National Foundation for Infectious Diseases: http://www.nfid.org/factsheets/diphtadult.html.

NINDS Aicardi syndrome information page. 2005. Retrieved March 8, 2005, from http://www.ninds.nih.gov/disorders/aicardi/aicardi.htm.

NINDS Canavan disease information page. 2005. Retrieved March 10, 2005, from http://www.ninds.nih.gov/disorders/canavan/canavan.htm.

NINDS Creutzfeldt-Jakob disease information page. 2001. Retrieved March 16, 2004, from the National Institute of Neurological Disorders and Stroke, National Institutes of Health: http://www.ninds.nih.gov/health_and_medical/disorders/cjd.htm.

NINDS spina bifida information page. 2001. Retrieved May 30, 2003, from the National Institutes of Health, The National Institute of Neurological Disorders and Stroke: http://www.ninds.nih.gov/health_and_medical/disorders/spina_bifida.htm.

NINDS temporal arteritis. 2001. Retrieved June 4, 2003, from the National Institute of Neurological Disorders and Stroke, National Institutes of Health: http://www.ninds.nih.gov/health_and_medical/disorders/vasculitis_doc.htm.

NOAH Albinism. 2002. National Organization for Albinism and Hypopigmentation. Retrieved March 8, 2005, from http://www.albinism.org/publications/what_is_albinism.html.

*Nocardiosis.* 2004. *CDC*, Retrieved November 12, 2004, from the National Center for Infectious Diseases, Division of Bacterial and Mycotic Diseases. Centers for Disease Control and Prevention: http://www.cdc.gov/ncidod/dbmd/diseaseinfo/nocardiosis_t.htm.

Noecker, R. 2003. Glaucoma. *eMedicine*, Retrieved November 11, 2004, from: http://www.emedicine.com/aaem/topic224.htm.

NORD-Aarskog Syndrome. 2005. National Organization for Rare Disorders (NORD). Retrieved February 27, 2005, from http://www.rarediseases.org/search/rdbdetail_abstract.html?disname=Aarskog% 20Syndrome.

NORD-Aase Syndrome. 2003. National Organization for Rare Disorders (NORD). Retrieved February 27, 2005, from http://www.rarediseases.org/search/rdbdetail_abstract.html?disname=Aase%20Syndrome.

*Norovirus.* 2003. *CDC*, Retrieved November 12, 2004, from the National Center for Infectious Diseases, Respiratory and Enteric Viruses Branch. Centers for Disease Control and Prevention: http://www.cdc.gov/ncidod/dvrd/revb/gastro/norovirus-qa.htm.

OASIS. 2005. Asperger's syndrome. Retrieved March 8, 2005, from Online Asperger Syndrome Information and Support: http://www.udel.edu/bkirby/asperger/.

Ocampo, V. 2004. Cataract, senile. *eMedicine*, Retrieved November 11, 2004, from: http://www.emedicine.com/oph/topic49.htm.

Odeke, S. 2003. Hashimoto thyroiditis. *eMedicine*, Retrieved November 11, 2004, from: http://www.emedicine.com/med/topic949.htm.

Ohio State University. 1996. *Angiostrongylus cantonensis. Graphic Images of Parasites*, Retrieved November 12, 2004 from the College of Biological Sciences: http://www.biosci.ohio-state.edu/~parasite/angiostrongylus.htm.l.

Okulicz, J., & Jozwiak, S. 2002. Lentigo. *eMedicine*, Retrieved November 11, 2004, from: http://www.emedicine.com/derm/topic221.htm.

Okulicz, J., & Schwartz, R. 2005. Ichthyosis vulgaris, hereditary and acquired. *eMedicine*. Retrieved March 13, 2005, from http://www.emedicine.com/derm/topic678.htm.

Opisthorchiasis. 2004. *DPDx*, Retrieved November 12, 2004, from the National Center for Infectious Diseases, Division of Parasitic Diseases. Centers for Disease Control and Prevention: http://www.dpd.cdc.gov/dpdx/HTM.L/opisthorchiasis.htm.

Owens, T. 2004. Trench mouth. *MedlinePlus*, Retrieved March 15, 2005, from the U.S. National Library of Medicine and the National Institutes of Health: http://www.nlm.nih.gov/medlineplus/ency/article/001044.htm.

Papilloma. 2002. Retrieved May 29, 2003, from The Voice Disorders Center at the Massachusetts Eye and Ear Infirmary, Harvard Medical School Teaching Hospital: http://www.voicedisordercenter.meei.harvard.edu/disorders/papilloma.html.

*Paragonimiasis.* 2004. *DPDx*, Retrieved November 12, 2004, from the National Center for Infectious Diseases, Division of Parasitic Diseases. Centers for Disease Control and Prevention: http://www.dpd.cdc.gov/dpdx/HTM.L/Paragonimiasis.htm.

Parkinson's disease backgrounder. 2001. Retrieved June 10, 2003, from the National Institute of Neurological Disorders and Stroke, National Institutes of Health: http://www.ninds.nih.gov/health_and_medical/pubs/parkinson's_disease_backgrounder.htm.

Parmar, M. 2002. Glomerlulonephritis, acute. *eMedicine*: Retrieved June 9, 2003, from http://www.emedicine.com/med/topic879.htm.

*Parvovirus B19 (fifth disease).* 2003. *CDC*, Retrieved November 12, 2004, from the National Center for Infectious Diseases, Respiratory and Enteric Viruses Branch. Centers for Disease Control and Prevention: http://www.cdc.gov/ncidod/dvrd/revb/respiratory/parvo_b19.htm.

Paulino, A., & Coppes, M. 2003. Wilms tumor. *eMedicine*, Retrieved November 11, 2004, from: http://www.emedicine.com/ped/topic2440.htm.

Peng, S. 2004a. Fibromyalgia. *MedlinePlus*, Retrieved November 11, 2004, from the U.S. National Library of Medicine and the National Institutes of Health: http://www.nlm.nih.gov/medlineplus/ency/article/000427.htm.

Peng, S. 2004b. Rheumatoid arthritis. *MedlinePlus*, Retrieved November 10, 2004, from the U.S. National Library of Medicine and the National Institutes of Health: http://www.nlm.nih.gov/medlineplus/ency/article/000431.htm.

Peng, S. 2004c. Systemic lupus erythematosus. *MedlinePlus*, Retrieved November 10, 2004, from the U.S. National Library of Medicine and the National Institutes of Health: http://www.nlm.nih.gov/medlineplus/ency/article/000435.htm.

Peng, S. 2003a. Chronic gouty arthritis. *MedlinePlus*, Retrieved November 11, 2004, from the U.S. National Library of Medicine and the National Institutes of Health: http://www.nlm.nih.gov/medlineplus/ency/article/000424.htm.

Peng, S. 2003b. Kawasaki disease. *MedlinePlus*, Retrieved November 10, 2004, from the U.S. National Library of Medicine and the National Institutes of Health: http://www.nlm.nih.gov/medlineplus/ency/article/000989.htm.

Phaeohyphomycosis. 2004. Retrieved on November 17, 2004, from the University of Adelaide, Australia: http://www.mycology.adelaide.edu.au/Mycoses/Opportunistic/Phaeohyphomycosis/.

*Pinworm infection.* 1999. *DPD*, Retrieved November 12, 2004, from the National Center for Infectious Diseases, Division of Parasitic Diseases. Centers for Disease Control and Prevention: http://www.cdc.gov/ncidod/dpd/parasites/pinworm/factsht_pinworm.htm.

Plague. 2001. Retrieved July 19, 2003, from the National Center for Infectious Diseases, Division of Vector-Borne Infectious Disease. Centers for Disease Control and Prevention: http://www.cdc.gov/ncidod/dvbid/plague/index.htm.

*Pneumocystis carinii* pneumonia. 2003. Retrieved July 26, 2003, from the National Center for Infectious Diseases, Division of Parasitic Infections. Centers for Disease Control and Prevention: http://www.cdc.gov/ncidod/dpd/parasites/pneumocystis/default.htm.

Polenakovik, H., & Polenakovik, S. 2004. Strongyloidiasis. *eMedicine*, Retrieved November 11, 2004, from: http://www.emedicine.com/med/topic2189.htm.

Poliomyelitis. (n/d). Retrieved July 26, 2003, from the National Immunization Program, Centers for Disease Control and Prevention: http://www.cdc.gov/nip/publications/pink/polio.pdf.

Pons, M. 2001. Macular degeneration. *eMedicine*, Retrieved November 11, 2004, from: http://www.emedicine.com/aaem/topic295.htm.

Postellon, D. 2003. Turner syndrome. *eMedicine*, Retrieved November 11, 2004, from: http://www.emedicine.com/ped/topic2330.htm.

Pre-eclampsia. (n/d). Retrieved July 25, 2003, from the Action on Pre-Eclampsia Promoting Safer Pregnancy: http://www.apec.org.uk/apec_what.html.

Price, D., & Wilson, S. 2001. Epidural hematoma. *eMedicine*: Retrieved June 5, 2003, from http://www.emedicine.com/EMERG/topic167.htm.

Prostatitis: Disorders of the prostate. 2003. Retrieved March 17, 2004, from the National Kidney and Urologic Diseases Information Clearinghouse (NKUDIC), National Institute of Diabetes and Digestive and Kidney Diseases (NIDDK), National Institutes of Health: http://kidney.niddk.nih.gov/kudiseases/pubs/prostatitis/.

Psittacosis. 2003. Retrieved from the National Center for Infectious Diseases, Division of Bacterial and Mycotic Diseases. Centers for Disease Control and Prevention: http://www.cdc.gov/ncidod/dbmd/diseaseinfo/psittacosis_t.htm.

*Pubic lice infestation.* 2004. *DPD*, Retrieved November 12, 2004, from the National Center for Infectious Diseases, Division of Parasitic Diseases. Centers for Disease Control and Prevention: http://www.cdc.gov/ncidod/dpd/parasites/lice/factsht_pubic_lice.htm.

Q fever. 2003. Retrieved July 26, 2003, from the National Center for Infectious Diseases, Division of Viral and Rickettsial Diseases, Viral and Rickettsial Zoonoses Branch. Centers for Disease Control and Prevention:http://www.cdc.gov/ncidod/dvrd/qfever/index.htm.

Rabies. 2001. Retrieved July 26, 2003, from the National Center for Infectious Disease, Division of Viral and Rickettsial Diseases, Viral and Rickettsial Zoonoses Branch. Centers for Disease Control and Prevention:http://www.cdc.gov/ncidod/dvrd/rabies/.

Radebold, K. 2003. Zollinger-Ellison syndrome. *eMedicine*, Retrieved November 11, 2004, from: http://www.emedicine.com/ped/topic2472.htm.

Rai, A., & Weisse, M. 2002. Diphyllobothriasis latum infection. *eMedicine*. Retrieved March 12, 2005, from http://www.emedicine.com/ped/topic597.htm.

Ratner, A. 2003. Rubella. *MedlinePlus*, Retrieved November 11, 2004, from the U.S. National Library of Medicine and the National Institutes of Health: http://www.nlm.nih.gov/medlineplus/ency/article/001574.htm.

Rein, D. 2003. Hyperemesis gravidarum. *MedlinePlus*, Retrieved November 11, 2004, from the U.S. National Library of Medicine and the National Institutes of Health: http://www.nlm.nih.gov/medlineplus/ency/article/001499.htm.

Rennert, N. 2004a. Chronic thyroiditis. M*edlinePlus*, Retrieved November 10, 2004, from the U.S. National Library of Medicine and the National Institutes of Health: http://www.nlm.nih.gov/medlineplus/ency/article/000371.htm.

Rennert, N. 2004b. Hypothyroidism. M*edlinePlus*, Retrieved November 10, 2004, from the U.S. National Library of Medicine and the National Institutes of Health: http://www.nlm.nih.gov/medlineplus/ency/article/000353.htm.

*Respiratory syncytial virus.* 2003. CDC, Retrieved November 12, 2004, from the National Center for Infectious Diseases, Respiratory and Enteric Viruses Branch. Centers for Disease Control and Prevention: http://www.cdc.gov/ncidod/dvrd/revb/respiratory/rsvfeat.htm.

Respiratory syncytial virus. 1997. In Peter G., ed. *Red Book: Report of the Committee on Infectious Diseases.* 24th ed. Elk Grove Village, IL: American Academy of Pediatrics; 1997: 443.

Revilla, F., & Grutzendler, J. 2004. Huntington disease. *eMedicine*, Retrieved November 11, 2004, from: http://www.emedicine.com/neuro/topic81.htm.

Rhabdomyosarcoma. 2002. Retrieved May 29, 2003, from the Pediatric Oncology Resource Center: http://www.acor.org/diseases/ped-onc/diseases/rhabdo.html.

Rhinitis. 2000. Retrieved March 16, 2004, from the American College of Allergy, Asthma, and Immunology: http://allergy.mcg.edu/advice/rhin.html.

Riaz, K., & Forker, A. 2003. Hypertensive heart disease. *eMedicine*: Retrieved June 4, 2003, from http://www.emedicine.com/med/topic3432.htm.

*Rift valley fever.* 2004. CDC, Retrieved November 12, 2004, from the National Center for Infectious Diseases, Special Pathogens Branch. Centers for Disease Control and Prevention: http://www.cdc.gov/ncidod/dvrd/spb/mnpages/*dispages*/rvf.htm.

Robertson, G. 2003. What is diabetes insipidus. Retrieved March 12, 2005, from the Diabetes Insipidus Foundation: http://www.diabetesinsipidus.org/whatisdi.htm.

Rocky Mountain spotted fever. 2000. Retrieved July 26, 2003, from the National Center for Infectious Diseases, Division of Viral and Rickettsial Diseases, Viral and Rickettsial Zoonoses Branch. Centers for Disease Control and Prevention: http://www.cdc.gov/ncidod/dvrd/rmsf/index.htm.

Roland, P. 2004. Otosclerosis. *eMedicine*. Retrieved March 14, 2005, from http://www.emedicine.com/ped/topic1692.htm.

*Rotavirus.* 2003. CDC, Retrieved November 12, 2004, from the National Center for Infectious Diseases, Respiratory and Enteric Viruses Branch. Centers for Disease Control and Prevention: http://www.cdc.gov/ncidod/dvrd/revb/gastro/rotavirus.htm.

Roth, K. 2003. Alkaptonuria. *eMedicine*, Retrieved November 11, 2004, from http://www.emedicine.com/ped/topic64.htm.

Roy, H. 2004. Episcleritis. *eMedicine*. Retrieved March 12, 2005, from http://www.emedicine.com/oph/topic641.htm.

Ryan, E. 2004. Libman-Sacks endocarditis. *eMedicine*, Retrieved November 11, 2004, from: http://www.emedicine.com/med/topic1295.htm.

Sampson, H., Mendelson, L., and Rosen, J. 1992. Fatal and near-fatal anaphylaxis reactions in children. *New England Journal of Medicine.* 327: 380–384.

Santen, S. 2001a. Cholangitis. *eMedicine*: Retrieved June 7, 2003, from http://www.emedicine.com/EMERG/topic96.htm.

Santen, S. 2001b. Cholecystitis and biliary colic. *eMedicine*: Retrieved June 7, 2003, from http://www.emedicine.com/EMERG/topic98.htm.

Santen, S. 2001c. Cholelithiasis. *eMedicine*: Retrieved June 7, 2003, from http://www.emedicine.com/EMERG/topic97.htm.

SARS. 2003. Retrieved July 20, 2003, from the Centers for Disease Control and Prevention: http://www.cdc.gov/ncidod/sars/factsheet.htm.

Sawyer, M. 2003. Achalasia. *eMedicine*, Retrieved November 11, 2004, from: http://www.emedicine.com/radio/topic6.htm.

Schaefer, G. 2002. Ehlers-Danlos syndrome. *eMedicine*, Retrieved November 11, 2004, from: http://www.emedicine.com/ped/topic654.htm.

Schaffert, A. 2003. Ankylosing spondylitis. *eMedicine*, Retrieved November 11, 2004, from: http://www.emedicine.com/neuro/topic15.htm.

Scheimann, A. 2003. Prader-Willi syndrome. *eMedicine*, Retrieved November 11, 2004, from: http://www.emedicine.com/ped/topic1880.htm.

Scheinfeld, N. 2004. Henoch-Schoenlein purpura. *eMedicine*, Retrieved November 11, 2004, from: http://www.emedicine.com/ped/topic3020.htm.

*Schistosomiasis.* 2004. *DPD*, Retrieved November 12, 2004, from the National Center for Infectious Diseases, Division of Parasitic Diseases. Centers for Disease Control and Prevention: http://www.cdc.gov/ncidod/dpd/parasites/schistosomiasis/factsht_schistosomiasis.htm.

Schwartz, R. 2004. Bacillary Angiomatosis. *eMedicine*, Retrieved November 12, 2004, from: http://www.emedicine.com/derm/topic44.htm.

Scoggins, T. 2004. Reiter syndrome. *eMedicine*, Retrieved November 11, 2004, from: http://www.emedicine.com/emerg/topic498.htm.

Scoliosis. 2002. Retrieved June 1, 2003, from the Mayo Clinic: http://www.mayoclinic.com/invoke.cfm?objectid=7DBFF2C2-87DE-43DE-8FB57941FC1AC5F6.

Scully, C. 2005. Leukoplakia, oral. *eMedicine*. Retrieved March 13, 2005, from http://www.emedicine.com/derm/topic227.htm.

Segu, V. 2004. Gynecomastia. *eMedicine*, Retrieved November 11, 2004, from: http://www.emedicine.com/med/topic934.htm.

Seldon, S. 2001. Seborrheic dermatitis. *eMedicine*: Retrieved May 29, 2003, from http://www.emedicine.com/derm/topic396.htm.

Shah, A. 2004. Myasthenia gravis. *eMedicine*, Retrieved November 11, 2004, from: http://www.emedicine.com/neuro/topic232.htm.

Shah, S. 2002. Aortic coarctation. *eMedicine*, Retrieved November 11, 2004, from: http://www.emedicine.com/med/topic154.htm.

Shaikh, U. 2003. Lymphadenitis. *eMedicine*, Retrieved November 11, 2004, from: http://www.emedicine.com/ped/topic32.htm.

Sharma, G. 2004a. Atrial myxoma. *eMedicine*, Retrieved November 11, 2004, from: http://www.emedicine.com/med/topic186.htm.

Sharma, G. 2004b. Sinusitis. *eMedicine*, Retrieved November 11, 2004, from: http://www.emedicine.com/ped/topic2108.htm.

Sharma, S., & Thomson, G. 2004c. Wegener granulomatosis. *eMedicine*, Retrieved November 11, 2004, from: http://www.emedicine.com/med/topic2401.htm.

Sherif, A., & Perez, N. 2004. Diverticulitis. *eMedicine*. Retrieved March 12, 2005, from http://www.emedicine.com/med/topic578.htm.

Shields, T. 2002. Raynaud syndrome. *eMedicine*, Retrieved November 11, 2004, from: http://www.emedicine.com/aaem/topic375.htm.#section~when_to_go_to_the_hospital.

Shigellosis. 2003. Retrieved July 26, 2003, from the National Center for Infectious Disease, Division of Bacterial and Mycotic Diseases. Centers for Disease Control and Prevention: http://www.cdc.gov/ncidod/dbmd/diseaseinfo/shigellosis_g.htm.

Shukla, P. 2002. Meckel diverticulum. *eMedicine*, Retrieved November 11, 2004, from: http://www.emedicine.com/ped/topic1389.htm.

Sidhaye, A. 2004a. Gigantism. *MedlinePlus*, Retrieved November 11, 2004, from the U.S. National Library of Medicine and the National Institutes of Health: http://www.nlm.nih.gov/medlineplus/ency/article/001174.htm.

Sidhaye, A. 2004b. Graves' disease. *MedlinePlus*, Retrieved November 11, 2004, from the U.S. National Library of Medicine and the National Institutes of Health: http://www.nlm.nih.gov/medlineplus/ency/article/000358.htm.

Sidhaye, A. 2004c. Osteitis fibrosa. *MedlinePlus*, Retrieved November 10, 2004, from the U.S. National Library of Medicine and the National Institutes of Health: http://www.nlm.nih.gov/medlineplus/ency/article/001252.htm.

Sidhaye, A. 2004d. Osteomalacia. *MedlinePlus*, Retrieved November 10, 2004, from the U.S. National Library of Medicine and the National Institutes of Health: http://www.nlm.nih.gov/medlineplus/ency/article/000376.htm.

SIDS. 2001. Retrieved May 30, 2003, from the Centers for Disease Control and Prevention, National Vaccine Program Office: http://www.cdc.gov/od/nvpo/fs_tableVII_doc5.htm.

Singh, G. 2001. Dacryoadenitis. *eMedicine*, Retrieved November 11, 2004, from: http://www.emedicine.com/oph/topic594.htm.

Smallpox. 2002. Retrieved July 26, 2003, from Public Health Emergency Preparedness & Response, Centers for Disease Control and Prevention: http://www.bt.cdc.gov/agent/smallpox/overview/disease-facts.asp.

Smith, D. 2003a. Diphyllobothriasis. *MedlinePlus*, Retrieved November 11, 2004, from the U.S. National Library of Medicine and the National Institutes of Health: http://www.nlm.nih.gov/medlineplus/ency/article/001375.htm.

Smith, D. 2003b. Giardiasis. *MedlinePlus*, Retrieved November 11, 2004, from the U.S. National Library of Medicine and the National Institutes of Health: http://www.nlm.nih.gov/medlineplus/ency/article/000288.htm.

Smith, D. 2003c. Hymenolepiasis. *MedlinePlus*, Retrieved November 11, 2004, from the U.S. National Library of Medicine and the National Institutes of Health: http://www.nlm.nih.gov/medlineplus/ency/article/001378.htm.

Smith, D. 2003d. Leprosy. *MedlinePlus*, Retrieved November 10, 2004, from the U.S. National Library of Medicine and the National Institutes of Health: http://www.nlm.nih.gov/medlineplus/ency/article/001347.htm.

Smith, D. 2003e. Listeriosis. *MedlinePlus*, Retrieved November 10, 2004, from the U.S. National Library of Medicine and the National Institutes of Health: http://www.nlm.nih.gov/medlineplus/ency/article/001380.htm.

Smith, D. 2003f. Salmonella enterocolitis. *MedlinePlus*, Retrieved November 10, 2004, from the U.S. National Library of Medicine and the National Institutes of Health: http://www.nlm.nih.gov/medlineplus/ency/article/000294.htm.

Soliman, E. 2004. Tourette syndrome. *eMedicine*, Retrieved March 15, 2005, from http://www.emedicine.com/med/topic3107.htm.

Spoonemoore, K. 2002. Catscratch disease. *eMedicine*, Retrieved November 11, 2004, from: http://www.emedicine.com/derm/topic69.htm.

*Sporotrichosis*. 2004. *DBMD*, Retrieved November 12, 2004, from the National Center for Infectious Diseases, Division of Bacterial and Mycotic Diseases. Centers for Disease Control and Prevention:http://www.cdc.gov/ncidod/dbmd/*diseaseinfo*/sporotrichosis_g.htm.

Srinivas, N. 2004. Barrett esophagus. *eMedicine*, Retrieved November 11, 2004, from: http://www.emedicine.com/radio/topic73.htm.

*STARI: Southern tick-associated rash illness*. 2001. *CDC*, Retrieved November 12, 2004, from the National Center for Infectious Diseases, Division of Vector-Borne Infectious Diseases. Centers for Disease Control and Prevention: http://www.cdc.gov/ncidod/dvbid/stari/index.htm.

Steefel, L. 1999. Color blindness. *The Gale Encyclopedia of Medicine*. Retrieved May 30, 2003, from http://www.findarticles.com/cf_dls/g2601/0003/2601000336/p1/article.jhtml.

Steele, M. 2004. Carpal tunnel syndrome. *eMedicine*. Retrieved March 10, 2005, from http://www.emedicine.com/emerg/topic83.htm.

Stewart, D. 2004a. Aarskog Syndrome. *MedlinePlus*. Retrieved November 24, 2004, from the U.S. National Library of Medicine and the National Institutes of Health: http://www.nlm.nih.gov/medlineplus/ency/article/001654.htm.

Stewart, D. 2004b. Galactosemia. *MedlinePlus*, Retrieved November 11, 2004, from the U.S. National Library of Medicine and the National Institutes of Health: http://www.nlm.nih.gov/medlineplus/ency/article/000366.htm.

Stewart, D. 2004c. McCune-Albright syndrome. *MedlinePlus*, Retrieved November 10, 2004, from the U.S. National Library of Medicine and the National Institutes of Health: http://www.nlm.nih.gov/medlineplus/ency/article/001217.htm.

Stewart, D. 2004d. Niemann-Pick. *MedlinePlus*, Retrieved November 10, 2004, from the U.S. National Library of Medicine and the National Institutes of Health: http://www.nlm.nih.gov/medlineplus/ency/article/001207.htm.

Stewart, D. 2003a. Aase Syndrome. *MedlinePlus*. Retrieved February 27, 2005, from the U.S. National Library of Medicine and the National Institutes of Health: http://www.nlm.nih.gov/medlineplus/ency/article/001662.htm.

Stewart, D. 2003b. Apert syndrome. *MedlinePlus*. Retrieved March 8, 2005, from the U.S. National Library of Medicine and the National Institutes of Health: http://www.nlm.nih.gov/medlineplus/ency/article/001581.htm.

Stewart, D. 2003c. Chediak-Higashi syndrome. *MedlinePlus*. Retrieved March 9, 2005, from the U.S. National Library of Medicine and the National Institutes of Health: http://www.nlm.nih.gov/medlineplus/ency/article/001312.htm.

Stewart, D. 2003d. Cri du chat syndrome. *MedlinePlus*. Retrieved March 9, 2005, from the U.S. National Library of Medicine and the National Institutes of Health: http://www.nlm.nih.gov/medlineplus/ency/article/001593.htm.

Stewart, D. 2003e. Down Syndrome. *MedlinePlus*, Retrieved November 11, 2004, from the U.S. National Library of Medicine and the National Institutes of Health: http://www.nlm.nih.gov/medlineplus/ency/article/000997.htm.

Stewart, D. 2003f. Ehlers-Danlos syndrome. *MedlinePlus*, Retrieved November 11, 2004, from the U.S. National Library of Medicine and the National Institutes of Health: http://www.nlm.nih.gov/medlineplus/ency/article/001468.htm.

Stewart, D. 2003g. Klinefelter syndrome. *MedlinePlus*, Retrieved November 10, 2004, from the U.S. National Library of Medicine and the National Institutes of Health: http://www.nlm.nih.gov/medlineplus/ency/article/000382.htm.

Stewart, D. 2003h. Krabbe disease. *MedlinePlus*, Retrieved March 13, 2005, from the U.S. National Library of Medicine and the National Institutes of Health: http://www.nlm.nih.gov/medlineplus/ency/article/001198.htm.

Stewart, D. 2003i. Marfan syndrome. *MedlinePlus*, Retrieved November 10, 2004, from the U.S. National Library of Medicine and the National Institutes of Health: http://www.nlm.nih.gov/medlineplus/ency/article/000418.htm.

Stewart, D. 2003j. Morquio syndrome. *MedlinePlus*, Retrieved March 13, 2005, from the U.S. National Library of Medicine and the National Institutes of Health: http://www.nlm.nih.gov/medlineplus/ency/article/001206.htm.

Stewart, D. 2003k. Noonan Syndrome. *MedlinePlus*, Retrieved November 10, 2004, from the U.S. National Library of Medicine and the National Institutes of Health: http://www.nlm.nih.gov/medlineplus/ency/article/001656.htm.

Stewart, D. 2003l. Osler-Weber-Rendu syndrome. *MedlinePlus*, Retrieved November 10, 2004, from the U.S. National Library of Medicine and the National Institutes of Health: http://www.nlm.nih.gov/medlineplus/ency/article/000837.htm.

Stewart, D. 2003m. Rubinstein-Taybi syndrome. *MedlinePlus*, Retrieved November 10, 2004, from the U.S. National Library of Medicine and the National Institutes of Health: http://www.nlm.nih.gov/medlineplus/ency/article/001249.htm.

Stewart, D. 2003n. Russell-Silver syndrome. *MedlinePlus*, Retrieved November 10, 2004, from the U.S. National Library of Medicine and the National Institutes of Health: http://www.nlm.nih.gov/medlineplus/ency/article/001209.htm.

Stewart, D. 2003o. Treacher-Collins syndrome. *MedlinePlus*, Retrieved March 15, 2005, from the U.S. National Library of Medicine and the National Institutes of Health: http://www.nlm.nih.gov/medlineplus/ency/article/001659.htm

Stewart, D. 2003p. Turner syndrome. *MedlinePlus*, Retrieved November 10, 2004, from the U.S. National Library of Medicine and the National Institutes of Health: http://www.nlm.nih.gov/medlineplus/ency/article/000379.htm.

Stewart, D. 2003q. Von Gierke disease. *MedlinePlus*, Retrieved November 10, 2004, from the U.S. National Library of Medicine and the National Institutes of Health: http://www.nlm.nih.gov/medlineplus/ency/article/000338.htm.

Stewart, D. 2003r. Waardenburg syndrome. *MedlinePlus*, Retrieved November 10, 2004, from the U.S. National Library of Medicine and the National Institutes of Health: http://www.nlm.nih.gov/medlineplus/ency/article/001428.htm.

Stone, C. 2004a. Bacterial gastroenteritis. *MedlinePlus*, Retrieved November 11, 2004, from the U.S. National Library of Medicine and the National Institutes of Health: http://www.nlm.nih.gov/medlineplus/ency/article/000254.htm.

Stone, C. 2004b. Blind loop syndrome. *MedlinePlus*. Retrieved March 9, 2005, from the U.S. National Library of Medicine and the National Institutes of Health: http://www.nlm.nih.gov/medlineplus/ency/article/001146.htm.

Stone, C. 2004c. Cirrhosis. *MedlinePlus*, Retrieved November 11, 2004, from the U.S. National Library of Medicine and the National Institutes of Health: http://www.nlm.nih.gov/medlineplus/ency/article/000255.htm.

Stone, C. 2004d. Colorectal polyps. *MedlinePlus*, Retrieved November 10, 2004, from the U.S. National Library of Medicine and the National Institutes of Health: http://www.nlm.nih.gov/medlineplus/ency/article/000266.htm.

Stone, C. 2004e. Crohn's disease. *MedlinePlus*, Retrieved November 11, 2004, from the U.S. National Library of Medicine and the National Institutes of Health: http://www.nlm.nih.gov/medlineplus/ency/article/000249.htm.

Stone, C. 2004f. Diverticulitis. *MedlinePlus*, Retrieved November 11, 2004, from the U.S. National Library of Medicine and the National Institutes of Health: http://www.nlm.nih.gov/medlineplus/ency/article/000257.htm.

Stone, C. 2004g. Esophagitis. *MedlinePlus*, Retrieved November 11, 2004, from the U.S. National Library of Medicine and the National Institutes of Health: http://www.nlm.nih.gov/medlineplus/ency/article/001153.htm.

Stone, C. 2004h. Zollinger-Ellison syndrome. *MedlinePlus*, Retrieved November 10, 2004, from the U.S. National Library of Medicine and the National Institutes of Health: http://www.nlm.nih.gov/medlineplus/ency/article/000325.htm.

Stone, C. 2003a. Enteritis. *MedlinePlus*, Retrieved November 11, 2004, from the U.S. National Library of Medicine and the National Institutes of Health: http://www.nlm.nih.gov/medlineplus/ency/article/001149.htm.

Stone, C. 2003b. Gilbert's syndrome. *MedlinePlus*, Retrieved November 11, 2004, from the U.S. National Library of Medicine and the National Institutes of Health: http://www.nlm.nih.gov/medlineplus/ency/article/000301.htm.

Strauss, L. 2002. Ewing sarcoma. *eMedicine*, Retrieved November 11, 2004, from: http://www.emedicine.com/radio/topic275.htm.

*Strongyloidiasis*. 2004. *DPDx*, Retrieved November 12, 2004, from the National Institute for Infectious Diseases, Division of Parasitic Diseases. Centers for Disease Control and Prevention:http://www.dpd.cdc.gov/dpdx/HTM.L/Strongyloidiasis.htm.

Swetter, S. 2004. Malignant melanoma. *eMedicine*. Retrieved March 13, 2005, from http://www.emedicine.com/derm/topic257.htm.

Takayasu's Arteritis Foundation. (n/d). Retrieved June 4, 2003, from http://www.takayasu.org.

Tan, W. 2004. Mesothelioma. *eMedicine*, Retrieved November 11, 2004, from: http://www.emedicine.com/med/topic1457.htm.

Tang, W., & Young, J. 2002. Myocarditis. *eMedicine*. Retrieved March 13, 2005, from http://www.emedicine.com/med/topic1569.htm.

Tegay, D., & Fallet, S. 2004. Krabbe disease. *eMedicine*. Retrieved March 13, 2005, from http://www.emedicine.com/ped/topic2892.htm.

Tetanus. (n/d). Retrieved July 26, 2003, from the Centers for Disease Control and Prevention: http://www.cdc.gov/nip/publications/pink/tetanus.pdf.

Toxoplasmosis. 2003. Retrieved July 26, 2003, from the National Center for Infectious Diseases, Division of Parasitic Infections. Centers for Disease Control and Prevention: http://www.cdc.gov/ncidod/dpd/parasites/toxoplasmosis/factsht_toxoplasmosis.htm.

Trench mouth. 2004. Mayo Clinic. Retrieved March 15, 2005, from http://www.mayoclinic.com/invoke.cfm?objectid=8DFF2890-D41B-4AC6-978DFD7879D7C474&dsection=1.

*Trichuriasis*. 2004. *DPDx*, Retrieved November 12, 2004, from the National Center for Infectious Diseases, Division of Parasitic Diseases. Centers for Disease Control and Prevention: http://www.dpd.cdc.gov/dpdx/HTM.L/Trichuriasis.htm.

Tsoi, L. 2002. Esophagitis. *eMedicine*: Retrieved June 7, 2003, from http://www.emedicine.com/EMERG/topic175.htm.

Tuberculosis. 2003. Retrieved July 26, 2003, from the National Center for HIV, STDs, and TB Prevention, Division of Tuberculosis Elimination. Centers for Disease Control and Prevention: http://www.cdc.gov/nchstp/tb/faqs/qa.htm.

Tuberculosis. 2002. Retrieved March 16, 2004, from the World Health Organization: http://www.who.int/mediacentre/factsheets/fs104/en/.

Tuberculosis resources. (n/d). Retrieved July 26, 2003, from the Department of Biomedical Informatics at Columbia University: http://www.cpmc.columbia.edu/tbcpp/.

Tularemia. 2002. Retrieved July 26, 2003, from the National Center for Infectious Diseases, Division of Vector-Borne Infectious Diseases. Centers for Disease Control and Prevention: http://www.cdc.gov/ncidod/dvbid/misc/tularemiaFAQ.htm.

Turiansky, G. 2002. Eumycetoma (fungal mycetoma). *eMedicine*, Retrieved November 11, 2004, from: http://www.emedicine.com/derm/topic147.htm.

Types of seizures. 2003. Retrieved July 25, 2003, from the Epilepsy Foundation: http://www.epilepsyfoundation.org/answerplace/Medical/seizures/types/

Typhoid fever. 2001. Retrieved July 26, 2003, from the National Center for Infectious Disease, Division of Bacterial and Mycotic Diseases. Centers for Disease Control and Prevention: http://www.cdc.gov/ncidod/dbmd/diseaseinfo/typhoidfever_g.htm.

Ulcerative colitis. 2003. Retrieved June 7, 2003, from the National Digestive Diseases Information Clearinghouse, National Institutesof Health:http://www.niddk.nih.gov/health/digest/pubs/colitis/colitis.htm.

Update 2002: Bovine spongiform encephalopathy and variant Creutzfelt-Jacob disease. 2002. Retrieved July 26, 2003, from the National Center for Infectious Diseases, Division of Viral and Rickettsial Diseases. Centers for Disease Control and Prevention: http://www.cdc.gov/ncidod/diseases/cjd/bse_cjd.htm.

Upton, S. 2001. Cyclospora cayetanensis. *Parasitology laboratory*, Retrieved November 12, 2004, from Kansas State University, Biology Division: http://www.ksu.edu/parasitology/cyclospora/cyclospora.html.

Uwaifo, G. and Sarlis, N. 2004. McCune-Albright Syndrome. eMedicine. Retrieved May 29, 2005, from http://www.emedicine.com/med/topic3194.htm.

Valentini, R. 2004. Goodpasture syndrome. *eMedicine*, Retrieved November 11, 2004, from http://www.emedicine.com/ped/topic888.htm.

Valero, S. 2004. Retinopathy, Diabetic, Proliferative. *eMedicine*, Retrieved November 11, 2004, from: http://www.emedicine.com/oph/topic415.htm.

Valley, V., & Fly, C. 2002. Pericarditis and cardiac tamponade. *eMedicine*: Retrieved June 4, 2003, from http://www.emedicine.com/EMERG/topic412.htm.

Van Rijn, R., & McHugh, K. 2004. Ricketts. *eMedicine*. Retrieved March 11, 2005, from http://www.emedicine.com/radio/topic610.htm.

Vanni, R. 2002. Uterus: Leiomyoma. *Atlas of Genetics and Cytogenetics in Oncology Haematology*. Retrieved May 29, 2003, from http://www.infobiogen.fr/services/chromcancer/Tumors/leiomyomID5031.html

Varicella disease (chickenpox). 2003. Retrieved July 26, 2003, from the National Immunization Program, Centers for Disease Control and Prevention: http://www.cdc.gov/nip/diseases/varicella/.

Varicose veins. 2003. Retrieved June 4, 2003, from the Mayo Clinic: http://www.mayoclinic.com/invoke.cfm?id=DS00256.

*Vibrio parahaemolyticus.* 2004. *DBMB*, Retrieved November 12, 2004, from the National Center for Infectious Diseases, Division of Bacterial and Mycotic Diseases. Centers for Disease Control and Prevention: http://www.cdc.gov/ncidod/dbmd/diseaseinfo/vibrioparahaemolyticus_g.htm.

*Vibrio vulnificus.* 2004. *DBMB*, Retrieved November 12, 2004, from the National Center for Infectious Diseases, Division of Bacterial and Mycotic Diseases. Centers for Disease Control and Prevention: http://www.cdc.gov/ncidod/dbmd/diseaseinfo/vibriovulnificus_g.htm.

Viral Hepatitis A. 2003. Retrieved July 22, 2003, from the National Center for Infectious Diseases, Division of Hepatitis. Centers for Disease Control and Prevention: http://www.cdc.gov/ncidod/diseases/hepatitis/a/index.htm.

Viral Hepatitis B. 2003. Retrieved July 22, 2003, from the National Center for Infectious Diseases, Division of Hepatitis. Centers for Disease Control and Prevention: http://www.cdc.gov/ncidod/diseases/hepatitis/b/index.htm.

Viral Hepatitis C. 2003. Retrieved July 22, 2003, from the National Center for Infectious Diseases, Division of Hepatitis. Centers for Disease Control and Prevention: http://www.cdc.gov/ncidod/diseases/hepatitis/c/index.htm.

*VISA/VRSA-vancomycin-intermediate/resistant staphylococcus aureus.* 2003. *CDC*, Retrieved November 12, 2004, from the National Center for Infectious Diseases, Division of HealthCare Quality Promotion. Centers for Disease Control and Prevention: http://www.cdc.gov/ncidod/hip/ARESIST/visa.htm.

Vuguin, P., & Perez, N. 2002. Pheochromocytoma. *eMedicine*. Retrieved March 14, 2005, from http://www.emedicine.com/ped/topic1788.htm.

Webner, D. 2003. Varicose veins. *MedlinePlus*, Retrieved November 10, 2004, from the U.S. National Library of Medicine and the National Institutes of Health: http://www.nlm.nih.gov/medlineplus/ency/article/001109.htm.

Weiner, D. 2001. Pediatrics, Reye Syndrome. *eMedicine*, Retrieved November 11, 2004, from: http://www.emedicine.com/emerg/topic399.htm.

Wener, K. 2004a. Actinomycosis. *MedlinePlus*, Retrieved November 11, 2004, from the U.S. National Library of Medicine and the National Institutes of Health: http://www.nlm.nih.gov/medlineplus/ency/article/000599.htm.

Wener, K. 2004b. CMV-pneumonia. *MedlinePlus*, Retrieved November 10, 2004, from the U.S. National Library of Medicine and the National Institutes of Health: http://www.nlm.nih.gov/medlineplus/ency/article/000664.htm.

Wener, K. 2004c. Ebola hemorrhagic fever. *MedlinePlus*, Retrieved November 11, 2004, from the U.S. National Library of Medicine and the National Institutes of Health: http://www.nlm.nih.gov/medlineplus/ency/article/001339.htm.

Wener, K. 2004d. Ehrlichiosis. *MedlinePlus*, Retrieved November 11, 2004, from the U.S. National Library of Medicine and the National Institutes of Health: http://www.nlm.nih.gov/medlineplus/ency/article/001381.htm.

Wener, K. 2004e. Endocarditis. *MedlinePlus*, Retrieved November 11, 2004, from the U.S. National Library of Medicine and the National Institutes of Health: http://www.nlm.nih.gov/medlineplus/ency/article/001098.htm.

Wener, K. 2004f. Gas gangrene. *MedlinePlus*, Retrieved November 11, 2004, from the U.S. National Library of Medicine and the National Institutes of Health: http://www.nlm.nih.gov/medlineplus/ency/article/000620.htm.

Wener, K. 2004g. Herpes genital. *MedlinePlus*, Retrieved November 10, 2004, from the U.S. National Library of Medicine and the National Institutes of Health: http://www.nlm.nih.gov/medlineplus/ency/article/000857.htm.

Wener, K. 2004h. Leishmaniasis. *MedlinePlus*, Retrieved November 10, 2004, from the U.S. National Library of Medicine and the National Institutes of Health: http://www.nlm.nih.gov/medlineplus/ency/article/001386.htm.

Wener, K. 2004i. Pneumocystis carinii pneumonia. *MedlinePlus*, Retrieved November 10, 2004, from the U.S. National Library of Medicine and the National Institutes of Health: http://www.nlm.nih.gov/medlineplus/ency/article/000671.htm.

Wener, K. 2004j. Poliomyelitis. *MedlinePlus*, Retrieved March 14, 2005, from the U.S. National Library of Medicine and the National Institutes of Health: http://www.nlm.nih.gov/medlineplus/ency/article/001402.htm.

Wener, K. 2004k. Toxoplasmosis. *MedlinePlus*, Retrieved November 10, 2004, from the U.S. National Library of Medicine and the National Institutes of Health: http://www.nlm.nih.gov/medlineplus/ency/article/000637.htm.

Wener, K. 2003. Rheumatic fever. *MedlinePlus*, Retrieved November 10, 2004, from the U.S. National Library of Medicine and the National Institutes of Health: http://www.nlm.nih.gov/medlineplus/ency/article/003940.htm.

West Nile virus. 2003. Retrieved July 26, 2003, from the National Center for Infectious Diseases, Division of Parasitic Infections. Centers for Disease Control and Prevention: http://www.cdc.gov/ncidod/dvbid/westnile/wnv_factSheet.htm.

What is Leiomyosarcoma? 2001. Retrieved May 29, 2003, from the British Association of Cancer United Patients: http://www.cancerbacup.org.uk/questions/specific/sarcomas/sts/leiomyosarcoma.htm.

Wong, I. 2002. Uveitis, fuchs heterochromic. *eMedicine*, Retrieved November 11, 2004, from: http://www.emedicine.com/oph/topic432.htm.

Yaish, H. 2001. Thalassemia. *eMedicine*, Retrieved November 11, 2004, from: http://www.emedicine.com/ped/topic2229.htm.

Yakobi, R. 2001. Sarcoidosis. *eMedicine*, Retrieved November 11, 2004, from: http://www.emedicine.com/emerg/topic516.htm.

Yancey, L. 2001. Morning sickness. *eMedicine*, Retrieved November 11, 2004, from: http://www.emedicine.com/aaem/topic315.htm.

*Yellow Fever.* 2003. Retrieved November 10, 2004, from the National Center for Infectious Diseases, Divison of Vector-Borne Infectious Diseases. Centers for Disease Control and Prevention: http://www.cdc.gov/ncidod/dvbid/yellowfever/index.htm.

Yen, K., & Yen, M. 2001. Mucormycosis. *eMedicine*, Retrieved November 11, 2004, from: http://www.emedicine.com/oph/topic225.htm.

*Yersinia enterocolitica*. 2004. Retrieved November 10, 2004, from the National Center for Infectious Diseases, Division of Bacterial and Mycotic Diseases. Centers for Disease Control and Prevention: http://www.cdc.gov/ncidod/dbmd/diseaseinfo/yersinia_g.htm.

Young, C. 2002. Plantar fasciitis. *eMedicine*, Retrieved November 11, 2004, from: http://www.emedicine.com/sports/topic103.htm.

Zalewska, A. 2003. Boutonneuse fever. *eMedicine*, Retrieved November 11, 2004, from: http://www.emedicine.com/derm/topic759.htm.

Zeina, B. 2003. Pemphigus vulgaris. *eMedicine*, Retrieved November 11, 2004, from: http://www.emedicine.com/derm/topic319.htm.

Zhao, F., & Enzenauer, R. 2004. Conjunctivitis, neonatal. *eMedicine*, Retrieved March 14, 2005, from http://www.emedicine.com/oph/topic325.htm.

# Index